Peripheral Nerve

AMERICAN ENCOUNTERS/GLOBAL INTERACTIONS

A Series edited by Gilbert M. Joseph
and Penny Von Eschen

The series aims to stimulate critical perspectives and fresh interpretive frameworks for scholarship on the history of the imposing global presence of the United States. Its primary concerns include the deployment and contestation of power, the construction and deconstruction of cultural and political borders, the fluid meaning of intercultural encounters, and the complex interplay between the global and the local. American Encounters seeks to strengthen dialogue and collaboration between historian of U.S. international relations and area studies specialists.

The series encourages scholarship based on multi-archive historical research. At the same time, it supports a recognition of the representational character of all stories about the past and promotes critical inquiry into issues of subjectivity and narrative. In the process, American Encounters strives to understand the context in which meanings related to nations, cultures, and political economy are continually produced, challenged, and reshaped.

Peripheral
Nerve

HEALTH AND MEDICINE
IN COLD WAR LATIN AMERICA

Anne-Emanuelle Birn and Raúl Necochea López

DUKE UNIVERSITY PRESS
DURHAM AND LONDON
2020

Designed by Drew Sisk
Typeset in Portrait Text, Folio, and Rockwell
by Westchester Publishing Services

Library of Congress Cataloging-in-Publication Data
Names: Birn, Anne-Emanuelle, [date]. | Necochea López,
Raúl, editor.
Title: Peripheral nerve : health and medicine in cold war
Latin America / Anne-Emanuelle Birn and Raúl Necochea
López.
Other titles: American encounters/global interactions.
Description: Durham : Duke University Press, 2020. |
Series: American encounters/global interactions |
Includes bibliographical references and index.
Identifiers: LCCN 2019050692 (print) | LCCN 2019050693
(ebook) | ISBN 9781478008682 (hardcover) | ISBN
9781478009566 (paperback) | ISBN 9781478012221 (ebook)
Subjects: LCSH: Public health—Political aspects—Latin
America—History. | Medical policy—Latin America—
History. | Cold War—Social aspects—Latin America. |
Latin America—Foreign relations—Soviet Union. | Soviet
Union—Foreign relations—Latin America. | Latin America—
Foreign relations—United States. | United States—Foreign
relations—Latin America.
Classification: LCC RA395.L3 P47 2020 (print) | LCC RA395.L3
(ebook) | DDC 362.1098—dc23
LC record available at https://lccn.loc.gov/2019050692
LC ebook record available at https://lccn.loc.gov/2019050693

Cover art: Illustration and design by Drew Sisk.

AEB *To my beloved father, Richard, and cherished father-in-law, Leonid Pavlovich, who, having spent their lives and careers on "opposite" sides of the Cold War, never met but shared a love of literature and infused it in their progeny.*

RNL *This book is as old as my lively children, Tomás and Ansel, and half as old as my unfolding story with the amazing Erica Wood. This is for the three of them.*

CONTENTS

GILBERT M. JOSEPH

*Farnam Professor of History and
International Studies, Yale University*

The last twenty years have witnessed nothing less than the remaking of Latin American Cold War history, as the field has burgeoned into a veritable growth industry. For decades, study of the region's postwar conflict was dominated by mainstream diplomatic and foreign relations historians who conceived of it largely in bipolar terms and were preoccupied with grand strategy and U.S. policy and sources. Since about 2000, however, scholarship has been significantly reoriented by Latin Americanists who, without marginalizing international conflicts and rivalries, have more often approached the Cold War from the inside out—and often "from below." In the process they have begun to flesh out a distinctive *Latin American* Cold War, rather than merely studying the dynamics and collateral damage of superpower rivalry *in* a peripheral region. These scholars speak the region's languages and read voraciously across disciplines, employing tools and concepts from area studies, political and social history, anthropology, political science, cultural studies, and studies of technology, health, and medicine. They seek out (and work to declassify) new archival sources as well as pose new questions to older documentary collections. In part owing to more productive conversations with mainstream diplomatic historians and foreign relations scholars, more ambitious transnational and transregional analyses have emerged, steeped in multisited archival and oral history research strategies. Since the early 2000s, bolstered by the creation of new international research clusters, the organization of numerous conferences and symposia, and a series of collective volumes and special journal issues, a new self-identified generation of historians and international relations scholars with a penchant for "border crossings" has reshaped Latin American Cold War studies. Anne-Emanuelle Birn's and Raúl Necochea López's *Peripheral Nerve: Health and Medicine in Cold War Latin America* constitutes a signal contribution to this new watershed of scholarship.

As the book's title cleverly indicates, while Latin American countries ambiguously resided on the periphery and semiperiphery of Cold War–era theoretical imaginings, they invariably exhibited nerve, whether via quiet audacity or full-blown impudence. Such nerve also meant that Latin America's Cold War was rarely cold. Indeed, few periods in the region's history were as violent, turbulent, or transformative as the half century that ran roughly from the end of World War II through the early 1990s. One would have to go back to the early nineteenth-century wars of independence to find the same level of mass mobilization, revolutionary upheaval, and counterrevolutionary repression. Yet the international connections, organizational capacities, and technologies of death and surveillance at work in the late twentieth-century Cold War render that earlier cycle of violence almost quaint by comparison. Latin America's late great novelist Gabriel García Márquez graphically evoked this "outsized" and "unbridled reality" in his 1982 Nobel acceptance speech. Conjuring up a litany of grisly and apocalyptic events—the dirty wars, disappearances, and displacements of the 1970s and early 1980s that had turned Central America and South America's Southern Cone into killing fields and barrios—he told his Nobel audience that he had been obliged to develop a new literary genre, "magical realism," to assimilate the period's mind-boggling occurrences and, as he put it, "render our lives believable."

How do we account for such cataclysmic violence? To be sure, Latin America's past has always been marked by alternating cycles of social reform and intense conservative reaction, in which the influence, aid, and intervention of imperial powers have figured prominently. Even so, the dynamics of the Latin American Cold War were embedded in a particularly ferocious dialectic linking reformist and revolutionary projects for social change and national development, with the excessive counterrevolutionary responses they triggered, in the decades after World War II. This dialectic, which several of the contributors to *Peripheral Nerve* engrossingly document and which played out in intertwined domestic and international arenas of political, social, and cultural power, shaped Latin American life in the late twentieth century and, as the editors demonstrate in the epilogue, has "lingerings and echoes" in the new millennium. At a macro level, the Cold War was a struggle between two postwar "rookie" superpowers—the United States and the USSR—over shifting geopolitical stakes and ideological visions of how the world should be organized. But what ultimately gave the Latin American Cold War its "heat" were the politicization and internationalization of everyday life. On a variety of fronts across several decades, Latin American elites and newly expanded and empowered popular classes participated in local and national political contests over land, labor, the control of markets, the disposition of scientific, medical, and health resources, and what constituted citizenship itself—contests that rarely escaped the powerful undertow of the larger superpower conflict.

Peripheral Nerve advances our understanding of the region's Cold War in many consequential respects. Above all, it challenges the conventional historical narrative that, in health and medicine, as elsewhere, Latin America's Cold War history was circumscribed and constrained by the hegemonic dominance of the United States in its imperial "backyard." Rather, without negating the historical dynamics of U.S. power, the collection inflects what Anne-Emanuelle Birn describes in her introduction as the repeated "defiance of Latin American actors who sought alternative channels of health and medical solidarity" with the Soviet Union and its allies, and via South–South solidarities within and beyond Latin America. The book's examination of Latin America's relations with the Second World before, during, and after the Cold War redresses a serious imbalance in the burgeoning literature, while extending the new scholarship's appreciation of the regional struggle's "multivalent, multilevel nature," as Birn writes in her introduction.

At the same time, the collection is invaluable for the manner in which it deepens two particularly fertile veins in the new literature. First, there is the issue of Cold War chronology and temporality—the need to examine both the broader contexts and specific conjunctures in which Latin American state and society experienced the challenges and opportunities of life in revolutionary and counterrevolutionary times. Much of the new scholarship stresses the importance of applying a more encompassing frame of analysis to the Cold War decades (even as some wonder if the conflict ever really ended in the early 1990s, or morphed into an unsettling new phase that continues today). In an earlier collaboration among international scholars, *A Century of Revolution: Insurgent and Counterinsurgent Violence during Latin America's Long Cold War*, Greg Grandin and I argue that the region's Cold War decades should be placed in the broader context of Latin America's "revolutionary twentieth century," which simultaneously constituted a *"long* Cold War" (especially in North–South relations), articulating longer waves of revolutionary and counterrevolutionary phenomena. That was because Latin America's revolutionary twentieth century coincided with the rise of U.S. hemispheric and global hegemony, with both dynamics proceeding along parallel tracks, and each informing the shape the other took. This "century of revolution," which ran at least from the Mexican Revolution of 1910 (if not the political and social repercussions of the wars of 1898) to the Central American insurgencies of the 1980s, was effectively defined by sequential attempts by Latin American reformers to transcend what had become an unsustainable model of exclusionary nationalism, restricted political and social institutions and gender relations, persisting rural clientelism, and dependent export-based development. Although the experience of each country's involvement in this nearly century-long cycle of insurgent politics aimed at reform and liberalization, as well as each nation's relationship with the imperial hegemon, was *distinct*, many shared similar patterns of radicalized reform, followed not infrequently by revolution, civil war, and counter-revolutionary state terror. Moreover, each successive bid to transform society generated domestic experiences and international responses that shaped subsequent attempts.

Yet, within this *longue durée* of U.S. hemispheric hegemony and resistance to it, Grandin and I contend that the Cold War proper (c.1947–1990) constituted a particularly consequential juncture. This was evident in terms of the massive infusion of counterinsurgent aid and expert personnel, the dramatic narrowing of political space and options, and the manner in which a deadly combination of rational, precise counterinsurgent technologies (typically imported from the United States and its allies) and more vengeful local sentiments and tactics honed the new internal security state and the bureaucratic strategies of terror that undergirded it.

Although Birn and Necochea López do not explicitly engage the notion of a "long Cold War," they consistently argue against rigidly circumscribing the Cold War period. In her insightful introduction, Birn provides a fresh "prehistory" of the Cold War that not only recognizes the multivalent nature of U.S. power but also inflects Latin America's largely neglected connections with the Eastern Bloc, particularly in the area of health and medicine. She then usefully periodizes the early, middle, and later stages of the Cold War decades; indeed, these phases help to structure the three thematic sections of the collection.

Peripheral Nerve also contributes powerfully to what is likely the most important recent development in regional Cold War studies: the elaboration of its multistranded cultural dimension. For if the field has become a growth industry in the last fifteen years, its leading edge may well be efforts to tease out the complex, power-laden *cultural* processes, relationships, exchanges, and institutional forms that antedated and shaped the late twentieth-century conflict, and had consequences beyond its denouement. Although foreign diplomats and grand strategists, military juntas and intelligence apparatuses, leftist guerrillas and right-wing paramilitary forces, CIA-backed coups and covert operations have remained at the center of traditional accounts of the Cold War in Latin America, beneath or in the wake of the conflicts they orchestrated, the Latin American Cold War was waged by technocrats and experts—an array of scientists and engineers, doctors and health workers, agronomists and architects, scholars and economists. The webs of expertise they wove served to materialize the political ideologies and grand strategies of the era; moreover, as *Peripheral Nerve* fleshes out in some detail, such medical and scientific experts underwrote forms of resistance and shaped alternative solidarities and destinies that challenged imperial forces of both the Right and Left. One of the pleasures of this rich collection is that, apart from narrating fascinating, at times poignant, transnational stories of little-known Argentine psychiatrists, U.S. nurses, Cuban international health workers, and Brazilian parasitologists, it also provides glimpses into the medical and health-related careers of high-profile Latin American leaders such as Che Guevara, Salvador Allende, and Michelle Bachelet. In the process, the volume's contributors underscore the fact that the appeal of the superpowers' mass utopias was predicated on dreams of development and modernization that were appropriated in a variety of contexts and ways, often with different results. These dreams and aspirations fueled complex political and cultural struggles likely just as consequential as the paroxysms of insurgent and counterinsurgent violence the period witnessed. And these micro-struggles relied on a myriad of specialized, transnational experts and cultural intermediaries whose role in the region's Cold War is just beginning to receive its due.

To date, most studies of the region's cultural Cold War have focused on the usual subjects of cultural history—the intellectuals, students, artists, writers, and political and social thinkers who sought a higher profile in the conflict and often were important catalysts at diverse points on the ideological spectrum. Similarly, several studies of certain signature projects of "development" (like the Alliance for Progress) and critiques of the vexed concept itself have emerged and narrowed the gap between Latin Americanist scholarship and more robust interdisciplinary work on this theme for other areas of the Global South. But what *Peripheral Nerve* and some other new research argue compellingly is that the experts, technocrats, and cultural and political intermediaries behind these projects have routinely been elided. Only now are scholars beginning to flesh out their roles in various infrastructural, scientific, and environmental projects, medical clinics and communal health crusades, educational and housing missions, biological research and agricultural experiment stations. They contend that by examining these experts' concrete plans, travels, networks of collaboration, and manner of negotiating their work at both higher levels and at the grassroots—with national leaders, U.S. and Soviet Bloc agencies, transnational foundations and think tanks, and, not least, the local populations they studied and served—we can develop a more nuanced history of Cold War Latin America.

Another new edited volume, Andra Chastain and Timothy Lorek's *Itineraries of Expertise: Science, Technology, and the Environment in Latin America's Long Cold War*, like *Peripheral Nerve*, makes particularly important contributions in this regard. Both collections provide detailed analysis over decades of experts who were both peripatetic and locally situated, who often saw or portrayed themselves as "neutral," removed from politics, even as their work fed directly or indirectly into prevailing geopolitical agendas. In establishing these transnational dimensions of Cold War expertise, both works contribute to a Cold War history that is attentive to history's contingencies and capable of transcending frayed, dichotomizing paradigms of interpretation. Read together, these new volumes showcase how experts traversed a variety of boundaries: between the city and the countryside, between northern and southern nations, between Southern and Eastern Bloc destinations, and within the Global South. They demonstrate how experts' itineraries and collaborations tended to strengthen, but occasionally undermined and complicated the imperatives dictated by Cold War geopolitics. In the process, this new research forces us to reconsider other binaries in conventional Cold War studies: between so-called "developed" and "developing" nations, between the First (or Second) World and the Third World, and between the Global North and Global South. Congruent with recent turns in transnational studies, by highlighting multiple agents, sites, and scales of expertise during the Cold War, these new collections accentuate a blurring of the "local" and the "foreign," especially where the production of knowledge is concerned.

Yet another collection published in Italy and then in Argentina, edited by Italian cultural historian Benedetta Calandra and her Argentine colleague Marina Franco, attempts to assess the state of scholarship on *La Guerra Fría Cultural en América Latina*. Like *Peripheral Nerve* and *Itineraries of Expertise*, this international volume—which assembles a team of interdisciplinary scholars, mostly from Italy, Spain, and Latin America—stresses the *emerging* nature of studies on Latin America's cultural Cold War. Unlike the more robust bodies of work on Europe and the United States, studies of Latin America's Cold War cultures still remain modest and dispersed, with immense gaps. Nevertheless the collection's contributors (like those of *Peripheral Nerve* and *Itineraries of Expertise*) argue for a "long Cold War" in the cultural realm. They suggest that the pivotal political events and watersheds of the Cold War proper were *not* congruent with longer-running cultural and intellectual formations. The latter, they argue, date back at least to the positivist and progressive "civilizing" and "modernizing" missions of the early twentieth century, and then took an important turn in the 1940s and 1950s when a more muscular technocratic capacity, influenced substantially by New Deal mindsets and welfarist policies, gained ascendance throughout the hemisphere.

Without neglecting or whitewashing what they call "scandalous" high-profile episodes like the U.S. Department of Defense's manipulative, counter-insurgent use of social science research in initiatives like Project Camelot, the contributors to the Calandra and Franco volume prefer to tease out *nuances* in the deployment and resistance of imperial cultural power. They eschew just-so stories of hegemony and broad instrumentalist applications of "soft power," arguing instead for historicized, case-specific analyses of imperial contact zones, agents, and more contingent, even ambiguous forms of local reception. To cite one example, the essay by Chilean historian Fernando Purcell on the Peace Corps offers a fine-grained treatment of that organization that empha-sizes the multivalent relationships and often autonomous identities that U.S. Peace Corps volunteers forged with their host communities. Interestingly, other recent work reveals that a stream of former Peace Corps volunteers went on to long academic careers in Latin American studies that were characterized by an abiding critique of U.S. foreign policy, interventions, and the concept of "development" itself.

The new cultural history of the Latin American Cold War that these three recent collaborative volumes exemplify is distinguished, above all, by their ability to interrogate and cross the temporal, spatial, and methodologi-cal boundaries that conventional diplomatic and foreign relations scholarship set in place. The peripatetic experts and technocrats under scrutiny in these works spanned generations of knowledge production, traversed multiple levels and ideological divides of the world system, and in many instances *themselves* came to embody transnational identities and "hybrid nationalities of exper-tise." In this regard, an interesting feature of several of the essays in *Itineraries of Expertise* and *Peripheral Nerve* is the role that certain sites in the Global South, such as Mexico and Puerto Rico, and to a lesser extent Colombia, played in the creation of such hybrid identities, typically in the context of transitions from revolutionary and liberal welfare states to the neoliberal regimes that succeeded them. Mexico, Puerto Rico, and Colombia served as intermediary spaces and proving grounds for the kind of biological, medical, and agronomic research, and the type of social policies that would, in time, give rise to such institutional hallmarks of the regional and global Cold War as the Green Revo-lution and the Alliance for Progress.

There is much more that can be done by scholars to internationalize cul-tural (and political-economic) studies of the Latin American Cold War. As in many other societies belonging to the Global South, Latin American states and the intellectuals, scientists, medical, and health professionals that collaborated with or opposed them frequently sought to balance between the First and Second Worlds, defying bipolar imperatives when they could and, in the process, entertaining for a time the possibilities of an incipient nonaligned Third World project. The essay in *Peripheral Nerve* by Marco Ramos on the scientific encounters and *desencuentros* of anti-imperialist Argentine psychiatrists in the 1970s and 1980s is particularly illuminating in this regard. The rise and fall of *Tercermundismo* and connections with the Non-Aligned Movement in Mexico in the 1970s under populist president Luis Echeverría was emblematic of various ill-fated Latin American attempts, by governments and popular movements alike, to identify with a distinct Third World experience during the global Cold War. Yet another new collective volume, *Latin America and the Third World: An International History*, edited by international historians Thomas Field, Stella Krepp, and Vanni Pettinà, argues that, along with more recently decolonized nations in Africa, Asia, and the non-Hispanophone Caribbean, "Latin America must be treated as a fundamental participant in the Third World project," incorporating perspectives for understanding the region that have often been foreclosed by "the traditional Western Hemispheric or regional framing." In this respect, the editors seek to break out of what international historian Tanya Harmer has recently termed "the historiographical Monroe Doctrine." This, the new volume's contributors demonstrate, entails deeper research into Latin America's political-economic and cultural relations with the Socialist Second World and more attention to ThirdWorldist political and cultural formations like the 1966 Tricontinental Conference in Havana, Cuba, and the Organization of Solidarity with the Peoples of Asia, Africa, and Latin America (OSPAAL), founded in its wake. It also entails examination of economic projects such as the Organization of Petroleum Exporting Countries (OPEC) and the New International Economic Order, created in the 1960s and 1970s, respectively.

Peripheral Nerve provides many entry points for this kind of internationalist approach. It pioneers analysis of Latin America's relations with the Soviet Union and Eastern Bloc during the Cold War and encourages us to deepen our appreciation of the idea of Latin America's "alternative destinies and solidarities," as Birn refers to them in this volume's introduction, even in the "Giant's Backyard." One of the volume's more provocative contributions is its excavation of the origins during the Cold War (and even before) of South–South collaborations that have gained greater traction under the Pink Tide regimes of the first decades of this century. (Of course, some will question the coherence and staying power of such collaborations, both within and beyond the area of medicine and health, as the Pink Tide continues to ebb.)

The outlook for future work in Latin American Cold War studies is quite promising, and Birn and Necochea López map out an ambitious agenda for studies of health and medicine in the epilogue. Where Latin America's Cold War connections with the Eastern Bloc are concerned, this agenda will become more feasible as greater numbers of international scholars master Slavic languages and Mandarin, and as the governments of these authoritarian states open up more of their archives.

Elsewhere, however, there are even greater reasons for scholarly optimism. As some wounds heal, and as a horizon of life replaces one of death in several of Latin America's former killing zones (notwithstanding drug and gang violence in Central America's Northern Triangle and flickering insurgencies in Nicaragua, Colombia, and Venezuela), a greater variety of studies reconstructing the social and cultural histories and memories of the Latin American Cold War has emerged. As forensic and truth-telling processes play out, the climate for new encounters with the Cold War—undergirded by newly declassified documents and greater access to oral sources in Latin America and the United States—warms. The cresting wave of interdisciplinary scholarship—represented so richly in *Peripheral Nerve*—augurs the possibility of further dialogue between more traditional and newer approaches to the regional and global conflict, thereby advancing the burgeoning literature on the cultural Cold War. With the historical record increasingly accessible at a variety of global locations, and with historical amnesia challenged at the international and national levels, as well as at the grassroots, Latin American and U.S. students are rediscovering new aspects of their nations' political, social, cultural, and transnational histories during the second half of the twentieth century and beyond. This development has enlivened our calling as teachers as well as scholars, both in the North and the South.

This book was almost a decade in the making, the fruition of plans first mapped out in the context of Raúl's too-short postdoc with Anne-Emanuelle at the University of Toronto. A 2010 workshop held in conjunction with the (now) annual meeting of the Latin American Studies Association, and cosponsored by its Health, Science, and Society Section and the U of T's Latin American Studies Program and its Institute for the History and Philosophy of Science and Technology, spawned some of the chapters included here; others we were fortunate to gather subsequently. We are grateful to workshop participants, commentators, and comrades, among them Enrique Beldarraín Chaple, María Carranza, Katherine Centellas, Marcos Cueto, Mariola Espinosa, Sebastián Gil-Riaño, Teresa Huhle, Nikolai Krementsov, Lynn Morgan, Steve Palmer, Jason Pribilsky, Alex Puerto, Liz Roberts, Jeannie Samuel, Nicolás Sánchez-Guerrero, Mark Solovey, Gabriela Soto Laveaga, Sarah Tracy, and Adam Warren.

This book is in all senses a collective endeavor, and we are so honored to have contributions from such a stellar group of scholars, who responded to our many demands and delays with forbearance and understanding.

Utmost thanks to Mariajosé Aguilera, skillful and astute copyeditor, adviser, researcher, and historian-in-the-making, who in the course of this project rediscovered her own family's alternative solidarities across the Iron Curtain—an uncle from Nicaragua who studied veterinary medicine in Ukraine in the 1980s.

Deepest gratitude to Nikolai Krementsov for sharing his extensive knowledge of Cold War history, politics, and medicoscientific developments from multiple perspectives of the Curtain. His generosity and rigor in reviewing made, as always, for extensive improvements, if a few nerves and headaches along the way!

We are grateful for funding from the Canadian Institutes of Health Research (CIHR) grant #EOG-126976 ("Health Diplomacy at a Crossroads: Social Justice–Oriented South–South Cooperation in a Time of Global Change"), and from the Department of Social Medicine, the Simmons Scholars Program, and the Office of Research Development at the University of North Carolina, which together supported the preparation and publication of this volume.

We are delighted that our volume is part of the American Encounters/ Global Interactions series edited by Gilbert M. Joseph and Penny Von Eschen. Our enormous appreciation goes to Gil Joseph, who believed in and encouraged this project from the beginning and throughout *el camino*; to our Duke University Press editor, Gisela Fosado, who pushed and inspired us to produce a "furniture-moving" volume; to editorial associate Alejandra Mejía for her skill and speed in answering our questions; to Ellen Goldlust, project editor, for her levelheadedness and careful attention to minutiae and the big picture alike; and to copyeditors, printers, marketing, and other press staff. We are also grateful to the dozens of archivists and librarians whose work permitted the research and telling of these stories and to the anonymous reviewers who homed in on some key analytic and dialogic aspects that strengthened the book immeasurably.

And, of course, to our families, who lived under the shadow of this volume for far too long, *gracias por siempre*.

Alternative Destinies and Solidarities for Health and Medicine in Latin America before and during the Cold War

ANNE-EMANUELLE BIRN

In May 1944, Emilio Frugoni, a poet, professor, former senator, and founder of the Uruguayan Socialist Party, arrived in Moscow as Uruguay's first ambassador to the Soviet Union in eight years.[1] Frugoni was accompanied by his personal secretary as well as a scientific attaché, Dr. Lauro Cruz Goyenola, an active member of the Frente Popular (Popular Front) coalition and contributor to the pro-Soviet *Diario Popular*. In addition to serving as the aging Frugoni's personal physician, Cruz Goyenola was charged with studying the organization of Soviet health care and the country's system of scientific research. His mission proved trying, and this once "true believer" became disillusioned. Having spent only six months in Moscow, Cruz Goyenola suddenly resigned from his post in late October and returned to Montevideo.

This experience might have culminated in quiet disappointment but for one crucial factor: like many visitors to the USSR in the 1930s and 1940s, Cruz Goyenola penned a book about his travels. However, in contrast to the admiring reflections of most (regardless of their ideological orientation)—and violating diplomatic norms of discretion—Cruz Goyenola penned a diatribe, *Rusia por Dentro* (Russia from the Inside).[2] First issued in March 1946, this highly critical account of Soviet medicine and society appeared in almost a dozen editions over the next two years (shifting to a Buenos Aires press after a presidential sanction blocked further publication in Uruguay), igniting a furious polemic among intellectuals, political parties, journalists, and the Uruguayan public at large.[3] Scores of heated attacks and counteroffensives ensued in the form of pamphlets, newspaper articles, book-length tomes, and countless disputes and discussions in the ubiquitous cafés on both shores of the Río de la Plata.

Cruz Goyenola's book was released just two weeks after Winston Churchill's famed "Iron Curtain" speech in Fulton, Missouri. That the debates around *Rusia por Dentro* persisted for so long suggests *both* that the unfolding Cold War rapidly reverberated across Latin America *and* that Latin American (health) experts were charting their own course in the postwar era. Indeed, Latin American intellectuals' and politicians' staking of their early positions vis-à-vis world powers and power politics was not surprising—they had long experience in preemptively and adaptively defining their stance. *Rusia por Dentro*'s publication provided an effective platform for Uruguayans to deliberate upon the country's standpoint and orientation in the emerging Cold War—neither strictly favoring nor rejecting the United States or the USSR but instead considering the pros and cons of these divergent political allegiances, benefactors, and trading partners as well as deciding on the most auspicious welfare state, health and medicine, and scientific exemplars.

Enabling such broad-ranging deliberations in Uruguay and throughout the region was the latitude Latin American countries had long exerted in political, cultural, and scientific relations with one another (for example, through Latin American and Pan-American congresses and organizations)—albeit interrupted by tensions, conflict, and outright war—and with the leading world (imperial) powers. The latter comprised not only remnants of colonial connections with Portugal and Spain but also a range of other ties: with Britain, France, and Germany in economic, and certain political and cultural realms; with France, Germany, and Scandinavia in medical and scientific domains; and with the United States, given its ever-growing political, economic, social, medical, and technological tentacles, perhaps most vividly shepherded by the activities of the Rockefeller Foundation (RF) and the Pan American Health Organization.[4] By this time, Latin American countries had also begun to engage in commercial, political, and scientific areas with a newer player on the global scene: the Soviet Union.

The Soviet Union differed from all other locales in that it was the world's first purposefully constructed socialist state. Importantly, public health and medicine were not separate or separable from the overall Soviet model, but rather an integral part of the socialist system and its social policies, which also covered gender and ethnic rights, labor conditions, education, pensions, and protection of mothers and children. Of course, just as Americans and other Westerners both analyzed and caricatured the Soviet social system before and during the Cold War, it is essential to underscore the contrast between the ideal image of the public health system projected by the Soviets for external consumption and its actual implementation and administration in the Soviet

Union. This distinction is illustrated by the idealistic or critical perceptions of observers and visitors, such as those portrayed in *Rusia por Dentro*.

In sum, through these varied entanglements—which involved back-and-forth expert communications, conferences, and sponsored research—Latin American physicians, scientists, and social reformers did not simply digest European, North American, Soviet, and one another's ideas and approaches, but debated them furiously, forged their own variants suited to domestic problems, and projected them internationally.[5] This complex positionality persisted throughout the Cold War.

Like Cruz Goyenola's account of the Soviet Union, and the multilayered responses to it, this volume transcends and troubles dominant narratives of European influences on Latin America being (definitively) supplanted by U.S. influence in the post–World War II era by incorporating the role of the Cold War into the world of local, regional, and transnational public health and medicine within and across Latin America. Not only does the pioneering set of case studies herein show how Latin American actors used, rejected, and reshaped U.S. preferences and interventions, it also reveals a range of ties between Latin American actors and Soviet/Eastern Bloc counterparts, as well as with other Third World countries within and beyond the region, that served as an important part of national and regional health policy and medical developments.

A Historiographical Gaze

For four and a half decades, the Cold War was the central factor in global politics and society. It dominated foreign policy and guided domestic developments in industry, economics, the sciences, and education, while permeating the cultural life of the United States and the Soviet Union and their respective blocs—all with repercussions for virtually every other setting.

Moreover, the role of the two blocs (complicated by the ascendance of Maoism and the Sino-Soviet split starting in the late 1950s), as representing the contrasting ideologies of capitalism and communism (and the distinct forms of societal organization deriving from these worldviews), must be distinguished from the separate but imbricated question of geopolitical spheres of influence. Although both superpowers had such spheres of influence, the Soviet sphere extending beyond Eastern Europe to include a range of socialist countries and political movements in Asia and Africa (also predating the Cold War, via the Comintern),[6] no sphere of influence was more potent than that of the United States in Latin America (and parts of the Caribbean), dating back at least to the 1823 Monroe Doctrine (and before, but less formally asserted).[7] Not only has this shaped events in the region, but it has also influenced much of the historiographic literature:[8] historians of the Cold War period in Latin America have long been wearing U.S. "sphere of influence" blinders even if historical actors were not.

As the chapters in this volume identify, the conflict between the two super-powers was a fundamental factor—as well as an ever-present backdrop—in shaping, albeit not determining, Latin America's political and medical destiny in the post–World War II era. The turf wars and distrust between the U.S.-led and Soviet-led blocs played out in particularly contentious ways since Latin America was the traditional U.S. "backyard" and thanks to what was by the time of the Cold War most Latin American countries' more than century-long independence and insertion into the international arena. This was manifested in the decisions of Latin American health policy and medical leaders about whom to invite from abroad and how to engage them to participate in institution-building, professionalization, research, training, and policy design. In so doing—as illustrated by Katherine E. Bliss's chapter on an FBI-hunted left-wing nurse exiled from the United States whose contributions to a massive rural health project were welcomed by the Mexican government—Latin American actors both surreptitiously and explicitly pitted the superpowers against each other.

Such a transformation took different forms in different locales. While this volume focuses on Latin America, the larger historical—and historiographical—panorama is essential to our understanding of the range of health politics and practices analyzed in this collection. Far from mere contextual stage-setting, the Cold War served as a dynamic component of medical and health regimes that endure to this day, including the management of disease eradication campaigns, science funding mechanisms, population policies, the standing of medical experts, and corresponding subaltern mobilizations to offset environmental, political, and economic changes. For example, Nicole L. Pacino's chapter demonstrates how the RF's attempts to temper communist influences in Bolivia were as much, if not more, to protect its own standing in the years of (medical) McCarthyist leftist witch-hunting in the United States as to shape medical education in Bolivia.[9]

Latin America offers a propitious setting for multiple reasons.[10] Although Latin Americans inhabit a remarkable geographical, racial, political, and economic mosaic, they also share certain historical and cultural features, including a long period of Iberian colonialism, postcolonial economic dependency eventually centering on the United States, and diverse population origins, in addition to noteworthy, if sometimes fraught, institution building. The region's trajectory as a land of migrants, encompassing forced laborers from around the world, enslaved Africans, displaced Indigenous groups, and Chinese contract workers, as well as "voluntary" immigrants, likewise mattered in its openness and exposure to outside ideas.[11]

After World War II, the dominant economic development model in the region—import substitution, which bolstered national industries and elites—was facilitated by U.S. paranoia in the face of the Soviet model, and also championed by the Economic Commission for Latin America (ECLA; expanded in 1984 to include the Caribbean as ECLAC), a regional United Nations (UN) agency then on a mission to make the terms of trade fairer between Latin America and more industrialized countries. In parallel, at the global level, various Latin American countries played an influential role in the establishment and administration of key UN agencies, including the World Health Organization (WHO) and the United Nations Educational, Scientific, and Cultural Organization (UNESCO),[12] continuing a long tradition of engagement in international scientific and professional circles, albeit under a changed world order. In centering Cold War health and medicine experiences at the national and subregional level, this volume deals only tangentially with Latin American countries' Cold War engagement with UN agencies—certainly a worthwhile avenue of exploration in the future.[13]

Outside the formal realm of these agencies, many Latin American countries—other than Cuba—remained "observers" or were on the sidelines of the "Non-Aligned Movement" (NAM) of Third World countries into the 1970s and 1980s. Latin America had not formally participated in the movement's 1955 inaugural conference in Bandung, Indonesia, which focused on the recently decolonized world's aim of challenging neocolonialism. But by the late 1970s, Cuba asserted global leadership in the NAM's response to the capitalist-communist polarity.[14] Almost all Latin American countries were founding members of the G-77, formed in 1964 (Cuba joined in 1971), which challenged the U.S.-Soviet rivalry's stranglehold on geopolitics, trade patterns, and global governance at the UN, and contested the accompanying threats posed to national sovereignty.

These forms of collective resistance and cooperation, at times involving Eastern European countries and China, spanned health, humanitarian, and medical dimensions.[15] Given the long intraregional trajectory of cooperation in Latin American health and science, new variants of professional and social movement–driven South–South health solidarity emerged during the Cold War in the context of region-wide resistance to dictatorships, Central America's protracted civil wars, and social medicine aspirations. Revolutionary Cuba served as a key leader of health justice initiatives across borders—illustrated in this collection by Cheasty Anderson's chapter on Cuban-Nicaraguan health cooperation under the 1980s Sandinista regime.[16]

But this period was not only marked by civil society resistance: the Cold War also heightened longtime rivalries and generated new competition between countries, motivating governments and leading institutions to outperform one another—out of pride or opportunism. For instance, in the arena of demographic control, Andean countries were eager to stem rapid population growth more effectively than their neighbors, thereby garnering significant foreign aid, especially from the United States.[17] The health and development planning strategies that arose out of the Alliance for Progress—Washington's project for preventing a proliferation of Cuba-style revolutions—similarly engendered rival courting of resources as well as resentment amid Washington's attempts to orchestrate nonsocialist collective development approaches and political loyalties through all means necessary, including backing of repressive regimes.[18]

These large and small rivalries coexisted uncomfortably with the alternative relationships that certain governments, revolutionary groups, social movements, universities, scientists, and other actors forged and that involved technical, cultural, and educational exchanges between Latin America and Soviet Bloc countries and other regions of the Third World,[19] as explored further in the book's epilogue. As Marco Ramos argues in the case of psychotherapeutic innovations in Argentina, simultaneous and overlapping connections to varied partners with conflicting ideological stances and commitments gave rise to "*desencuentros*" (mismatches) in addition to inspiring "meetings of the mind." Gilberto Hochman and Carlos Henrique Assunção Paiva, meanwhile, show how a celebrated left-wing Brazilian parasitologist—and harsh critic of the political basis of rural misery and disease—parlayed his international connections and networks to at least partially inoculate himself against right-wing repression.

The Cold War period intersected with Latin America's accelerated health and medical state-building domestically, also entailing mounting engagement with international health initiatives. There is a burgeoning and dynamic literature on disease campaigns, public health agencies, health services organization, medical research, population control, and other health policy developments, as well as on social medicine and health and social justice movements spanning the region.[20] But mostly the Cold War itself has been omitted from this historiography. In the few instances in which the Cold War has received concerted attention, it has functioned as either a general backdrop or a rhetorical tool for discussions of (mostly) U.S.-influenced international health efforts.[21] Yet there are certainly hints of other axes of engagement. For example, following its revolution, Cuba turned to Czechoslovakia—the Eastern Bloc country with the best health indicators—as an exemplar for centralized health planning and decentralized administration of service delivery. Czech advisers helped organize early mass vaccination campaigns, and Cuban planners drew from the Czech polyclinic model, even as they debated different forms of adaptation.[22]

Together, these factors make a regional study of Cold War health and medicine in Latin America highly useful and compelling. The similarities and differences across settings influenced patterns of international engagement as the Cold War unfolded, sometimes, but not always, along national boundaries, exemplified by anticapitalist guerrilla movements that crisscrossed Central America, the Andes, and Southern Cone countries. The counterpoint between Latin America's common traits and its local peculiarities adds a rich layer of tension and complexity seldom found elsewhere in the world.

Placing Health and Medicine in Cold War Latin America

The first wave of post-1990 scholarly work on the Cold War focused, not surprisingly, on relations between the United States and the USSR, followed by studies on the effects of the Cold War on general political and cultural developments, mostly in Western/Northern industrialized contexts.[23] Though some scholars have stressed the importance of shifting the lens away from the United States and the USSR, until recently, this has been carried out mostly in relation to the superpowers' proxy wars, military interventions, and support for dictatorships repressing revolutionary movements in Third World countries.[24]

Beyond the political realm, historians of science have also begun to focus on the Cold War period.[25] Unifocal and bifocal studies have fastened our attention on a growing set of themes regarding scientific competition and secrecy, institution-building and opportunism, typical and unexpected collaborations, and the multiple loyalties testing health researchers, public health officials, and institutional leaders. But to date such work has not gone beyond Cold War specialists' traditional focus on the United States, the Soviet Union, and their major allies. This volume turns to health and medicine in Cold War Latin America as a particularly important site in which to analyze the strategies that different groups of local, foreign, and transnational actors used to manage the rivalry between the United States and the USSR to suit their own cultural dispositions; to further their professional, institutional, sociopolitical, national, and regional interests; and to fashion new alliances and shared agendas beyond the ambit of the rival superpowers.

Given the prevailing historiographic emphasis, two potent narratives continue to frame many studies of the "global" Cold War and, by extension, how it played out in Latin America and in specific domains, for example health and medicine. In one narrative, the main sphere of action involved the Eastern and Western Blocs, with other regions of the world falling into one camp or another in supporting roles—as allies, suppliers of key natural resources and expertise, and observational and laboratory outposts, often under conditions of brutal dictatorship and conflict (the role of the NAM remains underexplored in the historical literature). An accompanying narrative is that the United States used the Cold War as a justification to expand its preexisting and overbearing economic, political, and ideological interference in Latin America, its role so overshadowing interactions that it remained the principal (medical) interlocutor for the "dependent, defenseless" region, except in revolutionary settings (e.g., Cuba and Nicaragua).[26]

Present knowledge of and debates around the Cold War in Latin America, drawn from nascent scholarship on political and cultural developments,[27] clearly point to the importance of studying Cold War influences on areas such as health policymaking, medicine, medical education, and public health. Notwithstanding the deep relevance of—and potential challenges posed by— these realms to our understanding of Latin America's cultural and social life in the second half of the twentieth century, application of a Cold War lens to health and medical domains has been all but overlooked by scholars. Even the prizewinning synthesis *Medicine and Public Health in Latin America: A History*, undoubtedly reflecting the extant literature, overemphasizes U.S. hegemony and brings little nuance or consideration to the role of Soviet and Eastern European actors (or of nonaligned alliances and influences) or the multifarious proclivities of local players.[28]

The present volume is the first to address this significant gap. Its case studies of health and medicine in multiple Latin American settings illustrate the intricate negotiations exhibited in the Cold War period and attendant relations with the United States, the USSR, and other countries aligned with one of the rival blocs or deliberately nonaligned.[29] Development programs, ideologies of universalism proposed by the world's two superpowers, and technoscientific competition and leadership were all features of an era that influenced and was influenced by local and transnational events. One dimension that remains understudied is Latin America's interplay with China, including after the Cold War became tripolar in the 1960s. We pick up on this in the epilogue, where we begin to explore these interactions during the Cold War in addition to touching on the contemporary resurgence of Sino–Latin American South–South health cooperation.

To better contextualize the volume itself, we first highlight the underemphasized dimension of the periodization of the Cold War. This is significant even if one looks solely at the relations between the superpowers, let alone the unfolding of events in particular regions and arenas. The content and staging of this volume seek to underscore that the Cold War was a very complex, shifting, and sometimes labile era, with distinct sub-periods and characterized by waxing and waning tensions. As we will see just ahead, the years before the Cold War's first decade, as symbolically inaugurated by Churchill's 1946 speech, are central to understanding its trajectory through the late 1950s and early 1960s, the late 1960s to late 1970s, and the 1980s. Each of these subperiods is emblematized by a set of events and policy changes (e.g., the Berlin crisis, the Korean War, the Thaw, the Cuban Revolution and Cuban Missile Crisis, the Vietnam War, détente, the Thatcher–Reagan conservative turn, the Afghan war, the Gorbachev years, and the fall of the Berlin Wall) that also had resonance and repercussions in Latin America.

Yet many scholars, including of the history of Latin America and history of medicine, still treat the period as uniform and do not pay (sufficient) attention to these nuances.[30] This is particularly pertinent to Latin America because of the Cuban Revolution and what it represented regionally and transnationally—in terms of leftist and guerrilla movements that blossomed across the region in the 1960s and 1970s, the 1970 election of Salvador Allende, Central America's civil wars through the 1980s and the repressive U.S. backlash, as well as the intra–Latin American solidarities sparked by these developments. Questions of how the dynamics of the Cold War played out in medicine and public health are also highly germane. Two examples are Latin American countries' response to much of the Soviet Bloc's departure from the WHO from the late 1940s to the mid-1950s and the support of a disparate array of governments— from Nicaragua's Sandinistas to the Argentine dictatorship—for international health's reorientation from technical disease campaigns to a community-based approach to integrated primary health care, as articulated at the famed 1978 WHO-UNICEF Alma-Ata conference. (See the epilogue for further details.)[31] Subtle attention to periodization also changes the way we think about how and when global politics matters and when it takes a back seat to sovereign developments.

A Crucial Prehistory

Before preparing the immediate landscape of this volume, we pause on a vital and long-neglected precursor of the Cold War context: Soviet–Latin American (health) connections from the 1920s to the 1940s. The interwar years saw the flourishing of Latin American medical, labor, political, and social policy networks regionally and globally, sometimes operating in the guise of progressive "social medicine" interchanges.[32] To be sure, the Pan-American and especially Latin American movements starting in the late nineteenth century were vital, both in terms of regional interrelations and, crucially, in engaging with—and sidestepping—U.S. influences.[33] Post–World War I U.S. isolationism enabled a new level of interaction for Latin American countries on the international stage with such agencies as the League of Nations Health Organisation and the International Labour Office. International engagement also expanded beyond Western Europe to the newly born Soviet Union, an illustration of the possibilities, and perils, of socialist health and societal organization.

These connections involved travelers (bidirectionally) and the nurturing of more formalized bilateral relations, with Mexico-USSR ties as a foremost instance. This period and these connections harbor critical themes that help explain the overall rhythm and timbre of Cold War patterns, as well as explicating events and links raised by particular chapters in the collection.

As with the often-rigid circumscribing of the Cold War, overarching historiographic portrayals of the interwar years in Latin American public health and medicine—as marked principally by displacement of European contacts and influences with an ever-more prominent U.S. presence—merit countering.[34] In fact, this period reveals a vibrant world of give-and-take, one that would prove central to the alternative health solidarities that emerged during the Cold War: the little-studied interplay of experts from Latin America and Soviet Russia.[35] The conversations and flirtations of Mexicans, Argentines, Brazilians, and others with Soviet communism are telling both of the willingness and interest of Latin Americans to escape the cultural, economic, and scientific yoke of European (neo)colonialism and North American imperialism and, more broadly, of the wide range of ideas and experiences with which Latin American state- and institution-building sought to engage, especially as most of the region's governments were in the process of founding public health and social security systems. Later on, these exchanges would translate into Third World solidarity through the NAM.

An initial phase of this engagement in the 1920s involved interchange of experiences between Latin America and the Soviet Union, largely via correspondence. As historians of medicine, public health, and science in the early Soviet Union have shown, the Bolshevik Revolution resulted in a large-scale centralization of social services, research funding, training, and regulations, with the state as the principal or sole patron of the new institutional architecture in these and many other fields.[36] But this was not simply a top-down endeavor and institutional overhaul. In the wake of terrible human loss in World War I and the influenza pandemic, and amid the Civil War's violence, chaos, and famine, the newborn Soviet Union witnessed the emergence of a host of new players with novel imaginings of how a revolutionary society might be organized in such varied realms as biology, literature and literacy, housing, and occupational health.[37]

Curiosity about these efforts traversed the globe, encouraged by the new Soviet regime. Almost immediately following the revolution, officials deployed public health as a tool of diplomacy, with the dual aim of learning from other countries and showcasing domestic developments.[38] There was worldwide interest in the Russian Revolution and its "results," including in the health and medical domains.[39] Intense European and U.S. attention was shared in other parts of the world, including in South Asia, among burgeoning anticolonial movements, and in Latin America.[40] Perhaps no country within Latin America paid closer heed than Mexico, whose own revolution predated the Bolshevik one but whose aspirations for national transformation had more limited reach.

In the wake of its violent and prolonged revolution (1910–1920s), Mexico saw the Soviet experience as a natural point of comparison. The two countries shared oppressive pasts of debt peonage; recent long, divisive, and bloody internal wars; and ambitious plans for building modern states, with both experiencing ongoing tensions between sidelining and (at least rhetorically) supporting Indigenous and "folk" culture. While each faced distinct challenges in unifying and rebuilding, both countries enjoyed the advantage of natural resources: by 1920, for example, Mexico had surpassed Russia to become the world's second largest petroleum producer after the United States, although the Mexican state did not wrestle control of its oil production from foreign owners until 1938.[41]

In terms of public health organization, Mexican authorities began to contact their Soviet counterparts almost the moment diplomatic relations were established in 1924; the former were especially keen to exchange publications and health education information.[42] This exchange seems to have continued steadily, and in the mid-1930s a Department of Public Health handbook for rural hygiene recommended that every health department in the country stock its library with sixteen general public health texts, including two from the Soviet Union.[43]

By the late 1920s and 1930s, numerous cultural and intellectual figures were traveling in both directions—from the Soviet Union, ballerina Anna Pavlova, writer-actor Vladimir Mayakovsky, and filmmaker Sergei Eisenstein all spent time in Mexico. Sojourners from Mexico to the Soviet Union included photographer Tina Modotti (after being expelled from Mexico in 1930, she spent several years in the USSR) and artist David Alfaro Siqueiros (who became an agent for Stalin's secret police), to name but a few. Famed Mexican muralist Diego Rivera spent almost a year in the USSR in 1927–1928 (hurriedly leaving in the face of anti-Stalinist allegations) and returned almost three decades later to seek cancer treatment.[44] There were also Soviet scientific expeditions to Mexico involving geographers, oil engineers, and most famously, botanists and agronomists, including several expeditions to Yucatán headed by renowned botanist and geneticist Nikolai Vavilov in the early 1930s.[45]

Though Mexican doctors and health officials were frequent correspondents with their Soviet counterparts, they seem to have been too preoccupied with local affairs to engage in medical "tourism." Moreover, starting in 1921 and continuing for three decades, the RF's International Health Board organized an ambitious, cooperative public health program of disease control campaigns, rural health organization, and fellowship training, all of which sought to orient Mexican health authorities and personnel to their northern neighbor.[46]

Nonetheless, the arrival of Soviet ambassador Alexandra Kollontai to Mexico in 1926 portended the possibility of further public health exchange—particularly around feminist concerns of maternal and child health policy, birth control, and prostitution.[47] Her controversial stay animated Mexico's postrevolutionary discussions around social welfare, but her posting was too short-lived to yield lasting interchange.[48]

Importantly, as Daniela Spenser has put it, Mexico found itself part of an "impossible triangle" with the United States and the USSR. Mexico used its relationship with the Soviet Union to broaden its alliances and bolster its position against the United States. The United States periodically surfaced accusations that Bolshevism was rooting itself in Mexico and pressured Mexico to break diplomatic ties with the USSR. Mexico, for its part, waited until after the United States "softened its stance" toward Mexico's revolutionary program in 1927,[49] banning the Mexican Communist Party in 1929. The following year Mexico broke off relations with the Soviet Union due to complaints of subversive activities. In the 1930s, the otherwise left-leaning administration of Lázaro Cárdenas "refused to re-establish diplomatic relations with Moscow," famously offering refugee protection to Stalin's exiled rival Leon Trotsky at the urging of Diego Rivera, among others.[50]

Still, the land redistribution, labor and social policy, and state-building efforts of the Cárdenas era provide helpful insights into Soviet-Mexican medical ties. Cárdenas's 1934 platform—centered on his "Plan Sexenal" (Six-Year Plan)—echoed Stalin's "Five-Year Plans" for the Soviet economy, launched in 1928. A central plank of Cárdenas's Six-Year Plan was public education, including expanding access to vocational training. In 1936 Mexico's National Polytechnic Institute was founded with a mission similar to that of Soviet "Rabfak" (*rabochij fakul'tet*; workers' schools)—preparing workers lacking formal education to enter university.[51] Mexico's Polytechnic Institute soon became involved in training rural health workers.

Resonance with Soviet approaches to health and medicine made their way into policy through other channels as well. Cárdenas brought to Mexico City as his public health architects the Nicolaita group of radical physicians (so named for their institutional base at the Universidad Michoacana de San Nicolás de Hidalgo in Morelia, Michoacán), who headed his Department of Public Health when he was the governor of Michoacán. The Nicolaitas, bearing views ranging from humanist to socialist, helped craft two key Cardenista policies. The first was a plan for establishing integrated medical and social services on traditional *ejidos* (collective landholding arrangements)—not dissimilar to medical services developed on Soviet collectivized farms in the 1930s, albeit in rural Mexico medical staff became ejido employees and services were partially community-financed.[52] The second initiative involved redressing the shortage of medical personnel in rural areas through a new social service requirement. Each graduating doctor, nurse, and technician was to spend a minimum of six months working in a rural health post before receiving their degree. While these programs claimed multiple fathers, the most prominent was Nicolaita Dr. Enrique Arreguín Vélez, who had investigated Soviet rural health approaches via correspondence and publications.[53]

In 1938 it seemed that there would finally be an opportunity for Mexicans and Soviets to directly compare and learn from each other's experiences in the area of rural health. For several years, the League of Nations Health Organisation had been planning an International Rural Hygiene Congress to be held in Mexico, and Soviet public health officials were to be key participants. But the conference was abruptly cancelled. Former U.S. surgeon general and head of the Pan American Sanitary Bureau Dr. Hugh S. Cumming, who was deeply suspicious of Soviet involvement in Latin America, managed to derail the conference in behind-the-scenes maneuverings.[54] Other moments of rapprochement between some Latin American health specialists and Soviet and other left-leaning counterparts continued to feed distrust, resentment, and misunderstanding on the part of U.S. experts and politicians well into the Cold War.[55]

Ultimately, the Mexican-Soviet public health encounter was stunted by perennial U.S. fears of a Bolshevist stronghold in Mexico and by Mexico's official diplomatic stance and maneuverings. To be sure, the RF played a central role in this regard. Through the 1920s and 1930s foundation observers repeatedly analogized Mexico to the Soviet Union in terms of such "watchwords" as "socialization of health," "land and industry," "mass education," and "reconstruction." But by the early 1940s the RF reassured itself that despite the fact that the "anti-capitalistic and anti-church murals of Diego Rivera, Orozco, and other modernists are almost as common in Mexico as are the blatant Red posters in Moscow," the political cultures of the two countries differed markedly, with the Mexican masses interested not in ideology but in "material betterment" and not "particularly concerned over the system through which they get it."[56] Although decades of RF programs helped "crowd out" Soviet influences in the health arena, Soviet–Mexican relations picked up, if modestly, in the 1950s through pharmaceutical and cultural exchanges,[57] as explored in Gabriela Soto Laveaga's chapter.

Beyond Mexico, the twentieth century witnessed the founding in many Latin American countries of Communist and Socialist political parties and umbrella popular front coalitions,[58] many motivated by the "Second International" (international proletarian movement) and its Soviet successor, Comintern, and inspired by the USSR's social policies implemented following the Bolshevik Revolution. Even so, only a few Latin American countries established diplomatic ties with the USSR in the 1920s (e.g., two years after Mexico, Uruguay established official Soviet relations in 1926, but Argentina did so only in 1946; Brazil established relations in 1945 but suspended them in 1947, Colombia from 1935 to 1948, and Venezuela from 1945 to 1952, with the latter three countries reestablishing ties in the 1960–1970 decade). Still, there was correspondence back and forth, publications of comparative health and social statistics, and the interchange of official publications and scholarly materials in a range of fields between the USSR and many Latin American countries.[59]

Moreover, starting in the 1930s, a variety of Latin American physicians and social welfare advocates—envisioning a Soviet welfare state utopia as a blueprint for domestic reforms—were keen to witness the USSR's wide-reaching social policy accomplishments firsthand. As far as we can tell, the 1930s and 1940s saw at least two dozen Latin American medical visitors to the Soviet

Union from Argentina, Brazil, Chile, Colombia, Cuba, El Salvador, Mexico, Peru, Uruguay, and Venezuela (and likely elsewhere)—travels that accelerated after World War II. For the most part, these exchanges involved focused visits of several weeks to Moscow, Leningrad, Kiev, and other major cities.

Like European and North American visitors who flocked to the Soviet Union starting in the 1920s, Latin American observers included both the curious and the true believers.[60] They carried out surveys of the organization of public health services, medical schools, and research institutes, and many of them published book-length accounts of their experiences. In all likelihood, most Latin American travelers and observers in this period were unaware of the Great Terror—Stalin's purges starting in 1936—and of the hardships of displacement under land collectivization. Or perhaps the visitors viewed these developments—as in the case of the Industrial Revolution in Western Europe— as an inevitable phase in the Soviet Union's modernization trajectory.

A small number of Latin American doctors spent longer stints in the Soviet Union carrying out research or working as clinicians. Argentine orthopedic surgeon Lelio Zeno, for example, spent over six months in 1932 working in the Moscow emergency clinic of the famed Soviet surgeon Sergei Judine. Zeno wrote a detailed book about the organization of Russian medicine shortly after his return to Buenos Aires,[61] and he returned to the Soviet Union several years later in preparation for a sequel. Maurício de Medeiros, a Brazilian physician, professor at the Rio de Janeiro Faculty of Medicine, and later minister of health under President Juscelino Kubitschek (1956–1958), traveled to the USSR in the late 1920s. A socialist (but not a communist), he penned a much-read travel journal (appearing in six editions!) in which he, like later medical visitors, marveled at Soviet socialist medicine and technology.[62] In 1935, a year for which VOKS (the Soviet cultural exchange agency) maintained detailed visitors' books, there were at least half a dozen medical visitors from Brazil (including Osório César of São Paulo, who published a series of volumes on Soviet medicine), Peru, Chile, and Argentina.[63] Several years earlier, Dr. Augusto Bunge, a well-known occupational and public health specialist and twenty-year Socialist Party representative in the Argentine Congress, spent two months in the USSR accompanied by a Buenos Aires journalist.[64] Although visits were suspended during World War II, interest did not abate, as indicated by the 1945 founding of the *Revista Cubana de Medicina Soviética*.

These exchanges served as important forerunners to Cold War–era visits by sympathetic observers, if not communist adherents, such as a group of Brazilian and Argentine doctors who toured health installations in Moscow, Leningrad, and Stalingrad in the early 1950s.[65] In this volume, Jadwiga E. Pieper

Mooney mines Chilean doctor Benjamín Viel's book *La Medicina Socializada y su Aplicación en Gran Bretaña, Unión Soviética y Chile*, based on his invited visit to the USSR in 1960, for insights about how Chileans adapted Soviet lessons to Chile's pressing sociomedical needs.[66]

In addition, up to several hundred other Latin American visitors not connected to health and medicine per se found their way to the USSR by the 1950s, and many of them raved about free Soviet health services among other features of Soviet society.[67] Among these were Argentine journalist Alfredo Varela, Uruguayan teacher Jesualdo Sosa, and a few years later Indigenous Bolivian intellectual Fausto Reinaga and Peruvian poet Gustavo Valcárcel; others, such as Brazilian philologist Silveira Bueno, presented more negative—sometimes virulent—views of what they saw, though health care organization was usually spared the vitriol.[68] While not the focus of this volume, marveling was (unevenly) reciprocated, especially following the Cuban Revolution.[69]

The books and popular articles interwar and early postwar Latin American visitors authored about (or that touched upon) Soviet public health services, medical schools, and research institutes, like *Rusia por Dentro*, entered into spirited national and regional debates about how to shape policies and institutions. Additional conduits for these ties crossing the interwar and postwar periods were Spanish Civil War health and medical refugees, many of whom spent a number of years in the Soviet Union before migrating to Mexico, Argentina, Cuba (especially in the context of the Cuban revolution), and other Latin American countries.[70]

After World War II, the curious Latin American gaze toward the Soviet Union became complicated and constrained by Cold War exigencies, particularly as Latin American countries were positioning themselves in the postwar world order.[71] Even so, medical and public health curiosity persisted, as attested to by medical school library holdings across the region, the lively engagement with Soviet Pavlovian psychiatry experts in Cuba, as Jennifer Lynn Lambe shows in her chapter, and the wide Latin American (women's) interest in Soviet psycho-prophylaxis methods of pain-free childbirth.[72]

In sum, Soviet and socialist medicoscientific developments and health organization were firmly on Latin America's "radar" on the eve of, as well as during, the Cold War, whether in laudatory terms, as articulated by most Latin American visitors of the time, or in denunciatory terms, as expressed by the disenchanted Cruz Goyenola.[73] It is thus impossible to understand the ebbs and flows of *Health and Medicine in Cold War Latin America*, or the array of agents and interlocutors involved, without this backdrop of several decades of curiosity, interchange, and domestic debates around the perceptions (and realities) of the Soviet Union's projected vision of its society, and health and medicine therein.

Yet, as the chapters in this volume demonstrate, we are still at an incipient place, methodologically and substantively, in understanding Soviet–Latin American interactions in any domain (exceptions being the work of Spenser and Rupprecht), let alone in the areas of health and medicine.[74] This is partly a question of training, with Latin Americanists typically proficient in Spanish and/or Portuguese and English, but rarely Russian or Chinese, and partly an issue of past and current access to—and dedicated research funding for exploring—archival materials in Russia, and even more so China, where politically motivated archival restrictions are a major impediment to historical research.

Such contemporary limitations, ironically, contrast with those of thousands of the primary actors in the past who, as explored in the epilogue, were trained in the Communist Bloc. Arguably, these linguistic and archival impediments for most historians of Latin America and of Latin American health and medicine have led to an overemphasis on the role of the United States in the region. This book alone is unable to transcend the skewed historiography: we do recognize that the chapters herein do not emphasize or extensively employ Russian/Soviet archives (nor any Chinese sources at all), and therefore do less than they might to reconstruct the Soviet side of the story and Soviet Bloc strategies and views on influencing the region, even as inferences can be made. While the chapters focus on reconstructing how Latin Americans navigated the Cold War political landscape on questions of medicine and health, we await future, more amply trained generations and greater availability of archival sources to break more definitively with North American myopia to tell other dimensions of the Cold War story.

Staging the Volume

Unpeeling successive historiographic skins—Cold War studies writ large, the Cold War's imprint on Latin America, and the varied and extensive health and medical developments that unfolded in the region in the mid- to late-twentieth century—this book breaks fresh ground in our understanding of how health and medical ideas and approaches, and their role in state-building in post–World War II Latin America, intersected with Cold War pressures and potentials.

As noted, the extant literature on Latin America during the Cold War period, especially in the health arena, focuses largely on—and as a result (over)emphasizes—the role of the U.S. government and various American go-betweens (philanthropies, academics, etc.) in shaping the era's politics, priorities, and practices. Conscious of the still-reigning imagery and interpretations of Latin America as U.S. "turf," the various chapters in this volume examine how Latin American nations both fit into and manipulated the larger Cold War schemata for health and medicine. This dynamic was apparent even in places, such as Puerto Rico, that were under near-complete U.S. political control, as Raúl Necochea López shows in his chapter. As such, just as the volume recognizes the importance of U.S. influences, contributors also analyze how local- and national-level phenomena contributed to Cold War dynamics.

Taking this a step further, the book as a whole challenges the constraining U.S.–Latin America historiographic scaffolding by chronicling the defiance of Latin American actors who sought alternative channels of health and medical solidarity with the Soviet Union and via South–South solidarities within and beyond Latin America, even as the surge of dictatorships in the mid- and late Cold War constricted experts' ability to manipulate or repel the dictates of authoritarian regimes' science and social welfare policies.[75] Further addressing omissions in the historiography, at least half the chapters explore in considerable depth the relations and interactions with Soviet actors, offering a complex portrayal of alternatives for a range of Latin American players. In addition, the volume engages with the Cold War era's multilayered framings of race and Indigeneity, which in some settings harked back to associations between rurality and "backwardness" whereas in others became associated with socialist struggles for economic justice. As such, this collection problematizes and enhances appreciation for the multivalent, multilevel nature of the Latin American Cold War as a significant perspective for studies of medicine and public health, international development, and international relations.

A range of intertwining themes are highlighted in particular chapters and throughout the volume. Building on interwar Latin American curiosity about the Soviet Union, a key theme is the development of strategic health and medical acquaintances between Latin Americans and Soviets, which served as a counterbalance to U.S. dominance while driving U.S. fears of communist inroads into Latin America's health and medical sectors. The presence of avowed health leftists across the region impelled U.S. surveillance of—and often targeted pressure on—these actors as well as direct repression by Latin American governments. Of course, some efforts were "preventive," with U.S. health and social welfare specialists charged with carrying out research and implementing projects to fend off the attractiveness of communism.

Medical education and the transmission of knowledge between health experts and the public stood out as especially contentious "interventions" in this regard. Yet many Latin American health scientists and professionals without particular ideological affinities were eager to explore Soviet medicine on par with U.S. developments. Finally, various Latin American administrations played the Soviets and Americans off one another, even as they pursued domestic health and welfare state-building interests. This counterposing was also reflected in health professionals' solidarity, as well as official health cooperation among Latin American countries, as a means of pursuing mutual goals of state-building, socialism, sovereignty, and/or staving off outside intervention. Though not always involving confrontation between the rival blocs, the Cold War served as both scene-setter and protagonist across Latin America in the arenas of health policymaking and medical practice and research.

The term "peripheral nerve" in the title alludes to the volume's content both word by word and as an expression. "Peripheral" or "periphery" refers to Cold War–era world systems theory, articulated by Immanuel Wallerstein and others, whereby countries are classified as being in the core, periphery, or semiperiphery depending on their location and role in the global geopolitical economy.[76] Accordingly, Latin American countries reside(d) in the periphery or semiperiphery, depending on their level of industrialization, organizational capacity, and, in the case of semiperipheral countries such as Brazil and Mexico, their subimperial roles dominating peripheral countries. "Nerve" here refers to impudence or even daring, certainly a feature of a range of left-wing or counterhegemonic social movements, governments, and individuals as discussed in particular chapters, from Puerto Rican nationalists to Nicaragua's early Sandinista administration to Salvador Allende in Chile. None of these actors enjoyed the backing of the United States, unlike the authoritarian groups and regimes abetted by the American behemoth. Finally, the title's compound noun offers a physiological metaphor: peripheral nerves serve as the bridge between the brain (and spinal cord) and the rest of the body, controlling "the functions of sensation, movement and motor coordination."[77] Peripheral nerves often cause the most insistent shock (pain) that makes the body take note, evoking the ways in which health and medicine actors and activities in Cold War Latin America, though often overlooked, created enormous shockwaves that affected both peripheral and core places and players.

These issues and perspectives are addressed in nine chapters and an epilogue spanning Latin American space and the different time periods of the Cold War—written by both seasoned and rising scholars from across the Americas. The volume is divided into three sections, bookended by this introduction and a contemplative epilogue. Throughout, we insert cross-references in the endnotes to show how the chapters "speak" to one another within and across the collection, also enabling comparisons to be made across countries and eras.

The first section, "Leftist Affinities and U.S. Suspicions," examines the opening wave of the Cold War, in which paranoia about Soviet infiltration in Latin America saw U.S. authorities and experts seek to delineate political dalliances with leftist influences in distinct settings. At the same time, the real and imagined threat posed by U.S. intrusion was anticipated by various Latin American actors, who gauged the drawbacks and benefits of pursuing their domestic—somewhat idiosyncratic—interests and inclinations, and sometimes acted on their calculations of risk to themselves and their social networks.

Katherine E. Bliss's chapter traces the FBI's decades-long pursuit in Mexico of Dutch-American community health nurse Lini de Vries, whose leftist/Communist sympathies inspired her to volunteer with antifascist forces in the Spanish Civil War in the 1930s and then forced her into exile in Mexico the following decade. De Vries's varied interests in anthropology and rural health led her to chart a variegated career in Mexico into the 1970s, with health authorities creatively engaging her expertise. Mexican political authorities, meanwhile, deftly protected her—and their independence from U.S. pressure.

Nicole L. Pacino's chapter moves into the terrain of U.S. health philanthropy in Latin America, as embodied in the RF's long-standing and broad-ranging health and medicine actions and influence in the region. Her chapter traces the tensions in the foundation's official assessment of the political and medical education landscape in 1950s revolutionary Bolivia, and its diffident retreat from funding leftist medical faculties for fear of contravening the U.S. government's anticommunist agenda.

Gabriela Soto Laveaga's chapter turns to the interaction between commercial and ideological realms, when U.S. pharmaceutical and political officials sought to forcibly wrest away Mexico's steroid production monopoly in the early Cold War period. Far from recoiling in the face of U.S. threats, the Mexican actors in this story adroitly responded to Soviet advances in cultural and educational arenas, ultimately enhancing both pharmaceutical and political relations with Soviet interlocutors.

The next trio of chapters, under the heading "Health Experts/Expertise and Contested Ideologies," explore how the role of health experts in state-building efforts was enmeshed with the exigencies of the Cold War's "middle years." Latin Americans used specialized knowledge, savoir faire, social networks, and institutional positions of power as forms of "cultural solidarity"—and as leverage to fulfill particular political and scientific interests. As the chapters in this section show, these pursuits involved intermediaries and adversaries in both the Capitalist and Communist Blocs, as well as within Latin America itself.

Raúl Necochea López analyzes how U.S.-directed fertility surveys in Puerto Rico, meant to establish a scientific baseline for subsequent family planning policymaking throughout Latin America, fundamentally depended on the patronage and labor of Puerto Ricans while antagonizing the "gringophobic" nationalist movement that flourished during the Cold War.

Gilberto Hochman and Carlos Henrique Assunção Paiva's chapter traces the life and times of esteemed Brazilian parasitologist Samuel Barnsley Pessoa, reflecting on how Pessoa's achievements and prestige made him into a leading observer of the sociopolitical underpinnings of the poor health conditions in rural Brazil and a vocal critic of the forces leading to ill health as well as a mentor to communist biomedical scientists who were targeted, harassed, and persecuted by the Brazilian military dictatorship in the 1960s.

Jennifer Lynn Lambe homes in on psychiatry in revolutionary Cuba, showing that despite official acceptance by the 1970s of Pavlovian experimental and physiological approaches, the leaders of Soviet-style Cuban psychiatry nonetheless faced the resistance and skepticism of their colleagues. The latter advocated a sophisticated and eclectic approach to the foreign psychiatric theories taken up in Cuba, including psychodynamic approaches and especially Freudian psychoanalysis.

The third section moves through later Cold War decades, focusing on "Health Politics and Publics, with and without the Cold War." It traces medical and health policy aspirations that—at one and the same time—reacted to, benefited from, accommodated, and resisted Cold War exigencies while charting national interests and objectives that went beyond the Cold War conflict.

Jadwiga E. Pieper Mooney documents Chilean health policymakers' abiding esteem for the ideas and practice of social medicine, especially under Salvador Allende's socialist- and social medicine–inclined political trajectory as a young health minister, senator, and, fatefully, elected president (1970-1973). From the 1930s through the 1970s, Allende and his like-minded colleagues and rivals, most notably Benjamín Viel, drew inspiration from European and Soviet models of care at the same time that they fashioned sui generis approaches to combine prevention and therapeutics. This demanded elaborate political negotiations to dodge the label of "socialized medicine" until Augusto Pinochet's U.S.-supported military coup and dictatorship buried these efforts (and purged many of its exponents).

Marco Ramos explains how Argentine psychiatrists engaged with First and Second World orientations toward their field and found both wanting. Peronist nationalism and leftward activism in the 1970s led psychiatrists in Buenos Aires to envision a future for their profession that was free from both U.S. and Soviet imperialism, among a populace that would stand in anticolonial solidarity with other Third World nations.

Delving further into the arena of South–South collaboration, Cheasty Anderson examines Cuban medical diplomacy in 1980s Nicaragua. Cuban assistance contributed to remarkable public health achievements by the revolutionary Sandinista regime, which in turn benefited Cuba's health solidarity values and politics. At the same time, the diffusion in Nicaragua of communist ideology through Cuban medical workers—an outcome that the United States suspected and feared—was belied by the everyday demands of medical work in remote areas and by the Cuban government's indisposition to allow its health personnel's contact with local populations to extend beyond clinical encounters.

Finally, in the epilogue, Birn and Necochea López address the meaning and repercussions of these variegated experiences from the worlds of health and medicine, both during and since the Cold War. Notwithstanding the heavy hand of the United States, Latin America was "in the vanguard," not only through its persistent struggles to break with repressive regimes but also in seeking alternatives to neoliberal globalization, with greater or lesser success. Cold War–era health initiatives were thus destiny-forging, enabling Latin American health actors to position themselves both favorably and distinctively in the post–World War II order, as well as amplifying their voices more widely. Moreover, the alternative solidarities that were often a necessity in the Cold War years became an opportunity in their aftermath. Given that this volume is the first to attempt to grapple with this subject, many areas await historical investigation: the epilogue proposes a set of further avenues for exploration.

As a whole, this volume seeks to dislodge the simplistic unidirectional and unidimensional picture of the Cold War—and the implications for health and medicine—by transcending naive depictions of the competition between the superpowers and prevalent portrayals of relations between the United States and the USSR and their "satellites." Instead, we present, from the perspective of Latin American settings, a complex, multifaceted set of accounts of multidirectional, tangled connections among all the players, each pursuing their own agendas, and mobilizing and utilizing whatever resources—institutional, cultural, military, material, and so forth—other players had to offer in the Cold War context.

Notes

1   Frugoni, *De Montevideo*.
2   Cruz Goyenola, *Rusia por Dentro*. Eric Ashby, who was Australia's scientific at-
    taché to the USSR in 1945, not long after Cruz Goyenola departed, experienced
    similar obstacles but stayed on for a year and managed to conduct an extraordi-
    nary number of interviews and site visits once he became familiar with the pro-
    cess. He produced a highly favorable account of Russian science: Ashby, *Scientist
    in Russia*. See also Kershaw, "French and British Female Intellectuals."
3   See, for example, "Cuanto Vale la Mentira"; "Al Margen de Rusia por Dentro."
4   Matthew Brown, *Informal Empire in Latin America*; Matthew Brown and Paquette,
    Connections after Colonialism; Bulmer-Thomas, *Economic History of Latin America*;
    Carrillo, "Patología del Siglo XX"; Marcos Cueto and Palmer, *Medicine and Public
    Health in Latin America*; Joseph, LeGrand, and Salvatore, *Close Encounters of Empire*;
    Carlos Vargas, Sarmento, and Oliveira, "Cultural Networks." See also Birn, *Mar-
    riage of Convenience*; Marcos Cueto, *Valor de la Salud*.
5   Birn, "Uruguay on the World Stage"; Bizzo, "Agências Internacionais e Agenda
    Local"; Borowy, *Coming to Terms with World Health*; Carter, "Social Medicine and
    International Expert Networks"; Souza, "Between National and International
    Science and Education."
6   See, for example, Vatlin, *Komintern*; Wolikow, *L'Internationale Communiste*. For
    Latin America, see Caballero, *Latin America and the Comintern*; Jeifets and Jeifets,
    "Comintern y la Formación"; La Botz, "Communist International"; Mayer, "À la
    fois influente et marginale."
7   This volume covers only the so-called Spanish Caribbean (with individual chap-
    ters on Puerto Rico and Cuba) because the Cold War dynamics in the (former)
    Caribbean colonies of the United Kingdom, France, and the Netherlands played
    out rather differently, with distinct regional alliances and historical legacies that
    go beyond the scope of this collection.
8   Notable exceptions include Spenser, *Impossible Triangle*; Harmer and Riquelme
    Segovia, *Chile y la Guerra Fría Global*.
9   See Brickman, "Medical McCarthyism," 82–100.
10 Latin America is itself sometimes described as a Cold War construct; for further
    explication, see the epilogue.
11 Foote and Goebel, *Immigration and National Identities*.
12 Domingues and Petitjean, "International Science"; Maio, "Contraponto Paulista";
    Maio and Romero Sá, "Ciência na Periferia."
13 To date, even when taking a critical perspective, Cold War histories of inter-
    national health agencies (first and foremost WHO and UNICEF) have largely
    centered either on the exercise of U.S./Western power and ideology or on
    contestation from the context of decolonization, especially in South Asia. See,
    for example, Amrith, "Internationalising Health"; Bhattacharya, "Global and
    Local Histories of Medicine"; Packard, *History of Global Health*; Marcos Cueto,

Brown, and Fee, *World Health Organization*. Also notably sparse are historical analyses of Soviet involvement in WHO and in international health based on Soviet primary sources rather than on presumptions and Cold War caricatures. See Birn and Krementsov, "'Socialising' Primary Care?"; Krementsov and Birn, "Hall of Distorting Mirrors." Moreover, as Dóra Vargha argues, even those works with deeper historical understanding of the Communist world tend to overplay the influence of the Soviet Union. Largely overlooked are the role of Eastern Bloc countries, which actively pursued bilateral relations with health and medical specialists and policymakers both within Eastern Europe (building on long-standing scientific ties) and with countries in the Third World, both socialist (such as Cuba) and not (e.g., Argentina and Peru). Vargha, "Roots of Socialist International Health." These emerging works point to the importance of decentering UN agencies as the prime site of "the international" in Cold War–era international health.

14 McMahon, *Cold War in the Third World*; Prashad, *Darker Nations*.

15 Iacob, "Socialist Health Transfers"; Borowy, "Medical Aid"; Goure, "Latin America"; Hong, *Cold War Germany*.

16 Birn and Muntaner, "Latin American Social Medicine across Borders"; Feinsilver, "Fifty Years of Cuba's Medical Diplomacy"; Kirk and Erisman, *Cuban Medical Internationalism*.

17 Necochea López, *History of Family Planning*; Pieper Mooney, *Politics of Motherhood*.

18 Loureiro, "Alliance for Progress"; Pires-Alves and Maio, "Health at the Dawn of Development"; Caballero Argáez et al., *Alberto Lleras Camargo y John F. Kennedy*; Field, *From Development to Dictatorship*.

19 See, for example, Basbaum, *No Estranho País dos Iugoslavos*; Garrard-Burnett, Lawrence, and Moreno, *Beyond the Eagle's Shadow*; Rupprecht, *Soviet Internationalism after Stalin*.

20 Armus, "Disease in the Historiography of Modern Latin America"; Birn and Necochea López, "Footprints on the Future"; Carter, "Social Medicine and International Expert Networks"; Espinosa, "Globalizing the History of Disease"; Granda, "Algunas Reflexiones"; Necochea López, "Gambling on the Protestants"; Tajer, "Latin American Social Medicine."

21 Marcos Cueto, "International Health."

22 Danielson, *Cuban Medicine*.

23 Leffler and Painter, *Origins of the Cold War*; Light, *From Warfare to Welfare*; Lowen, *Creating the Cold War University*; Mikkonen and Koivunen, *Beyond the Divide*; Solovey, *Shaky Foundations*; Solovey and Cravens, *Cold War Social Science*; Whitaker and Marcuse, *Cold War Canada*.

24 Antic, Conterio, and Vargha, "Conclusion"; Babiracki and Jersild, *Socialist Internationalism in the Cold War*; Engerman, "Second World's Third World"; Fink, *Cold War*; Gaddis, *We Now Know*; Katsakioris, "Soviet-South Encounter"; Vargha, "Socialist World in Global Polio Eradication"; Vargha, *Polio across the Iron Curtain*; Borowy, "Health-Related Activities"; Pieper Mooney and Lanza, *Decentering Cold*

War History. See also Namikas, *Battleground Africa*; Schmidt, *Foreign Intervention in Africa*; Westad, *Global Cold War*.

25　See, for example, Farley, *Brock Chisholm*; Hecht, *Entangled Geographies*; special issue of *Isis*, "New Perspectives on Science and the Cold War," 101, 2 (2010); Krementsov, "In the Shadow of the Bomb"; Krementsov, *The Cure*; Leopold, *Under the Radar*; Leslie, *Cold War and American Science*; Needell, *Science, Cold War and the American State*; Oreskes and Krige, *Science and Technology in the Global Cold War*; Reinhardt, *End of a Global Pox*; Rudolph, *Scientists in the Classroom*; Solovey, "Science and the State," 165–70; Jessica Wang, *American Science in an Age of Anxiety*; Zuoyue Wang, *In Sputnik's Shadow*; Wolfe, *Competing with the Soviets*.

26　This theoretical stance as well as the historical scholarship it has spawned have been cogently critiqued by Pastor and Long, "Cold War and Its Aftermath," 263. See also Coatsworth, "Cold War in Central America," 201–21.

27　Brands, *Latin America's Cold War*; Cowan, *Securing Sex*; Darnton, *Rivalry and Alliance Politics*; Ford, *Childhood and Modernity*; Roberto García and Taracena Arriola, *Guerra Fría*; Grandin, *Last Colonial Massacre*; Harmer, *Allende's Chile*; Iber, *Neither Peace nor Freedom*; Joseph, "Border Crossings"; Joseph and Spenser, *In from the Cold*; Karl, "Reading the Cuban Revolution"; Kirkendall, *Paulo Freire*; Manke, Březinová, and Blecha, "Conceptual Readings"; Parker, *Hearts, Minds, Voices*; Pedemonte, "Cuba, l'URSS et le Chili"; Pettinà, *Historia Mínima*; Pettinà and Sánchez Román, "Beyond U.S. Hegemony"; Rabe, *Killing Zone*; Reeves, "Extracting the Eagle's Talons"; Spenser, *Espejos de la Guerra Fría*; Mor, *Human Rights and Transnational Solidarity*.

28　Marcos Cueto and Palmer, *Medicine and Public Health in Latin America*. See also Marcos Cueto, *Cold War, Deadly Fevers*; Suárez-Díaz, "Molecular Basis of Evolution and Disease," which similarly view the Cold War almost exclusively from within the U.S. ambit of ideologies and imperatives. An important exception to this tendency is Lambe, *Madhouse*.

29　Though our contributors touch only lightly on Chinese–Latin American Cold War medical engagement, China's role in South–South health cooperation is an important topic of analysis. See Friedman, *Shadow Cold War*; Rothwell, *Transpacific Revolutionaries*.

30　Calandra and Franco, *Guerra Fría Cultural*; Schoultz, "Latin America."

31　See Marcos Cueto, Brown, and Fee, *World Health Organization*; Garfield and Williams, *Health Care in Nicaragua*; Testa, "¿Atención Primaria o Primitiva?"

32　Angell, "Left in Latin America"; Birn and Muntaner, "Latin American Social Medicine across Borders"; Carr, "Pioneering Transnational Solidarity"; Herrera González, "Confederación de Trabajadores de América Latina."

33　Almeida, "Circuito Aberto"; Birn, "Nexo Nacional-Internacional"; Marcos Cueto, *Valor de la Salud*; Guy, "Pan American Child Congresses."

34　Marcos Cueto and Palmer, *Medicine and Public Health in Latin America*.

35　This point has been made cogently by Susan Solomon and colleagues regarding long-standing and animated interwar ties between the Soviet Union and both Eastern and Western European countries as shaping continuing interchange in the Cold War period. See Solomon, *Doing Medicine Together*; Solomon, Murard, and Zylberman, *Shifting Boundaries of Public Health*.

36 Krementsov, "Promises, Realities, and Legacies"; Starks, *Body Soviet*.

37 Krementsov, *Revolutionary Experiments*; Stites, *Revolutionary Dreams*.

38 Solomon, "Thinking Internationally, Acting Locally."

39 David-Fox, *Showcasing the Great Experiment*; Jones, *Radical Medicine*; Solomon, "Perils of Unconstrained Enthusiasm"; Krementsov and Solomon, "Giving and Taking across Borders"; Sigerist, *Socialized Medicine in the Soviet Union*; Studer, "Voyage en URSS et son 'retour.'"

40 See special issue of *Historia Crítica* 64 (2017): https://histcrit.uniandes.edu.co /index.php/es/revista-no-64.

41 Jonathan Brown, *Oil and Revolution in Mexico*.

42 L. R. Ochoa to Presidente del Departamento de Higiene y Salubridad en Rusia, January 20, 1924, State Archive of the Russian Federation (Gosudarstvennyi arkhiv Rossiiskoi federatsii—GARF), folder A482, file 35, afair 57, list 21.

43 Departamento de Salubridad Pública, Oficina Central de Higiene Rural y de Servicios Sanitarios en los Estados y Territorios, "Organización y funcionamiento de los servicios sanitarios en los estados y territorios," February 1936, Mexico City, instructivo 10.

44 In between, he may have been a sometime informant to U.S. authorities. See, for example, Robert G. McGregor Jr., memorandum of conversation, January 29, 1940, National Archives and Records Administration, Washington, DC, Diaries of Henry Morgenthau Jr., April 27, 1933–July 21, 1945, book 238; memorandum for Miss Perkins, February 1, 1940, National Archives and Records Administration, President (1933–1945: Roosevelt), President's Secretary's File (Roosevelt Administration), 1933–1945, box 194. On Rivera's medical treatment in the Soviet Union, see also Soto Laveaga's chapter in this volume.

45 Richardson, *Mexico through Russian Eyes*.

46 Birn, *Marriage of Convenience*.

47 Bliss, *Compromised Positions*; Porter, *Alexandra Kollontai*.

48 Cárdenas, *Historia de las Relaciones entre México y Rusia*; Richardson, *Mexico through Russian Eyes*.

49 Spenser, *Impossible Triangle*, back cover.

50 Blasier, *Giant's Rival*, 23. Trotsky arrived in Mexico in January 1937 and was assassinated in August 1940, following an earlier attempt on his life by muralist Siqueiros and a band of hitmen who riddled his house with bullets. That the Stalin-Trotsky rivalry ended so brutally in Mexico serves as a kind of forerunner to the Cold War rivalries that played out violently in Latin America.

51 In 1929, National University of Mexico professor Antonio Castro Leal wrote a letter to Soviet commissar of education Anatolii Lunacharskii, saying that he wanted to replicate Rabfak in Mexico. Lunacharskii sent him the information. Rossiiskii Tsentr Khraneniia i Izucheniia Dokumentov Noveishei Istorii (Russian Center for Storage and Study of Documents on Modern History), collection 142 (Lunacharskii's collection), inventory 1, folder 779, lists 48, 50.

52 Gadnitskaia and Samsonenko, "Meditsinskoe Obsluzhivanie v Povsednevnosti Lolkhoznoi Derevni"; Samsonenko, "Staffing and Efficiency of Medical Personnel"; Samsonenko, *Kollektivizatsiia i Zdravookhranenie.*

53 Kapelusz-Poppi, "Physician Activists"; Agostoni, "Médicos Rurales."

54 Memoirs of Hugh Smith Cumming Sr., p. 565, Manuscripts Department, University of Virginia Library, Charlottesville, Cumming Family Papers, box 5, folder 6922.

55 Less formal exchanges may also have played a role. For instance, Soviet influences may have been transferred through Mexico to other settings, such as Costa Rica, which was developing its social security system in the 1940s (personal communication with Steven Palmer, October 2010). Gauging such flow-through effects proves, needless to say, a considerable challenge.

56 Robert Lambert, "Visit to Mexico," March 1–14, 1941, Rockefeller Archive Center, Sleepy Hollow, NY, record group 1.1. series 323, box 13, folder 95.

57 See Keller, *Mexico's Cold War;* Pettinà, "¡Bienvenido Mr. Mikoyan!"

58 On influential communist and socialist movements in Latin America, see, for example, Gleijeses, *Shattered Hope;* Joseph and Grandin, *Century of Revolution.*

59 For example, the Uruguay-based International American Institute for the Protection of Childhood (founded in 1927) and its *Bulletin* maintained vibrant correspondence and journal exchange with Soviet counterparts. See Birn, "Little Agenda-Setters."

60 David-Fox, *Showcasing the Great Experiment.* For a rather stereotyped Cold War–era depiction from the U.S. position, see Margulies, *Pilgrimage to Russia.*

61 Zeno, *Medicina en Rusia.*

62 Medeiros, *Rússia.* See also Tôrres, "O Inferno"; Tôrres, "Visões do 'Extraordinário'"; Filho, "Uma Outra Modernidade," 102–21.

63 César, *Medicina na União Soviética;* César, *Onde o Proletariado Dirige;* César, *Que É o Estado Proletário?;* César, "Proteção da Saúde Pública."

64 See Bunge, *Continente Rojo;* Recalde, *Higiene y el Trabajo.* On left-wing Argentine visitors to the Soviet Union, see also Saítta, *Hacia la Revolución.*

65 Lobato and Machado, *Médicos Brasileiros na U.R.S.S.;* Silva, *Rússia Vista.*

66 Viel, *Medicina Socializada.*

67 Rupprecht, *Soviet Internationalism after Stalin.*

68 Jesualdo, *Mi Viaje a la U.R.S.S.* In the early 1960s, Jesualdo helped found and served as dean of the University of Havana's School of Education. See also Reinaga, *Sentimiento Mesiánico;* Valcárcel, *Medio Siglo de Revolución Invencible;* Valcárcel, *Reportaje al Futuro;* Varela, *Periodista Argentino;* Bueno, *Visões da Rússia;* Tôrres, "Relatos de Viagem de Brasileiros à URSS." Argentine diplomat Andrés de Cicco recounts the secrecy, fortress-like restrictions, and decrepit conditions he encountered at the Soviet Academy of Sciences in 1947 in *Un Año en Moscú.* In this period, numerous Latin American editions of works by European visitors were also published: see, for example, Rico, *En los Dominios del Kremlin.*

69 See, for example, Gorsuch, "Cuba, My Love."

70 Igual, "Médicos Republicanos Españoles Exiliados"; Igual, "Neurociencias"; Florencio Villa Landa, "Mi Vida," personal collection of Florencio Villa Landa, 491–515; Young, "To Russia with 'Spain.'"

71 Holanda, *Como Seria o Brasil Socialista?*; Rupprecht, "Globalisation and Internationalism."

72 See, for example, Miranda, *Educación y Servicios Médicos*; Shabanov, *Enseñanza Médica en la Unión Soviética*. See also the hundreds of Russian-language, mostly Soviet-era public health and medical books described in Facultad de Medicina, *Ediciones Soviéticas de Medicina Exhibidas*. Velvovsky and Nikolayev's psycho-prophylaxis (and drug-free) childbirth methods that were disseminated in the West in the 1950s (and famously appropriated by French doctors Lamaze and Vellay) came to Latin America more directly. A Spanish-language translation of Velvovsky's *Parto sin Dolor* (Childbirth without Pain) was a bestseller throughout Latin America in the 1950s and 1960s. See also Michaels, *Lamaze*.

73 David-Fox, *Showcasing the Great Experiment*.

74 For an engaging first-person recollection of mostly U.S.-based Latin American-ists with the Soviet Academy of Science's Institute of Latin America, see Bartley, "Cold War and Latin American Area Studies."

75 Amparo Gómez, Canales, and Balmer, *Science Policies and Twentieth-Century Dictatorships*.

76 See, for example, Wallerstein, *World-Systems Analysis*.

77 "Peripheral Nerve Injury," Johns Hopkins Medicine, accessed December 17, 2019, https://www.hopkinsmedicine.org/health/conditions-and-diseases/peripheral -nerve-injury.

Part I

Leftist Affinities and U.S. Suspicions

1

Under Surveillance

Public Health, the FBI,
and Exile in Cold War Mexico

KATHERINE E. BLISS

By 1949, the Cold War was well underway. In Europe, the United States and Western allies intensified the airlift of supplies to occupied Berlin in a successful effort to end the Soviet blockade. To the shock of U.S. authorities, the Soviets detonated their first nuclear device. In China, Mao Zedong and the People's Liberation Army achieved victory over the Chinese Nationalists and secured the triumph of the Chinese Communist Revolution. And in Washington, D.C., members of Congress held hearings on the role of the new United Nations in international affairs and continued to focus their attention on the threats they believed Americans with ties to foreign governments posed to national security.[1]

Across the United States, the impact continued to be felt from the publicity surrounding the July 1948 testimony before the House Un-American Activities Committee (HUAC) of Elizabeth Bentley, who in 1945 had confessed to the Federal Bureau of Investigation (FBI) that she had been a Communist and longtime Soviet spy. In her testimony, Bentley had named Lee Fuhr, a nursing student at Columbia University's Teachers College, as the one who had recruited her for party membership. The FBI had maintained discreet surveillance of Fuhr, a young widow, since her travel to Spain in 1937 to serve as a nurse with the Loyalist-supporting American Medical Brigade. But following Bentley's initial contact with the FBI in 1945 (which remained secret until her testimony to the HUAC in 1948), the bureau had begun more aggressively tracking the nurse, now remarried and known as Lini Stoumen, to question her directly about her relationships with known or suspected Communists. By the late fall of 1949 the stresses of the Bentley publicity, the dissolution of her second marriage, and the inconvenience of being under constant surveillance by the FBI led the forty-four-year-old Stoumen to flee the United States.

In December of that year, the public health specialist packed her bags and headed across the border to Mexico with her three-year-old daughter, taking her mother's maiden name, de Vries, as her own as she started a new life.

Initially landing in Cuernavaca, a city of some forty-three thousand located in the state of Morelos, just outside Mexico's Central Valley, de Vries secured work as an English teacher and then as a nursing instructor before moving to the southern state of Oaxaca in 1952. From 1956 to 1958 she developed health education programs for Indigenous communities situated within the Papaloapan Basin before moving to the city of Jalapa (or Xalapa) to teach at the Universidad Veracruzana. In 1963 she retired from the university and returned to Cuernavaca to attend to her own health issues, open a guesthouse, and write a memoir, *Up from the Cellar*, to offer her own version of life at the crossroads of public health and public scrutiny during the peak years of the Cold War.

While the Mexican government found in de Vries an intrepid community health worker, rewarding her effort to deliver health education to villagers in some of the nation's most remote Indigenous communities by presidential decree in 1962, the U.S. government viewed de Vries and her work in Mexico as a threat to its national interests. Indeed, for FBI analysts who scrutinized her activities in Mexico between 1950 and her death in 1982, de Vries was a principal member of what they believed to be the American Communist Group in Mexico and was integral to planning an "escape route" for U.S.-based Communists during the Korean War years. As Cuba's revolutionary regime moved into the Soviet orbit in the early 1960s, the bureau became convinced that de Vries used her contact with teachers and students to foment anti-American and pro-Cuba sentiment south of the border. For her part, de Vries portrayed herself as a nurse-educator and struggling single mother dedicated to social justice and international understanding.

Taking these conflicting views of de Vries and her work in community health as a point of departure, this chapter examines the intersection of politics and public health in Mexico as global Cold War tensions played out within the U.S. sphere of influence in Latin America. Over the past two decades, historians of U.S.–Latin American relations have called for researchers to build on earlier examinations of formal diplomatic activities and military strategies in studying how the United States attempted to consolidate its regional political hegemony in the mid-twentieth century.[2] Urging scholars to move beyond the "view from Washington" and utilize sources from newly available archives in the former Soviet Union and China, as well as Latin America, to examine multiple aspects of the struggle, researchers have also pushed for greater attention to grassroots mobilizations and to the ways in which social groups, and individuals themselves, experienced the processes of surveillance, repression, and exile.[3] This analysis contributes to the growing literature regarding the "informal" aspects of international relations—including in the realms of education, medicine, and the arts—by analyzing de Vries's life and work in Mexico in the shadow of the U.S. government's Cold War policies. This chapter sheds light on the importance of public health initiatives within the Mexican government's own efforts to promote economic development and its faith in the potential of technical solutions to resolve the challenges of population growth and food insecurity in the mid-twentieth century. At the same time, it demonstrates the extraterritorial reach of the FBI, a U.S. law enforcement agency; the collaboration of the Mexican government and the U.S. intelligence forces in carrying out surveillance on an American nurse and mother during a period of Cold War tensions; and the extraordinary interest of the U.S. national security apparatus in the private life and activities of a self-exiled woman who defined herself as an idealist committed to both improving public health and enhancing U.S.-Mexican relations.

From the Mills to Madrid

Born Lena Moerkerk in 1905 to Dutch immigrant parents in Paterson, New Jersey, de Vries, who was known by her Dutch nickname, Lini, dropped out of school at age twelve to work in the local silk mills to help support her parents and younger sister.[4] By her own account, de Vries's childhood was a bitter one, influenced both by the rigid adherence to the Dutch Reformed Protestantism of her mother, who had converted to Christianity from Judaism upon emigrating from Holland, and by the belief that she was not the biological daughter of her mother's husband, Moerkerk, but instead the child of a man named Bernard Pollock, to whom her mother had once been engaged.[5] Unlike many of her peers in the close-knit immigrant community, de Vries sought to escape the life of a "mill dolly," and as a teenager she worked as a telephone operator before training as a vocational nurse.[6]

In 1928 de Vries married Port Chester, New York, dairy owner Wilbur Fuhr, whom she met in the hospital while she was recovering from a case of acute rheumatic fever when she was still a nursing student. She gave birth to a daughter, Mary Lee, in 1930, just months before her husband died of a blood infection, leaving de Vries a widow at the age of twenty-five. Seeking to escape the influence of her staunchly Methodist mother-in-law and to pursue higher education, de Vries moved to New York City in the early 1930s to study advanced nursing at Columbia Teachers College.[7]

While working and studying in New York, de Vries joined the Columbia University chapter of the American League against War and Fascism and served as its representative at Teachers College. When not in classes at Columbia, de Vries studied anthropology at the New York Workers School, which members of the Communist Party (CP) had established in 1923 on the Lower East Side to provide an inexpensive introduction to Marxist thought and the social sciences to working-class residents of the city. It was through her classes at the Workers School that de Vries "began to realize I was a humanist, a liberal, and an individualist. I firmly believed in man's rights and wanted to have a society where man could reach his potential regardless of race, color, creed or financial status."[8] She claimed to have formally joined the CP in 1935.[9]

De Vries's contact through nursing with New York City's most impoverished communities led to her growing awareness of the connection between public health and political engagement. In 1936 she began working for family planning pioneer Margaret Sanger's Birth Control Clinical Research Bureau, sometimes to the consternation of her party friends, who believed her focus on providing women with contraception was politically misplaced and detracted from broader support for class struggle. Later, in her memoir, she wrote, "Visiting home after home, it was obvious that there was an improvement in family life when the fear of an unwanted pregnancy was removed. The data piling up also proved this. I was enthusiastic about family planning, but my comrade Communist Party members took me to task. Their position was, 'Why waste time on teaching birth control when the answers to society's ills lie in teaching Marxism?'"[10]

Shortly after she began working with Sanger, de Vries had another opportunity to link her passions for public health and political engagement. Her affiliation with the American League against War and Fascism had exposed her to the controversy in Spain and plight of the Spanish Republican cause. In January 1937 de Vries volunteered to work with a hospital unit attached to the American Medical Bureau to Aid Spanish Democracy, because, as she later recalled, "No one else went when I was trying to get them to go—so I went myself."[11] De Vries found her time in Spain providing medical care to the international brigades to be inspiring, a critical step in strengthening her belief that public health was connected to larger political causes. The American Medical Bureau counted on more than one hundred doctors, nurses, and other health workers and collaborated with other international volunteer groups in Spain; many participants, like de Vries, were CP members.[12]

Upon her return to the United States in May 1937, de Vries embarked on a weeklong tour sponsored by the Communist newspaper, *The Daily Worker*, to raise awareness about the Spanish cause.[13] Deciding afterward to apply her nursing skills to impoverished populations within the United States, de Vries pursued employment as a nurse and health educator in New Mexico, Washington, D.C., Puerto Rico, Chicago, and then Los Angeles, working for state-level organizations, the Works Progress Administration (WPA), and the U.S. Department of Agriculture. Her career during this period was marked by positions of increasing responsibility in the areas of family and community health and a deepening commitment to social justice. Over the years de Vries had become more philosophical about political engagement and the connection between her ideals and CP membership. She observed in her memoir that by the time she arrived on the West Coast in the early 1940s she no longer considered herself a party member, writing, "Something had happened to me in Spain. I no longer saw politics as all black or all white. I saw the shades of gray between. I was tired of talking 'isms.' . . . Many of the communists in the United States seemed more like dictators to me. I began wondering if I were a communist. What was I?"[14]

Even before the Bentley story became public, de Vries had begun facing personal difficulties. In 1945 she married photographer and army correspondent Lou Stoumen, whom she had met in Puerto Rico. Not only did she suffer a debilitating miscarriage a year after giving birth to their daughter, Toby, in 1946, but she subsequently required emergency surgery to repair a life-threatening hernia. In 1947 her marriage to Stoumen began to founder when he brought his younger lover to live in the Los Angeles house he shared with de Vries, Toby, and Mary Lee, who was finishing high school.[15] But Bentley's public revelations about her history of engagement with the CP clearly worsened de Vries's personal situation.[16] Bentley had stated to public officials that "during the fall of 1934, while I was at Columbia, I met one Lee Fuhr, nee Meekirk [sic], who was living in the same house that I was, and after I got to know her she took me to various affairs, and eventually I determined she was engaged in the Communist movement. . . . I recall that sometime in March 1935 I became a regular member of the Communist Party and I was sponsored by Professor [name blacked out] and Miss Lee Fuhr."[17]

In her memoirs, de Vries vigorously denied that she had been responsible for Bentley having become a Communist, acknowledging that she had known Bentley in New York but writing that Bentley "finally . . . joined the [American League against War and Fascism], but she never did a thing. The grubby jobs, like running off a leaflet or making a speech at some meeting, she turned down."[18]

In the aftermath of Bentley's testimony, the FBI intensified its review of de Vries's past work and current associations, gathering information about her political activities to build a case that as an employee for the WPA and the U.S. Department of Agriculture in the early 1940s de Vries had violated the 1939 Hatch Act, which prohibits employees of U.S. executive-branch agencies from engaging in political activities.[19] In an interview with FBI agents at the Los Angeles Field Division on June 17, 1946, de Vries was asked whether she was currently or had ever been a member of the CP. She replied, "No, when I hit New York I got a lot of new ideas at Columbia—it was like a new world opening to me. I was probably a leftist." But when pressed to declare whether she associated with Communists in Los Angeles, de Vries admitted that she had attended public health meetings in the Westlake area of Los Angeles at which Communists might have been present.[20]

As her marriage fell apart and the FBI intensified its scrutiny of her associations and activities, de Vries and daughter Toby temporarily moved to New Mexico to stay with friends de Vries had made a decade earlier while working with rural schoolteachers to improve maternal health in the impoverished northeastern corner of the state. It was in New Mexico that de Vries began to prepare for a permanent relocation south of the U.S.-Mexico border.

Exiles, Engineers, and Health Education

The public health situation de Vries encountered in Mexico in 1949 differed markedly from that in the United States, both in terms of political organization and with respect to diseases and health conditions of interest. Between 1910 and 1920 Mexico experienced what has been described as one of the deadliest conflicts of the twentieth century. Enhancing political participation, protecting the rights of peasants and workers, improving social and economic conditions, and reducing the influence of the Catholic Church were stated goals of the Mexican Revolution. By the postrevolutionary reform phase (1920 to 1940), the effort to improve public health also became a high priority. Government activities during this period were characterized by the development of new agencies to address urban and rural health issues; a focus on maternal and child health; and high-profile campaigns targeting specific diseases such as syphilis, malaria, and hookworm.

Mexican public health specialists had long interacted with and drawn inspiration from foreign counterparts, and in the nineteenth century many Mexican doctors and *higienistas*, as public health experts were called, had trained in France and Germany. However, in the context of turn-of-the-century Pan Americanism and greater inter-American cooperation on health, Mexican health specialists increasingly looked to the United States for advice on technical issues.[21] In the early years of the century prominent Mexican higienista Eduardo Liceaga had supported U.S.-sponsored efforts to create a mechanism for regional health cooperation, which led to the founding of the Washington, D.C.–based Pan American Sanitary Bureau in 1902.[22] Later, in the 1920s, even as U.S.-Mexico relations remained tense over the refusal of the United States to establish formal diplomatic ties with the revolutionary government, Mexican public health officials welcomed American academic researchers, as well as personnel from such U.S. philanthropic organizations as the Rockefeller Foundation, who provided expertise on disease eradication campaigns.[23] This kind of health collaboration would continue into the 1930s, despite the fact that Mexico nationalized foreign-owned oil companies, including the holdings of Standard Oil, the very corporation that had provided the resources for the Rockefeller Foundation's endowment in the first place.[24] Mexican public officials were particularly keen to use public health improvements as a way of promoting economic development and cultural modernization, key priorities within the postrevolutionary reform agenda.[25]

De Vries knew little about health, politics, or social conditions in Mexico before her arrival in 1949, her decision to move there influenced more by her ability to speak some Spanish and by the fact that it was possible to travel there without a passport (the U.S. Department of State had kept her passport when she returned from Spain) than by any long-standing personal connection to the country.[26] After arriving in Cuernavaca in December, de Vries stayed with Spanish Civil War refugee Constancia de la Mora, who ten years earlier had published the best-selling memoir *In Place of Splendor*, detailing her conservative, Catholic upbringing and rejection of her class privilege in embracing the Spanish Loyalist cause.[27] As de Vries settled into her new life in Mexico, she fraternized with Spanish refugees, many of whom were doctors and medical professors involved in Mexican public health programs, as well as other self-exiled American leftists in Cuernavaca.[28] It was in Cuernavaca that she decided to use the surname de Vries, explaining, "Since a real question exists as to whether Moerkerk is my biological father or Pollack, I chose to sign LM de Vries."[29]

Although she was surrounded by close contacts and had numerous opportunities for social interaction, de Vries wrote in her memoir that she deplored the high number of foreigners and tourist atmosphere in Cuernavaca and sought a place where she could be more engaged in the public health work she loved. The FBI had established an office within the U.S. embassy in Mexico City in 1939, and it is possible that de Vries worried about informants, even among the community of self-exiled American leftists in Cuernavaca, which included artists, intellectuals, and entrepreneurs, some of whom had been formally engaged in CP politics in the United States, and some of whom may have left home to avoid being subpoenaed to testify against friends or acquaintances regarding their political activities.[30] If she were nervous about informants, those concerns appear to have been justified.[31]

Information provided to the FBI by visitors to Cuernavaca, as well as residents, led agents to conclude that de Vries actively supported the ideals of international communism. One American tourist who had vacationed in Cuernavaca and met de Vries in 1951 wrote to FBI director J. Edgar Hoover, "Doubtlessly, you and members of your department are aware that there are a number of Americans there who give a great deal of support to the Communist ideals, including Lee Fuhr (Lini Morkerk Stoumen de Vreis [sic]), and whatever other name she might have. . . ."[32] The fact that de Vries associated with American, as well as foreign, Communists, was further cause for concern: one agent noted that de Vries "has established a well-organized cell in Mexico, is acting as a liaison in getting others to come to Mexico; and is preparing the place as a hideout in case of necessity."[33] The author of a July 1951 report noted that de Vries "is also connected with other very important Communist elements, both in Mexico City and in Cuernavaca, Morelos. . . . [S]he has excellent contacts in Mexico with the Spanish communists and she is also well connected with the Mexican Communists."[34] By February 1952 the Bureau designated the de Vries case as "one of the 10 most important cases pending in the Mexico City office," with de Vries believed to be "planning an escape route" for U.S.–based Communists in the event of a conflict with the Soviet Union.[35]

The passion de Vries felt for public health work must also have played a role in her decision to leave Cuernavaca and move to southern Mexico. In the summer of 1952 de Vries and daughter Toby relocated to Oaxaca, where de Vries opened a guesthouse and taught English and nursing to university students from Indigenous communities in the Sierra de Juárez. Yet her move to Oaxaca proved no obstacle to continued FBI surveillance. In August of that year the FBI sent a special agent to the state capital for several days to report on her daily activities.[36] The author of an October 1952 report on de Vries observed that "her financial situation appears to be somewhat precarious," and noted that one informant relayed that de Vries was apparently so nervous about being under surveillance that she now allowed only personal friends to stay as paying guests at her boardinghouse.[37]

While the bureau may have been concerned that de Vries was using her work as a nursing teacher as a cover for spreading communist propaganda, it was apparently also worried that her visitors, particularly those believed to

Katherine E. Bliss

work for U.S. government agencies, might be involved in communist conspiracies. The 1952 visit of Joseph Willem Ferdinand Stoppelman, a Dutch-born naturalized U.S. citizen who worked for the International Broadcasting Service in New York, to de Vries's house sparked considerable concern for the FBI because Stoppelman had at one point applied for a job at the Voice of America, the shortwave radio service for news and music that served as the overseas propaganda arm of the U.S. government.[38] Likewise, the 1953 visit of Sam Eskin to the de Vries guesthouse aroused suspicion because Eskin, a folk singer, had performed at an event seven years earlier in Los Angeles, California, organized by People's Songs. The latter had been cited by the California Committee on Un-American Activities.[39] Further, according to an informant, Eskin claimed to be "collecting folk song material for the Library of Congress," which led the FBI to inquire as to whether the singer was connected with that institution.[40] The same year, when a visitor to the de Vries guesthouse parked an early 1950s Chevrolet with New Mexico license plates on the street for several days, the FBI's Mexico City office "requested that the Albuquerque Office endeavor to determine the identity of the registered owner of the above vehicle, and when same is done, to check their indices and advise whether the registered owner, or lawful possessor, of this automobile is known to have engaged in Communist activities in New Mexico."[41]

As the FBI investigated de Vries's ties with nursing students and American tourists, she herself was contemplating her next professional engagement in public health. In *Up from the Cellar* de Vries noted that she initially learned about the Papaloapan Commission from her nursing students, many of whom had been born in communities affected by the Mexican government's ambitious plans to dam the Papaloapan River. In the early 1940s, as Mexican leaders had grown concerned over the twin challenges of population growth and declining agricultural production, officials originated a plan to transform the tropical watershed from a swampy coastal wasteland into a national breadbasket and source of hydroelectric power. Devastating floods in the fall of 1944 had catapulted the Papaloapan River Basin—which encompassed parts of the southeastern states of Oaxaca, Puebla, and Veracruz—to national attention, leading to broad public discussion regarding how to capitalize on the potential of this sparsely inhabited area.[42] The 1910 Revolution had promised agrarian reform and a brighter future for Mexicans of all social classes, and the 1917 Constitution's aim of reviving traditional agricultural cooperatives took hold under the left-leaning populist presidency of Lázaro Cárdenas (1934–1940). However, by the 1940s public officials became gravely concerned that Mexico's existing agricultural resources could not sustain the nation's growing population.[43] In central and northern states, Mexican officials sought Rockefeller Foundation support for the development of high-yield hybridized crops, including corn and wheat, that would be resilient in the region's climate. In the more densely populated South, federal projects focused on making more land available through watershed management approaches.[44] Believing that the relatively uninhabited river basin, which encompassed an area of approximately seventeen thousand square miles, could be converted into housing and tillable land for a growing Mexican population, the national government in 1947 had created a federal commission "patterned after the [1930s Tennessee Valley Authority] of the United States" to begin work to make the watershed suitable for agriculture and habitation.[45]

During the Miguel Alemán (1946–1952) presidency, the Mexican government appropriated an estimated $200 million in federal funds for what was billed as the world's largest tropical reclamation project. Already home to an estimated two hundred thousand people, including members of various Indigenous groups whose survival depended on subsistence agriculture, the region, officials hoped, would accommodate up to six hundred thousand new residents—migrants from Mexico's densely settled central regions—once the project was complete. To prepare for the transformation of the area, officials relocated up to twenty-five thousand culturally isolated Mazatecs, whose traditional lands would be flooded by the damming of the Río Tonto, a Papaloapan tributary. Federal authorities anticipated that migrants from other parts of Mexico would be able to accelerate the cultivation and export of such products as banana, cacao, coffee, sugarcane, rubber, coconuts, vanilla, and pineapples and perhaps reduce the region's economic reliance on the management of livestock vulnerable to foot-and-mouth disease.[46] In an area in which land was predominantly held and farmed communally, officials also sought to incentivize settlement of highland areas, enticing colonos (homesteaders) with private grants of land to use for planting corn, coffee, and tobacco.[47]

Among the principal challenges associated with damming the Papaloapan River and inducing people to relocate to the basin were the region's abysmal health conditions. Thanks to the area's heat, humidity, and tropical climate, diseases such as malaria, intestinal parasites, hookworm, and mal de pinto, sometimes also known as pinta—a bacterial skin infection that caused victims to lose pigmentation and could lead to more serious complications, including paralysis—were leading causes of ill-health.[48] Onchocerciasis, or river blindness, spread by the black fly, was particularly onerous, despite national-level campaigns since the 1930s to eradicate it.[49]

It was during a tour of some of the commission's engineering facilities in 1956 that de Vries was inspired to propose training rural schoolteachers to provide health education to students and their families in the most remote regions.[50] In this, de Vries drew on her experience working with teachers in New Mexico to improve maternal health, reasoning that in Oaxaca, as in New Mexico, teachers were likely to have at least some background in science. The effort was also consistent with postrevolutionary pedagogical approaches. There were also factors compelling her to leave the relative stability of the state capital. The ongoing FBI surveillance in the city of Oaxaca may have made her anxious to find work in a rural area. But political tensions at Benito Juárez University in Oaxaca, where de Vries had been teaching, may also have prompted her interest in changing jobs. She noted in her memoir that her good relationship with the outgoing rector in 1956 almost certainly meant that de Vries, along with the rector's other close friends and colleagues, would be fired by the incoming university administrator.[51]

Drawing on her nursing training at Columbia and her elective coursework in anthropology at the Workers School, de Vries argued for extending health education to rural communities, a view that coincided with the populist perspective on development embraced by the Papaloapan Commission leadership, many of whom had worked with Lázaro Cárdenas during his presidency and in the early 1940s once he returned to his home state of Michoacán.[52] It also resonated, to some extent, with the intercultural approach to health care advanced by physician and anthropologist Gonzalo Aguirre Beltrán, who from the late 1940s through the 1950s oversaw health operations for Mexico's Instituto Nacional Indigenista (INI), which managed activities in the Papaloapan area. But whereas Aguirre Beltrán and INI colleagues emphasized that Indigenous and Western beliefs about the origins of disease or poor health had to be given equal consideration in the development of programs to improve well-being, de Vries, like many Mexican health experts at the time, viewed Western medicine as superior to Indigenous health practices and beliefs in the Papaloapan Basin.[53] De Vries wrote that

> the medical practices that existed could be considered the worst that had come across from Europe in the 16th century and that which they remembered from their own culture [sic]. There were herb specialists, bone-setters, empiric midwives, witchcraft specialists, and "curanderos," all blended with the incense and smell of smoking herbs and copal. Medicine was a mixture of bits of Christian chants, Indian herbs, and medieval

medicine with the unknown destructive bacteria world smirking in their security.[54]

Aguirre Beltrán and de Vries may have differed somewhat in their views on the relative value of Western and Indigenous health perspectives, but their commitment to using schools to transmit new ideas and values coincided.[55] Upon learning that both of the commission engineers "hated to go into the region to prepare for road building" because "they were afraid of the black fly [the vector for onchocerciasis], which developed in rapids" and despaired over how to accomplish the "impossible task of teaching" for the changes that would come to the Papaloapan Basin as a result of the dams, new roads, and electricity, de Vries wrote that she "heard [herself] offering three days a week as a volunteer on 'How to Teach for Health Through the School Program and the Rural Teachers.'"[56] Despite her decidedly modernist and Western point of view, she would also portray her work as bridging an intellectual chasm between the engineers, who espoused a decidedly technocratic approach to preparing Indigenous communities for "modern life," and anthropologists, who advocated teaching in local languages and adapting health lessons to local cultural attitudes and practices.[57]

Frequently trekking far into the mountains, on trips that could take four days of twelve-hour shifts on muleback to arrive at the most remote Mixe, Zapotec, and Mazatec communities, de Vries began meeting with teachers for three days at a time to devise a plan for communicating health practices to children and their families. Drawing on her experience working with rural teachers in New Mexico, she grappled with basic questions: "How could we impart scientific knowledge to the existing yerbera, huesero, brujo and partera (herb-lady, bonesetter, witch doctor and midwife)? How could this new knowledge be integrated with the official structure of the school program, extending only through the third grade? Could health instruction be threaded through the public school curriculum's focus on reading, writing, arithmetic, civics, geography and science?"[58] In addition, de Vries worked closely with staff at the INI (founded in 1948) to develop theatrical scenarios in which the spread of disease was dramatized in Indigenous languages by children or papier-mâché figures acting the part of bacteria or spirochetes.[59]

Over the course of 1956 de Vries reported regularly on her public health activities to commission health and education officials, providing meticulous notes regarding her travels and work. While de Vries spent little time in her memos reflecting on her engagement with local healers and medical practitioners, her reports do suggest that the work was well received by local communities, many of which provided lodging and food to her and the other visiting educators at no charge and celebrated the group's arrival with music, dances, and sports events.[60] De Vries's memos and recollections also offer insight about the top-down nature of health programs in Mexico and the political fragmentation that could inhibit coordination among them. For example, shortly after she was hired by the commission, the project's head engineer, Estanislao Jiménez Díaz, sent letters introducing de Vries to directors at other agencies operating health programs in the Papaloapan Basin, including the INI, the Secretaría de Salubridad y Asistencia, and the National Anti-Malaria Commission (CNEP), among others. His request that each institution "provide Sra. de Vries what she may need from your organization to carry out her work successfully" suggests that in his experience, interagency cooperation on health was not always guaranteed and that he hoped to help de Vries establish a positive relationship with her health colleagues in other organizations.[61]

The agencies' diverse approaches to health sometimes compromised program outcomes, as de Vries's experience contracting malaria attests. In 1955 Mexico launched a national antimalaria campaign, with funding from UNICEF and the Pan American Health Organization (PAHO), in conjunction with the World Health Organization's global malaria-eradication campaign, which was announced in Mexico that year.[62] Following guidance from the national campaign, the Papaloapan Commission sprayed the pesticide DDT on walls in homes and public buildings to kill mosquitoes.[63] But the agencies differed on whether to require personnel to protect themselves against malaria infection. Employees of the internationally funded CNEP, which "criticized traditional medicine as a primitive and superstitious cultural trait," were required to take antimalaria medication, while federal workers devoted to other health projects, such as those associated with the domestically funded Papaloapan Commission, apparently were not.[64] Indeed, in her memoir, de Vries confessed that she had not even been aware of malaria prophylaxis before falling ill when she was in the field. She noted,

> And I would have to expect recurrences [of malaria], all because a mosquito had bitten me two weeks before at Nuevo Paso Nacional, a mosquito who had not read the [commission] sign saying that the area had been sprayed with DDT. . . . If only we had worked by the same rules as the Commission for the Eradication of Malaria. Their workers had to take preventive pills twice a week. If they got malaria, they were fired. Why hadn't anyone told me of those preventive pills?[65]

When de Vries wasn't suffering from malaria or other tropical ailments, she carried out work that went well beyond teaching rural *maestros* about disease prevention. Some of this work involved advocating for improved infrastructure to benefit the communities in the watershed; for example, in July 1956 de Vries wrote to Jiménez Díaz regarding her visit to the impoverished *pueblo* of Valerio Trujano, noting, "I think that it would be possible to accomplish a great deal in this community; with the enthusiasm and motivation of the people, for example, it would be possible to introduce potable water. . . . [T]he improvement of the pueblo depends on the introduction of water."[66] Given that de Vries was frequently one of the only outsiders who made it to the communities, villagers used their contact with her to pass along petitions for other benefits from the Papaloapan Commission. In June 1956 she reported to her commission supervisors that an agricultural official in the community of San Pedro Chicozapote had requested incubators to grow chicks and wood to build beehives in order to improve economic prospects for the population he served.[67]

In 1958 the untimely death of Raúl Sandoval, the commission's executive director and de Vries's supervisor, led to changes in commission leadership that prompted de Vries to resign her position. Describing her meeting with the new director, she wrote, "And then came the new man, appointed by the President to take over where Raúl Sandoval had left off. Listening to him once, twice, observing the changing attitudes, I decided I wanted to get out. From greatness we had fallen to pettiness."[68] But she also attributed her departure to health reasons: "There is a time to stay with a job and a time to leave it. That was my time to leave. Physically, in particular, it was time to leave. In the past I had felt bright enough from the neck up, but now I was weak all over. I felt every one of my 52 years."[69]

Later that year, de Vries relocated to Jalapa in the state of Veracruz to work with Aguirre Beltrán, who had been appointed rector of the Universidad Veracruzana. Having been won over to the intercultural approach to health the INI and Aguirre Beltrán advocated, she developed and taught new courses in medical anthropology and launched a program for foreign students. To earn additional income, she opened a guesthouse and tourist shop "to sell arts and crafts and to begin to sell some of my own collection from the mountains."[70]

Students, Suspicion, and Surveillance

During the late 1950s and 1960s, Mexico's posture with respect to Cold War politics and anticommunism was multifaceted. In international fora the Mexican government portrayed itself as carrying out the legacy of the Revolution of 1910 and defended the right of people to organize politically—and to take up arms—for social change. Within the Organization of American States, for example, the government vigorously defended its foreign policy of nonintervention, known as the Carranza Doctrine, which had been elaborated by President Venustiano Carranza (1917–1920) in response to repeated U.S. interference in Mexico's internal affairs, from the U.S.-Mexican War to the occupation of the port of Veracruz in 1914.[71] But on the domestic front, one party, the Partido Revolucionario Institucional, had a monopoly on political power. Popular movements involving peasants and labor were systematically repressed or co-opted and incorporated into party-associated organizations, and the Mexican Communist Party had been banned since 1929. From the 1940s through the 1970s the Mexican government both cooperated with U.S. intelligence agencies in spying on official representatives of communist regimes, including the USSR (with which Mexico had suspended diplomatic relations between 1930 and 1942), and tolerated U.S. intelligence efforts to maintain surveillance on Americans living in Mexico who were suspected of being CP members.[72]

U.S. intelligence agencies had a long history of operating in Mexico, dating to the early days of the Mexican Revolution, when FBI field offices placed along the border "concentrated on smuggling, neutrality violations, and intelligence collection."[73] Following the establishment of the bureau's office in Mexico City, the first Mexico station of the Central Intelligence Agency (CIA) opened in the Federal District in 1949, with a focus on "apparent violations of the Monroe Doctrine," according to the inaugural station chief, E. Howard Hunt.[74] Mexican agencies, such as the Dirección Federal de Seguridad (DFS), which was modeled on the FBI, collaborated with U.S. intelligence agents in maintaining surveillance on Americans suspected of being Communists.[75] But with a public opinion poll in 1956 showing that most Mexicans were neutral when asked about the significance of the threat of communism to Mexico's national security, U.S. diplomats frequently complained that Mexican officials did not take the threat seriously.[76]

In the late 1950s and early 1960s, the FBI continued to maintain surveillance on de Vries's activities in Mexico, and the documents released to her daughter Mary Lee in 1999 and 2001 suggest that the Mexican government also took an interest in de Vries's life.[77] In 1958, months of paralyzing transportation strikes across the country led the Mexican government to claim that foreign radicals and extremists were involved in a plot to destabilize the country. In late August and early September, student-led protests over an increase in capital-area bus fares gave way to demonstrations by members of the petroleum workers' union and teachers. The arrest of teachers' union leader Othón Salazar provoked massive demonstrations on September 6, leading the administration of President Adolfo Ruiz Cortines to carry out a "highly publicized program of arresting and deporting foreign agitators, who allegedly were involved in the civil disturbances that took place in Mexico City."[78] The Mexico City daily, *Excelsior*, reported on September 10 that "Lini Fuhr" had been among nine foreigners expelled from the country.[79] And on September 12 the *Chicago Tribune* reported that a "Lini Fohr" was on a list of nine "red agitators" who were arrested in Mexico and flown to San Antonio and Los Angeles.[80] But the *Excelsior* coverage of the deportations on September 12 made no mention of de Vries, and an FBI report later that month noted that "although only three American security subjects were deported under this program, considerable irresponsible newspaper publicity was given to the matter" and that de Vries's name had been erroneously included "among numerous others" in the Mexico City daily newspapers.[81] A confidential informant in Jalapa advised a bureau agent that, following the publicity, "the subject [de Vries] left the town of Jalapa, Veracruz, Mexico and proceeded to Oaxaca, Oaxaca for a visit until her fear of possible arrest and deportation from Mexico had passed."[82]

De Vries's role in managing the Universidad Veracruzana's student exchange programs from 1958 to 1963 apparently justified continued FBI attention because of her extensive contact with, and potential to influence, young Americans. Already concerned over the role of teachers and university students in supporting the 1958 labor unrest in Mexico, by 1961 U.S. officials viewed Mexican student mobilization in support of revolutionary Cuba with special concern and worried that campus activities could influence young Americans studying abroad to embrace leftist political ideologies.[83] In 1961 one informant told the FBI that "the summer school for foreign students at the University of Veracruz had the reputation in Jalapa of being a meeting place for American students who were more interested in discussing communism than the study of Spanish."[84]

Considering the importance of the FBI's Mexico City office as a staging point for U.S. operations in response to Cuban political developments during the early 1960s, reports of de Vries's attendance at rallies supporting Cuba's Fidel Castro and the Cuban Revolution must have confirmed for agents monitoring her that she was devoted to fomenting anti-American sentiment among the students with whom she interacted. An FBI assessment classified as "Secret" noted that "her curio shop named Tianguis is a meeting place of alleged national communists and foreigners" and that "many students and artists (exact identities unknown) have met the subject at her curio shop, where on occasion anti–United States and pro–Fidel Castro Ruz statements have been made."[85] Yet the refusal of Mexican president Adolfo López Mateos (1958–1964) to bow to U.S. demands that Mexico withdraw diplomatic recognition and support from the new regime in Cuba may have also contributed to the bureau's increasing anxiety over any Americans believed to be supporters of the Cuban cause.[86]

Two events may have prompted de Vries to relocate from Jalapa to Cuernavaca by 1963.[87] The first was the poor reception of the Spanish-language publication of her memoir, *El Zótano*, whose title referred to the cellar where she claimed that her mother had locked her up when she misbehaved as a child. In the book de Vries also alleged that she had been sexually abused by the family minister and that she believed her mother had always mistreated her because she viewed de Vries as the product of an extramarital sexual relationship. Perhaps alluding to the book's revealing nature, a reviewer for one local magazine referred to the author as "Bikini" M. de Vries and poked fun at the memoir's tone and confessional approach. One informant told the FBI that prior to the book's publication de Vries had been "highly regarded by 'decent people' [in Jalapa] but is now loathed," perhaps because her exposure of family secrets of a sexual nature were too risqué for socially conservative Jalapa society.[88]

Another factor was that de Vries had finally been naturalized as a Mexican citizen. Soon after her 1949 arrival in Cuernavaca, de Vries began applying for Mexican citizenship, gathering recommendations from former employers and working with politically connected lawyers and elected officials to plead her case. In the early 1960s her effort to acquire citizenship gained steam, with a series of petitions directed to President López Mateos himself. In April 1961 governor of Veracruz Antonio M. Quirasco wrote López Mateos in support of her citizenship petition, saying that "Sra. de Vries has completely assimilated into the Mexican milieu as a writer, social worker, and nurse-educator, and her contributions to our University have been of great value and significance."[89] The high-profile campaign appears to have paid off; in December 1961, López Mateos decided to confer citizenship upon de Vries, making her one of only a handful of people at that point to have been granted Mexican citizenship by presidential decree. In *Up from the Cellar* de Vries described the feeling of becoming a Mexican citizen as one of liberation: "On May 10, 1962, while I was working in Jalapa, Veracruz, President Adolfo López Mateos signed the decree making me a Mexican citizen! All the fears of the FBI seemed to lift off my shoulders. Suddenly I felt free. I was home."[90]

Memories, Mentoring, and Medical Challenges

Her Mexican citizenship secure, in the mid-1960s de Vries shifted her focus from health education and university administration to teaching and writing a memoir of her work at the frontlines of public health and development within the context of Cold War surveillance. In Cuernavaca she served on the anthropology faculty at the University of Morelos and ran an Institute of Mexican Studies out of her home, which once again doubled as a gift shop and boardinghouse.[91] Always a reliable correspondent, in her later years she exchanged letters with numerous close friends and family members, along with acquaintances and admirers of her work.[92] She devoted considerable time to mentoring young academics, primarily women, who were interested in Mexico. Following her naturalization as a Mexican citizen, FBI surveillance seems to have tapered off, with yearly updates offering little more than de Vries's address and occupation.

However, the Mexican government, through the DFS, intensified its surveillance of de Vries. Amid unverified reports that she was the leader of student protests at the Universidad Veracruzana in the fall of 1966, the DFS leadership requested a summary of her activities in Mexico, which detailed her immigration petitions, professional positions, and friendship with Communists from Mexico and abroad.[93] The DFS summary of her time in Cuernavaca noted that upon relocating to the city de Vries "continued her close association with American Communists in Mexico and that some of them pass their vacations in her guest house, and that her house is known among Communist elements in the United States as a safe place to stay when they are visiting Mexico."[94]

During the 1970s, de Vries affiliated in Cuernavaca with the Centro Intercultural de Documentación (CIDOC), founded by a former priest and outspoken critic of Western development and foreign-assistance models, Ivan Illich. Embracing his view that the study of foreign languages and cultures should focus on fostering solidarity and partnership among citizens of different nations, rather than vertical relationships of imperialism and oppression, she shared resources and contacts from her own Institute of Mexican Studies with Illich and supported CIDOC operations for several years.[95] Although she taught medical anthropology at CIDOC until the mid-1970s, it is not clear whether de Vries shared Illich's views, published in 1974 in a series of lectures, articles, and a book, *Medical Nemesis*, that the "medical professional practice has become a major threat to health."[96] De Vries concentrated much of her time in her later years on developing a new version of her memoir for U.S. audiences. For several years she regularly corresponded with her agent, Harriet Kimbro, about finding a publisher for the manuscript, while also helping friend and fellow Medical Brigade nurse Fredericka Martin organize an archive related to U.S. health workers involved in the fight in Spain. At the same time, her health was beginning to fail as she approached her eighth decade, and from 1976 onward she battled multiple health complications, including parasites, hernias, diverticulitis, abdominal abscesses, emphysema, and what was eventually diagnosed as celiac disease, or nontropical sprue.[97]

Later in the decade, de Vries finally secured a multiyear visa to the United States and visited friends and family to celebrate and publicize her memoir, *Up from the Cellar*, which was released by the Minneapolis-based feminist Vanilla Press in 1979.[98] She also sought medical treatment for some of her worsening health problems. Traveling to Ridgewood, New Jersey, where her parents were buried and where her sister Betty worked as a nurse, de Vries had surgery to repair uterine prolapse in 1982. She died at the hospital nine days later at age seventy-seven of cerebrovascular complications.

Conclusion

The life of Lini de Vries—nurse, educator, and self-described idealist/humanist—sheds light on intersections of health and politics in the context of the Cold War in multiple ways. De Vries's travel to Spain to serve as a volunteer nurse with the international brigades supporting the Spanish Loyalists in the 1930s cemented for her the sense that health-related work was an inherently political act. This experience sparked her interest in working with impoverished populations in the U.S. Southwest, Puerto Rico, and California but also led to her surveillance by the FBI under suspicion of being a Communist. When "spy queen" Elizabeth Bentley fingered de Vries as the person who had recruited her to the CP, de Vries drew on her experience in Spain as she decided to make a new life in Mexico.

When considered from the perspective of Mexican domestic politics and the transformation of the Papaloapan River Basin to address concerns over population growth and food insecurity, de Vries's experience educating Indigenous groups sheds light on how Mexican officials selectively adapted international development models, using the U.S. Tennessee Valley Authority project as a template for controlling floods and opening up arable land, but integrating Western and Indigenous approaches to health in fashioning outreach programs that were consistent with Mexico's postrevolutionary nationalism.

Finally, at the level of international relations, we can see de Vries's experience as expressive of the ambiguous and often tense relationship between the United States and Mexico when it came to Cold War cooperation. The Mexican government tolerated the activities of a U.S. agency in spying on a self-exiled citizen—and itself maintained surveillance of de Vries. However, in the midst of U.S.-Mexico tensions over political developments in revolutionary Cuba, President López Mateos made de Vries a citizen by presidential decree, even though she had previously been designated one of the FBI's top ten security concerns in Mexico.

Over the course of her life and work, de Vries's commitment to public health, social justice, and political freedom involved her in some of the mid-twentieth century's critical political episodes. For de Vries, public health was an entry point into the larger world of political struggle, but she paid in very personal ways for her commitment to health and humanitarian as well as civil activism. To her credit, she overcame many of these challenges by steadfastly practicing the health work she loved, teaching college students about health, as well as U.S.-Mexico relations, and mentoring a new generation of women interested in social conditions in Mexico. The experiences of Lini de Vries serve as a reminder of the many ways in which health became entangled in Cold War politics and how U.S. Cold War policies affected citizen and state aspirations for health in Mexico and across the Americas.

Notes

The author thanks Anne-Emanuelle Birn and Raúl Necochea López for their helpful edits and is grateful to Bill French, María Muñoz, Kathy Peiss, Monica Rankin, and John Tutino for their comments on earlier drafts. Grants from the Schlesinger Library at the Radcliffe Institute for Advanced Study, the Cold War Center at NYU's Tamiment Library, and the Robert F. Wagner Labor Archives provided travel and research support.

1   James Brown, *Printed Hearings of the House of Representatives.*
2   The foundational work in this respect is Joseph, LeGrand, and Salvatore, *Close Encounters of Empire.* See also Brands, *Latin America's Cold War*, 1–8; Grandin, *Empire's Workshop.*
3   See also Joseph, "What We Now Know and Should Know," 18, 29.
4   Extract from the Official Congregational Record of the Sixth Holland Reformed Church of Paterson, NJ, 1905, Lini M. de Vries Papers, 1910–2009, MC 573, box 1, folder 1, Schlesinger Library, Radcliffe Institute, Harvard University, Cambridge,

MA; de Vries, *Up from the Cellar*, 47–48. The participation of Dutch immigrant girls in the Paterson silk mills was common. See Sinke, *Dutch Immigrant Women*.

5   De Vries, *Up from the Cellar*, 29.

6   Transcript, Teachers College, 1943, de Vries Papers, box 1, folder 2.

7   De Vries completed her college degree in June 1943 (de Vries Papers, box 1, folder 2).

8   De Vries, *Up from the Cellar*, 154.

9   De Vries, *Up from the Cellar*, 157.

10 De Vries, *Up from the Cellar*, 164.

11 Blake Green, "The Angels of the Last Pure War," *San Francisco Chronicle*, February 10, 1977, clipping in de Vries Papers, box 1, folders 3, 5. See also Fredericka Martin Papers, box 6, folder 23, Tamiment Library, New York University, New York.

12 Lear, "American Medical Support."

13 Clark, "Lini Fuhr Is Back from Spain." She captured her memories of Spain in a novel, de Vries, *España 1937*.

14 De Vries, *Up from the Cellar*, 239.

15 De Vries, *Up from the Cellar*, 266, 287; personal communication from Mary Lee Baranger to the author, January 2015. For more information on Lou Stoumen, see "Lou Stoumen Is Dead."

16 Bentley, *Out of Bondage*. For analysis of Bentley's life and the impact of her testimony on Soviet espionage efforts in the United States, see Olmstead, *Red Spy Queen*.

17 FBI Report, El Paso, February 23, 1949 (covering January 5, 13, 14, 21, 27, 28, February 2, 3, 8, 14, 16, 17, 1949), de Vries Papers, box 1, folder 19.

18 De Vries, *Up from the Cellar*, 156.

19 De Vries, *Up from the Cellar*, 275.

20 FBI transcript of Los Angeles interview, July 16, 1946, de Vries Papers, box 1, folder 19.

21 See Marcos Cueto, *Valor de la Salud*. See also Carrillo and Birn, "Neighbours on Notice."

22 Marcos Cueto, *Valor de la Salud*, 38–44.

23 On U.S.-Mexico relations, see "Mexico and the Outside World."

24 Birn, *Marriage of Convenience*, 52, 225–26, 237.

25 Bliss, "For the Health of the Nation."

26 Albert Maltz also advised her to relocate to Mexico. Personal communication from Mary Lee Baranger to the author, June 10, 2015.

27 De la Mora, *In Place of Splendor*. See also Soledad Fox, "Memory and History."

28 On the Spanish refugee community in Mexico, see Fagen, *Exiles and Citizens*. Fagen notes that "during the 1940s and 1950s Mexico initiated major national health campaigns in which newly arrived Spanish physicians participated fully" (71).

29 Miscellaneous Notes, 1974–1977, de Vries Papers, box 2, folder 3.

30 Anhalt, *Gathering of Fugitives*, 39–70.

31 In response to a Freedom of Information Act (FOIA) request, in the late 1990s and early 2000s the FBI declassified and released some of its files on de Vries to her

daughter Mary Lee Baranger, who subsequently donated them to the Schlesinger Library at Harvard University. While all proper names and identifying information have been blacked out, it is clear that a number of people were providing bureau agents with information about de Vries and other American leftists living in Mexico in the 1950s.

32   FBI Interview with correspondent, July 30, 1951, de Vries Papers, box 1, folder 19.

33   Office memorandum to SAC, New York, from Director, FBI, Subject Lini Moerkerk Stoumen, July 30, 1951, de Vries Papers, box 2, folder 2.

34   FBI Report, September 1952, de Vries Papers, box 1, folder 19.

35   Self-Inspection Report, Mexico City Office, February 25, 1952, de Vries Papers, box 2, folder 2; de Vries Papers, box 1, folder 19.

36   FBI Report, October 9, 1952, de Vries Papers, box 1, folder 19.

37   Director, FBI, to SAC, December 16, 1952, de Vries Papers, box 1, folder 19; see also FBI Report, Los Angeles, October 1, 1952, de Vries Papers, box 2, folder 3.

38   Director, FBI, to Legal Attaché, Mexico City, May 1953, de Vries Papers, box 2, folder 3.

39   FBI Report, Mexico City, May 5, 1953, de Vries Papers, box 2, folder 3; see also FBI Report, Mexico City, May 12, 1953, de Vries Papers, box 2, folder 3.

40   Director, FBI, to Legal Attaché, Mexico City, May 1953, de Vries Papers, box 2, folder 3.

41   Legal Attaché, Mexico, to Director, FBI, March 10, 1953, de Vries Papers, box 2, folder 3.

42   Poleman, *Papaloapan Project*, 89–90.

43   See Tom Gill, *Land Hunger in Mexico*. Enrique Beltrán summarized many of these perspectives in a 1967 speech to the Escuela Nacional de Medicina Veterinaria y Zootecnia de la UNAM. See Beltrán, *Recursos Naturales*.

44   "100 Years: The Rockefeller Foundation." See also Fitzgerald, "Exporting American Agriculture"; Cotter, *Troubled Harvest*.

45   Winnie, "Papaloapan Project," 227; Garrison, "Reclamation Project," 60. See also Andrade Galindo and González, "Ex-Comisión del Papaloapan." On the use of the TVA as a development model, see Immerwahr, *Thinking Small*, 40–65.

46   Attolini, "Ganadería en la Cuenca del Papaloapan."

47   Garrison, "Reclamation Project," 62. See also "Basin Becomes Test Tube," 343; Galindo and González, "Ex-Comisión del Papaloapan," 43.

48   Winnie, "Papaloapan Project," 232; Carrillo, "From Badge of Pride."

49   De Vries, *Please, God, Take Care of the Mule*, 29. See also Carrillo, "From Badge of Pride"; Lewis, "Indigenista Dreams Meet Sober Realities."

50   De Vries, *Up from the Cellar*, 343. For the proposal, see de Vries Papers, box 7, folder 2.

51   De Vries, *Up from the Cellar*, 344.

52   See Kapelusz-Poppi, "Rural Health and State Construction." See also Agostoni, "Mensajeras de la Salud"; Arechiga, "Historia de la Salud."

53   The intercultural approach was first articulated at the first Congreso Indigenista Americano, which met in Pátzcuaro, Mexico, in 1940. See Marcos Cueto, *Salud Internacional*, 234. Aguirre Beltrán elaborated and refined the approach in an ad-

dress to the World Health Assembly in 1955. See Comisión Nacional del Desarrollo de los Pueblos Indígenas (CDI), Centro de Documentación, Fondo Documental 91/1955/12; Aguirre Beltrán, "Interpretation of Health Programs."

54 Essay on Teaching for Health, 1957, de Vries Papers, box 6, folder 5.

55 See Aguirre Beltrán, "Teoría y Práctica de la educación indígena," CDI, Centro de Documentación, Fondo Documental, 9/1953/5.

56 De Vries, *Please, God, Take Care of the Mule*, 29, 34.

57 De Vries, *Up from the Cellar*, 339. In many ways, de Vries's proposed method of teaching health through public schools resonated with health education approaches adopted in Mexico during the postrevolutionary period, when authorities sought to use schools to inculcate revolutionary ideals of nationalism and anticlericalism among the rural and urban populations alike. See Vaughan, "Nationalizing the Countryside."

58 De Vries, *Up from the Cellar*, 343; on her work in New Mexico, see 246–48.

59 De Vries, *Up from the Cellar*, 343. On the imperative to improve health conditions in rural areas, see also Anderson's and Hochman and Paiva's chapters in this volume.

60 Estanislao Jiménez Díaz to Dr. José Figueroa Ortiz, May 18, 1956, de Vries Papers, box 7, folder 3.

61 The letters of introduction reflect the diversity of federal and international agencies involved in the effort. See Letters, Miscellaneous, 1956, de Vries Papers, box 7, folder 3.

62 Miguel Bustamante et al., *Salud Pública en México*, 88–90.

63 See Marcos Cueto, *Cold War, Deadly Fevers*; Gómez-Dantés and Birn, "Malaria and Social Movements."

64 Marcos Cueto, *Cold War, Deadly Fevers*, 119.

65 De Vries, *Up from the Cellar*, 416.

66 Memo to Estanislao Jiménez Díaz, July 31, 1956, de Vries Papers, box 7, folder 6.

67 Memo to Estanislao Jiménez Díaz, July 31, 1956, de Vries Papers, box 7, folder 6. De Vries did not report whether his request was granted.

68 De Vries, *Up from the Cellar*, 418.

69 De Vries, *Up from the Cellar*, 419.

70 De Vries, *Up from the Cellar*, 419.

71 See Schuler, "Mexico and the Outside World."

72 See Jefferson Morley, *Our Man in Mexico*, 90–91, 123. Scott, whose formal title at the U.S. embassy was first secretary, regularly attended social events at which prominent Americans and Mexicans were present. In 1958 he attended an engagement party for *New York Times* Mexico correspondent Paul Kennedy. See "Town Topics"; Meisler, "Argument over Role of CIA"; Iber, "Managing Mexico's Cold War."

73 U.S. Department of Justice, Federal Bureau of Investigation, "Brief History."

74 Jefferson Morley, *Our Man in Mexico*, 85; National Security Archive, "Interview with E. Howard Hunt."

75 Padilla and Walker, "In the Archives."

76 Fein, "Producing the Cold War," 172; Schreiber, *Cold War Exiles in Mexico*, 2, 15.

77 A review of a "public version" of the file on de Vries maintained by the Dirección Federal de Seguridad (DFS), housed at the Archivo General de la Nación (AGN) in Mexico City and secured through a 2015 Infomex request, sheds light on the Mexican government's surveillance of de Vries and others in the so-called American Communist Group in Mexico (ACGM). AGN, DFS, Vries Stoumen, Lini M. de, file 1, folder 1; public version of classified file obtained August 26, 2015.

78 Legal Attaché to Director, FBI, de Vries Papers, October 22, 1958, box 2, file 5.

79 "Ya Expulsaron a Nueve," 1.

80 "Vows to Oust Red Agitators."

81 Legal Attaché, Mexico, to Director, FBI, October 22, 1958, de Vries Papers, box 2, folder 5; see also "México Expulsa a 40 Extranjeros," clipping in de Vries Papers, box 2, folder 5.

82 Legal Attaché, Mexico, to Director, FBI, October 22, 1958, de Vries Papers, box 2, folder 5.

83 See Zolov, "Cuba Sí, Yanquis No!," 215.

84 Special Agent in Charge, Los Angeles, to Director, FBI, September 7, 1960, de Vries Papers, box 2, folder 6. On fears of Communist infiltration of the education arena, see also Pacino's chapter in this volume.

85 Legal Attaché, Mexico, to Director, FBI, January 31, 1963, de Vries Papers, box 3, file 3.

86 On Mexico's diplomatic relationship with Cuba during this period, see Keller, "Foreign Policy for Domestic Consumption"; Arthur Smith, "Mexico and the Cuban Revolution," 73.

87 Internal Memo, FBI, October 29, 1963, de Vries Papers, box 2, folder 5.

88 Legal Attaché, Mexico, to Director, FBI, January 25, 1960, de Vries Papers, box 2, folder 5.

89 Antonio M. Quirasco to Adolfo López Mateos, April 12, 1961 (copy), de Vries Papers, box 3, folder 9.

90 De Vries, *Up from the Cellar*, 420.

91 Internal Memo, FBI, April 30, 1969, de Vries Papers, box 1, folder 19.

92 Martin Papers, box 6, folder 16.

93 AGN, DFS, Vries Stoumen, Lini M. de, file 1, folder 1; public version of classified file obtained August 26, 2015.

94 AGN, DFS, Vries Stoumen, Lini M. de, file 1, folder 1.

95 Interview with Gobi Stromberg, anthropologist and former assistant to de Vries, Cuernavaca, Mexico, October 22, 2015.

96 Illich, "Medical Nemesis," 918; Illich, *Medical Nemesis*.

97 Letter from Dr. Robert A. Mayers, May 3, 1978, de Vries Papers, box 3, folder 16.

98 U.S. Department of Justice Memo, April 1973, de Vries Papers, box 1, folder 19. On her earlier troubles securing a visa to enter the United States, see Los Angeles Special Agent in Charge to Director, FBI, October 1970, de Vries Papers, box 1, folder 19.

2

National Politics and Scientific Pursuits

Medical Education and the Strategic Value of Science in Postrevolutionary Bolivia

NICOLE L. PACINO

In August 1952, Dr. Johannes H. Bauer, a staff member of the Division of Medicine and Public Health of the Rockefeller Foundation (RF), visited Bolivia to conduct a survey of its medical schools. His final report, published in September 1952, disparaged Bolivia's medical education system's subpar equipment, instruction, and facilities, and suggested the RF should not pursue a relationship with its medical schools. He singled out the Universidad Mayor de San Simón in Cochabamba's medical school as "more of a joke than an institution of higher learning" because its students were too political and its rector, Dr. Arturo Urquidi Morales, was an "ardent communist."[1] He added that the medical school's dean and the majority of the university's students and faculty were also well-known communists.[2] Bauer's repeated references to communism indicates RF philanthropic aid to Bolivia was not solely focused on improving medical education, disseminating scientific knowledge, or advancing U.S. notions of modernity.[3] Rather, medical education surveys were a means to assess communism's influence in Bolivia during the Cold War.

During the Cold War, philanthropic aid closely reflected the U.S. objective of containing communism in its sphere of influence. Yet shared objectives did not necessarily translate into aligned approaches. In this chapter I consider how debates about medical education mirrored U.S. concerns about communism's influence in postrevolutionary Bolivia.[4] I first consider the on-the-ground situation in Cochabamba and use the "ardent communist" Urquidi as an example to show why Bauer considered Bolivian institutions unworthy of funding. I then examine Bauer's report to expose RF anxieties about Bolivia's revolutionary politics in relation to long-standing assumptions of U.S. cultural superiority and scientific elitism toward Latin America.[5] This assessment shows that Bauer used political ideology as a litmus test for scientific merit in a way that demonstrates how avid anticommunism in the U.S. in the 1950s led to the RF's "politicization of awards."[6] Finally, I compare RF and State Department assessments of Bolivian medical schools to show that State Department officials considered Bolivia's perceived communist threat an incentive for financial assistance rather than an area of concern. In doing so, I consider which factors most shaped RF decisions about Bolivian medical institutions: Was Bolivia considered too backward to merit RF financial assistance? Or did Urquidi's supposed political affiliations taint the entire medical education system? During the Cold War, the RF came to consider knowledge and institutions valuable only if they were free of communism's stigma, and Bauer asserted that political ideology sullied Bolivian medical schools. This case shows that the era's ideological tensions caused the RF's policy to shift from aligning with the State Department to significantly diverging from it, representing different conceptualizations of Bolivia's strategic value in the 1950s.

Background: Bolivia's Leftist Politics, RF Conservatism, and the Cold War

Bauer visited Bolivia just five months after the culmination of Latin America's second major twentieth-century revolution (following the Mexican Revolution of the 1910s–1920s). This successful social revolution brought the Movimiento Nacionalista Revolucionario (MNR) to power on April 9, 1952, after a military junta negated their legitimate electoral victory in 1951. Bauer's report must be considered in light of shifting RF priorities in the 1940s and 1950s, growing concern within the United States about communism's domestic and international influence, and U.S.-Bolivian relations after the 1952 revolution.

The MNR came to power with support from a diverse coalition of Bolivians, including miners, peasants, students, and the middle class. During 1952 and 1953, the MNR decreed universal suffrage, nationalized the tin-mining industry, and enacted redistributive agrarian reform. This "period of initial radicalism" changed the country's political and social landscape, and throughout the 1950s the MNR attempted to placate its radical peasant and working-class allies without alienating its more conservative, middle-class, and urban supporters. After 1956 the revolution became "restrained" as the MNR focused on consolidating power, fostering political loyalty, and courting U.S. financial assistance.[7]

At this time communism was not a dominant political ideology in Bolivia. Unlike Argentina, Mexico, Uruguay, and Brazil, which had active communist parties dating back to the 1920s, Bolivia had no formal Communist Party until decades later. Trotskyism's influence began in the 1920s and 1930s, when Bolivian radicals Tristán Marof and Guillermo Lora formed the Partido Obrero Revolucionario (Revolutionary Workers' Party, POR) after the disastrous Chaco War (1932–1935). In 1940, the Marxist-Leninist Partido de la Izquierda Revolucionaria (Party of the Revolutionary Left, PIR) was formed, but it was ideologically incoherent and not internationally recognized. A large segment of the PIR's membership broke away to form the Partido Comunista Boliviano (Bolivian Communist Party, PCB) in 1949. The PCB gained full international recognition and became Bolivia's first formal Communist Party, but its illegality forced members to operate underground until after the 1952 National Revolution. These parties' influence varied; whereas during the 1940s the POR helped develop a strong mine workers' movement, many of whose members participated in the 1952 revolution, the PIR's dogmatic pro-Soviet stance cost it followers, and the MNR effectively hijacked the PCB's agenda throughout the 1950s. None of these parties exercised major national political influence in the 1950s. Although they legally participated in all national elections after 1952, they never collectively garnered more than two percent of the vote, and none of their candidates were elected to national office. Combined membership was estimated at a high of five thousand in 1957.[8]

Each of these parties had a complicated relationship with the MNR in the revolutionary era. The PIR had an antagonistic history with the MNR dating back to the 1940s when they competed for working-class support. The PIR's splinter group, the PCB, helped the MNR win the 1951 presidential election and supported its revolution when a military coup prevented the MNR from taking office.[9] Despite supporting the MNR's revolution, the POR's policies were far more radical in orientation; it advocated carrying the revolution "all the way" by expropriating capitalist industries and hacienda lands. It expressed solidarity with Guatemala in the 1950s—where Jacobo Árbenz nationalized United Fruit company lands for redistribution—and suggested that Bolivia too would succumb to U.S. imperialist aggression if the MNR failed to overthrow capitalism. In 1954 the POR split into rival factions, both of which supported the Cuban Revolution while the MNR denounced it to demonstrate loyalty to the United States.[10] POR leaders continued to occupy strategic positions in the labor movement and had close relations with the MNR's Juan Lechín, head of the Central Obrera Boliviana (the Bolivian workers' union), although Lechín ultimately shaped the POR as a "radical appendage to *lechinismo*" that benefited the MNR more than the Communist Party.[11]

Throughout the 1950s the MNR increasingly targeted communist parties and sympathizers as threats to the nation in general and the revolution in particular. This campaign was a response to U.S. pressure to eliminate favorable conditions for communist parties to operate, but also allowed the MNR to stoke U.S. fears that their deposal would result in a government more sympathetic to communism. As a result, the PCB openly denounced the MNR by November 1953.[12] The rift between the MNR and PCB continued to grow, and in his 1960 congressional address President Hernán Siles Zuazo denounced the PCB's attempts to create political instability.[13]

Bauer likely would have been wary of Bolivia's shifting political and social context in the early 1950s given RF's subtle but significant role in promoting U.S. political ideology and economic interests abroad since the early twentieth century.[14] In 1913 the RF formed the International Health Commission (renamed the International Health Board in 1916 and International Health Division [IHD] in 1927) to expand its hookworm eradication programs from the southern United States to other countries. It launched its first disease control programs in Latin America in the 1910s and 1920s, targeting hookworm and yellow fever, with RF staff typically conducting detailed surveys of local health conditions as precursors to these programs' implementation. Through these campaigns the RF attempted to reform and modernize local health services and train public health specialists in U.S. medical practices. To this end, the RF provided more than seventeen hundred scholarships to Latin Americans (including sixteen Bolivians) to study agriculture, public health, and social sciences in the United States and parts of Latin America between 1917 and 1962.[15] These programs intended to demonstrate what U.S. philanthropy could achieve in the region, extol the virtues of the U.S. medical approach, and enforce a sense of cultural superiority at home. Additionally, these programs bolstered U.S. political hegemony abroad (although not explicitly under the State Department umbrella) and fostered close relations between the U.S. and Latin American governments through the RF's "hidden agenda" of promoting public health campaigns in regions where U.S corporations had economic interests.[16]

Despite the RF's extensive work in the region, it never sustained the commitment to Bolivia it did to other Latin American countries. The foundation's work in Bolivia began in 1932 when the Chaco War between Bolivia and Paraguay threatened successful yellow-fever eradication programs in Brazil. Its program concluded at the end of 1952 due to the International Health Division's closing in 1951. There are many reasons why the Bolivia office closed, including lack of success in its programs due to overexpansion and increasingly antagonistic relations between RF staffers and Bolivian doctors, both of which damaged the foundation's prestige.[17] Although the decision to close the La Paz office came before the 1952 revolution, growing political activism by women, Indigenous communities, and leftist organizations during the 1940s also played a role.[18] However, RF concern about Bolivian radical politics' potential impact on its programs was not unusual for this time. For instance, RF staffers in Mexico worried that the Cárdenas administration's Six-Year Plan (1934–1940)—an ambitious program focusing on agrarian reform, industrialization, education, and public health—would undermine RF programs. For this reason, the foundation agreed to limited but ongoing involvement with the Mexican government while remaining suspicious of Cárdenas's redistributive agenda.[19] The RF also decreased funding to Argentina during the Perón era (1946–1955) and closed its regional office in 1949 even though it had a long history of supporting Argentine physiology research.[20]

The RF's changing funding priorities also explain why its relationship with Bolivia came to an end in the early 1950s. By the 1940s, the foundation began to favor biomedical research and agricultural development over public health programs.[21] In Colombia, for example, RF priorities shifted from public health to agricultural programs in 1945, although it did launch a national nursing school in Bogotá in the 1940s.[22] It also began to focus on agricultural programs in Guatemala and Mexico at this time.[23] Furthermore, the RF preferred funding well-established research institutions in countries like Mexico and Brazil, which—depending on the timing—the foundation felt had "favorable" political conditions for programs to flourish.[24] At this juncture, foundation staffers considered Bolivia "too backward scientifically to receive much support from RF's new programs" because it lacked a renowned scientific community and political stability.[25]

As the RF sought worthy Latin American medical schools for investment in the 1940s and 1950s, it employed the same survey method used for decades. These surveys generally cited overenrollment, lack of full-time faculty positions, and limited laboratory training as evidence of scientific backwardness.[26] These concerns about Latin American medical schools mirrored Abraham Flexner's criticisms of North American medical education in his 1910 report. The Flexner Report, commissioned by the Carnegie Foundation, produced significant reforms, including state regulation of medical schools, rigorous academic and professional standards, and faculty engagement in medical research, which generated now-dominant ideas about medical education and practice in the United States. The Flexner Report also shaped the RF's medical policy in Latin America, resulting in a battle between "two conflicting academic and cultural traditions."[27] From the RF's perspective, Latin American medical schools, based on the French model, led to a lack of national cohesion in organization, curriculum, and licensing; conversely, the U.S. model promoted efficiency, professionalization, and national standards. Hence, the RF supported medical education in Latin America in an effort to overcome the problems that occurred when U.S.-trained Latin Americans returned to their home countries and to aid individuals who did not study medicine in the United States or Britain.

Another shift took place in RF attitudes about the relation between science and politics during the 1940s and 1950s. In the 1920s and 1930s the foundation occasionally supported people with leftist politics and socialist sympathies. Soviet scientists received RF grants at a time when the USSR and the United States did not have official diplomatic relations (although the RF informed the State Department of its decisions).[28] The foundation also assisted some avowed leftists whose work and research experience shaped their perspectives on social medicine and revolutionary politics.[29] By the 1950s, domestic concerns about communism led the RF to "a deliberate political decision not to support Communists abroad" because its leaders did not want to alienate U.S. politicians or risk prolonged investigations into their activities.[30] This shift, with the foundation more closely aligning with U.S. political and ideological interests, contextualizes Bauer's negative assessment of Urquidi's political leanings, which in the past might not have preoccupied the RF in the same way.

Bauer's 1952 decision that Bolivian medical schools were too "political" (meaning leftist) to merit RF funding was due in part to a history of U.S. government skepticism toward revolutionary movements and social change in Latin America and State Department concerns about containing communism abroad.[31] Given the similarities between the Bolivian revolution and the revolution already underway in Guatemala, which the U.S. government labeled communist, the State Department was initially wary of the MNR. The United States did not officially recognize Bolivia's new government until June 2, 1952—almost two months after the revolution. Nervousness about retaining U.S. support led Bolivian statesmen to distance themselves from communism and even exaggerate a potential communist threat to the government. For example, in 1953 President Víctor Paz Estenssoro asserted that the National Revolution was "the only means of combating communism."[32] Additionally, Víctor Andrade, Bolivian ambassador to the United States in 1944–1946, 1952–1958, and 1960–1962, worked to ensure that the Eisenhower administration understood the MNR's nationalist agenda.[33] The 1953 visit of Milton Eisenhower, brother of the U.S. president and a prominent university administrator, to La

Paz was a turning point for U.S.-Bolivian relations, after which the U.S. government decided that the MNR might have been leftist but certainly was not communist.[34] This distinction was particularly important as the State Department exaggerated the communist threat in Guatemala to justify a political coup against Árbenz in 1954.[35] Bolivia's MNR avoided the same fate because the U.S. government believed that it was not a threat to U.S. hegemony in the region and, as happened in Egypt, Ghana, and India, decided to support a nationalist regime to fend off a potential communist threat.[36]

To prevent the MNR from going "as far left as Guatemala," in President Eisenhower's words, the State Department supplied the MNR with "more Yankee aid dollars per Bolivian than for any other people on earth," amounting to $129 million between 1952 and 1959.[37] This unprecedented financial assistance to the MNR in the form of military materiel, economic stabilization, food aid, and social programs reflected the State Department's belief that it could thwart economic nationalism, tie Bolivia's economy directly to U.S. interests, and reduce communism's influence.[38]

The U.S. Agency for International Development (USAID) and its predecessor agency, the Institute of Inter-American Affairs (IIAA), oversaw nonmilitary aid beginning in 1942.[39] Between 1942 and 1961 roughly $3.1 million out of $111.2 million went directly to funding health and sanitation projects, including public health administration, disease control, and health education programs such as medical training for doctors and other health practitioners.[40] After 1961, the Kennedy administration's Alliance for Progress and the Peace Corps—Kennedy's proposed response to communism and the Cuban Revolution—specifically supported social programs.[41] As was also the case during the Kennedy administration, the MNR received State Department aid in the 1950s due to—not in spite of—the threat of communism.

Both Bauer's report and State Department correspondence about Bolivian communism in the 1950s indicated justified, if exaggerated, concerns. When Bauer concluded that the RF should not offer funding to Bolivia's medical schools despite shifting foundation interest toward medical research and professional education in the 1940s and 1950s, he did so within a broader context where Cold War–era concerns about communism affected the decisions of philanthropic organizations. Since RF officers had not hesitated to offer financial support to political radicals in the past, Bauer's decision to highlight communism's presence as a justification for denying funding to Bolivian schools suggests that the State Department's political concerns factored into these decisions. However, the State Department and the RF were not in agreement about how to address Bolivia's communist threat.

The "Ardent Communist" and Bolivian Radical Politics

Johannes M. Bauer's 1952 depiction of Dr. Arturo Urquidi Morales, the University of Cochabamba's rector, was a caricature: he was an "ardent communist" who was "strongly anti-American" and "frankly hostile" during the survey.[42] This one-dimensional model of a radical university leader and political activist demonstrated more about an artificial Cold War division of the world into supporters of capitalism and communism than any real understanding of Bolivia's political complexity. A closer look at Urquidi within the Bolivian context exposes how U.S. wariness of communism and RF apprehension about political activism at scientific institutions factored into funding decisions.

Urquidi was an educational leader, supporter of university reform, and the University of Cochabamba's rector on five separate occasions during the 1940s, 1950s, and 1960s.[43] He was a well-known Bolivian scholar with a history of leftist political activism regarding land reform and university autonomy. Trained as a sociologist, he was a prolific author of many books, pamphlets, and articles related to the country's agrarian condition, university autonomy, and education's civic mission in developing countries. His written work and public orations demonstrated Marxist sympathies, and in the 1940s he was a member of the PIR. However, he does not appear to have been active in the PCB or as a participant in ongoing transnational conversations about advancing communism in Bolivia in the 1950s and 1960s.

Due to his expertise on agrarian reform, President Víctor Paz Estenssoro appointed Urquidi to the Agrarian Reform Commission in 1953. Urquidi's reform proposal was based on his book *La Comunidad Indígena* (1941), which analyzed historical patterns of land use and argued that the state should reorganize Indigenous Bolivians into cooperatives to maximize their national economic contribution. While on the commission, he pushed the PIR vision of agrarian reform through mechanization and modernization of agriculture. By distributing land and organizing peasants into unions and militias loyal to the MNR, Urquidi believed they would become an engine of economic development and protectors of the revolution. This vision was supposed to create the conditions for a Marxist socialist revolution to occur. In reality, agrarian reform had the opposite effect, and peasant unions loyal to the MNR coopted *campesino* radicalism.[44] For this reason, even though Urquidi was one of the plan's architects, he critiqued its outcomes in *El Feudalismo en América y la Reforma Agraria Boliviana* (1966).[45]

Aside from his contribution to agrarian reform, Urquidi was a champion of university autonomy, and President Paz Estenssoro again asked him to serve on the National Education Reform Commission in 1955. Urquidi believed universities were "laboratories of thought" that should seek the "redemption and happiness of our people."[46] The modern university, he argued, performed a civic function, especially in the Third World. He thought universities should "train professionals and technicians, both theoretically and practically" to "prepare the Bolivian citizen to fight for national sovereignty to overcome Bolivian semi-feudalism and dependency" and "defend the nation's natural resources and cultural patrimony." Central to Urquidi's philosophy was the idea that reformers should "democratize the university . . . to strengthen relations between the university and the country's working masses."[47] This democratization process meant upsetting the status quo because Bolivian universities historically served the elite. Urquidi envisioned education as a way to fundamentally alter Bolivia's social and ethnic hierarchies, and growing worker and peasant activism after 1952 meant universities accepted a larger number of students from working-class and peasant backgrounds. This changing student demographic transformed universities into "channels of social mobilization" that were increasingly associated with student activism and radical politics after 1952.[48]

Though Urquidi was a polarizing figure for Bauer, Bolivian intellectuals respected his leadership. For example, Fernando Díez de Medina, a renowned Bolivian author who wrote for several newspapers, including *El Diario*, *La Razón*, and *Última Hora*, published a glowing endorsement of Urquidi's management of the University of Cochabamba in *Tribuna*, a La Paz–based newspaper, in 1951. "The miracle of this university," according to Díez de Medina, was "its helmsman, don Arturo Urquidi, a man of action and meditation, a modern role model . . . who devotes his energies to serving the youth. The socialists applaud him, the reactionaries detest him. But I do not see a Marxist: I see only a great Bolivian working effectively for a new society."[49] This view contrasted sharply with Bauer's, which described Urquidi as a scourge on intellectual development and scientific endeavors. To Díez de Medina, Urquidi's political leanings were irrelevant; to Bauer, they undermined the university's credibility.

Urquidi described himself as a "firm but incorruptible combatant" in defense of university autonomy.[50] Even though Bolivian universities won the right to institutional independence in the 1930s, Urquidi claimed they lived in a state of "permanent uneasiness" under the threat of state intervention and annulment of the autonomy guarantee. For this reason, he opposed governments that saw university autonomy as little more than protection for political dissidents.[51] Despite President Paz Estenssoro's assurances in 1952 that he would respect university autonomy, Urquidi's uneasiness was not unfounded.

At four o'clock on the morning of May 19, 1955, armed civilians organized by the MNR Comando Departamental—a provincial unit of the MNR party responsible for organizing and overseeing labor recruits, peasant unions, and urban party members that reported directly to the national party yet enjoyed considerable local autonomy—occupied the University of Cochabamba in a so-called "university revolution."[52] Although this occupation culminated in Urquidi's forced removal as rector, students and faculty responded with passive resistance and a general strike that compelled the government forces to withdraw after six months.[53]

Urquidi denounced the occupation as an assault on university freedom stemming from the MNR's discomfort with "the existence of respectable cultural centers capable of independently judging the actual historical moment in which the country exists." He saw this "violent occupation and subjugation of the university" as part of a preconceived, systematic plan to create a homogenous narrative of revolutionary change that eliminated any questioning of the MNR's leadership. In particular, he criticized the government's use of a communist threat as a pretext to subvert university autonomy, attack centers of independent thought, and orient Bolivia toward the United States for financial gain. He claimed the MNR's rationale for occupation was based on an "absurd story" that communists were trying to take over the university, and that MNR units strategically planted rifles around the university to support this story, a manipulation he called flagrant, insidious, and grotesque. He chastised the MNR leadership, arguing "whomever invokes communism to justify whatever absurdity simply reveals their own mental poverty and servility."[54] In his criticism of the MNR government, Urquidi drew upon nationalist and revolutionary rhetoric, declaring his mission to "incorporate the university into the country's productive process and increase [national] resources through our own effort" was cut short by the 1955 university occupation.[55] In doing so, he juxtaposed his own vision of revolutionary change with that of the MNR by criticizing their authoritarian tactics.

Urquidi's tireless defense of university autonomy coincided with his long-standing belief that underdevelopment adversely affected Bolivian education. In contrast to Bauer's explanations for the backwardness of Bolivian medical institutions, Urquidi claimed national universities suffered from lack of resources. He described these as "permanent characteristic[s] of Bolivian universities [where] logically, it is impossible to achieve greater efficiency in academic function, not to mention in scientific investigation." Although he acknowledged the "urgent necessity" to develop scientific knowledge in Bolivian universities, he argued they "lack the economic resources and the appropriate material means to carry out the kinds of investigation that would enrich our scientific heritage and national culture." Instead he suggested developing the social sciences to "arm the people in the struggle against oppression and dependency," rather than focus on the sciences, which were too expensive for poor Bolivian universities.[56]

While Urquidi's interest in developing the social sciences reflected his background as a sociologist, he also thought they would develop an explicit anti-imperialist critique among university students. This suggestion was also a way to circumvent the economic and technological dependence generated by developing capital-intensive physical and biological sciences. Moreover, he questioned whether foreign assistance helped national universities develop, and argued that foreign technicians' missions often failed because they lacked an understanding of the country and served imperialist objectives.[57] In doing so, Urquidi situated Bolivian universities' plight in a critique of economic and political dependency derived from the "colonial heritage" that kept Latin American countries from fulfilling their national potential.[58] His emphasis on Bolivia's educational struggles as "permanent" and insistence on programs of study that enhanced national culture echoed the *dependentista* critique of geopolitics—based on Argentine economist Raúl Prebisch's influential arguments—that were prevalent in Latin American leftist circles at the time. His insistence that universities should foster national culture as an anti-imperialist critique was unabashedly nationalist, but not necessarily communist.

Urquidi and Bauer fundamentally disagreed about the historical conditions that led to Bolivian universities' current state, how to foster intellectual growth, and Latin American universities' social function.[59] Urquidi was an apt straw man for Bauer, who used him as a scapegoat for the challenges facing Bolivian medical schools and the complex local conditions that Bauer did not or could not understand. Indeed, if Bauer wanted to single someone out at the University of Cochabamba as being a communist, there were plenty of people who did have the right characteristics. One was Ricardo Anaya, an economics professor and a PIR leader in the 1940s, who visited China in 1959 and subsequently lectured on China's agrarian reform.[60] Yet Urquidi was a convenient target due to his outspoken nature and prestigious position. He also represented many contradictory facets of Bolivian society. He was a Marxist, a onetime member of a Communist Party, and a promoter of democratizing the university. He cooperated with the MNR government, helping to design one of its signature reforms, but was also one of the revolution's greatest critics. His complicated identities and nuanced political positions made Urquidi an embodiment of Bolivian nationalism and messy revolutionary politics as well as a convenient symbol for Bolivian intellectual immaturity, which rationalized RF avoidance of Bolivian medical schools.

Myths and Realities of Bolivian Medical Education in Bauer's Report

Johannes H. Bauer arrived in Bolivia in August 1952 to survey medical schools and identify potential targets for RF cooperation. Medical education was a funding priority of the foundation in the 1940s and 1950s.[61] Bauer's report reflects long-standing assertions of U.S. cultural and scientific superiority, especially the idea that medical education in Latin America was backward and inferior to the U.S. model. However, it also highlights the political context of the Cold War, where avid anticommunist crusades affected philanthropic foundations' decisions. This context helps explain why Bauer described Urquidi as a one-dimensional Communist rather than a nuanced political activist, university leader, or Bolivian nationalist.

Bauer's survey of Bolivia's three medical schools in August 1952—the Universidad Mayor Real y Pontifical de San Francisco Xavier de Sucre (founded in 1624), the Universidad Mayor de San Andrés de La Paz (founded in 1830), and the Universidad Mayor de San Simón de Cochabamba (founded in 1832)—came a quarter century after the RF's initial survey of Bolivian medical education in 1926. Though Bolivian medical schools demonstrated improved quality of instruction and educational facilities, Bauer shared many of the same concerns raised in the earlier survey.[62] In Cochabamba, Bauer noted, lack of special entrance requirements meant only five percent of the students graduated, amounting to a "useless waste of time and effort both on the part of the student and the faculty." This overenrollment in the first year taxed the school's facilities and created a "hopeless" teaching situation. Only in the second year, "when most of the students who have failed to pass the necessary examination have been weeded out and the class reduced to a more manageable size," could actual laboratory work be done. In La Paz, Bauer described the small laboratories as "ill adapted for teaching purposes," the anatomy facilities as "especially unsatisfactory," and the physiology labs as "small, overcrowded, and lack[ing] necessary equipment." He also reported that professors did not hold full-time appointments and often worked additional jobs because they earned a measly twenty-five dollars per month on average.[63]

Bauer believed the structure of the entire educational system spelled failure for Bolivian universities. A 1932 national decree declared university autonomy, meaning that universities were regulated by individual provinces rather than the Ministry of Education or central government.[64] While universities followed general rules, their organization and curriculum varied significantly, and there were no national instructional or licensing standards. Bolivian medical professionals held that autonomy significantly improved medical education, although when practiced too rigidly, it prevented coordination between the different schools.[65] In contrast, Bauer saw autonomy as an obstacle to improving medical education.

Bauer believed these structural problems extended to the nation's elementary and secondary schools, which he assessed through information he requested from Dr. Nemesio Torres Muñoz, a Bolivian doctor who worked with the RF-supported Division of Rural Endemic Diseases.[66] In his report, Bauer criticized the lack of mandatory Spanish-language education in elementary schools because students learned their local languages (primarily Aymara and Quechua) before Spanish, which did not provide a foundation for success in higher education. He blamed the Indigenous population in part for this situation, claiming they were "suspicious and hostile toward the white man's schools, this being especially true of the Aimaras [sic], who are much more stubborn and warlike than the rather docile Quechuas."[67] He invoked these two pervasive stereotypes of Indigenous communities ostensibly to demonstrate the Bolivian educational system's challenges. In doing so, Bauer suggested that Indigenous languages were incompatible with the language of scientific or medical inquiry. He also overlooked (or was unaware of) the fact that Indigenous Bolivians might have legitimate suspicions of the government's educational agenda. During the late nineteenth and early twentieth centuries, Bolivian Liberals had promoted education to build a productive labor force, train military conscripts, and "civilize" Indigenous communities. In pursuit of these goals, schools generally offered a Spanish-only curriculum that marginalized ethnic differences and maligned Indigenous history in favor of a unified nationalist narrative.[68]

In his assessment of Bolivia's educational system, Bauer reproduced most of the conclusions of the earlier RF survey that had described medical education institutions as scientifically backward with inept faculty and antiquated curriculum. However, his 1952 assessment contained an added concern about communism, although there is no evidence in his officer's diary or final report that he was specifically asked to investigate this issue. He accentuated communism's influence at all levels of Bolivian society, from national politics to scientific pursuits. For instance, he claimed that "in the labor unions, the Communist element seems to be fairly strong, and there is considerable apprehension that the country may go communist altogether."[69]

As discussed earlier, neither of these claims is especially accurate. First, communism never had the same political sway in Bolivia as in other Latin American countries. Indeed, Bauer's insistence on communism's influence on Bolivian labor unions, which were headed by the MNR's Juan Lechín, was overstated.[70] Second, after taking power the MNR immediately declared that theirs was *not* a communist revolution. While Bauer may have mistaken communist parties' legality under the MNR government, including the POR's influence on the Central Obrera Boliviana, as an endorsement of communist ideology, the MNR repeatedly assured the United States of its commitment to democracy and capitalism. If anything, the MNR exaggerated the threat of communist subversion to gain political leverage and economic assistance throughout the 1950s.[71] Memos between U.S. diplomatic officials posted in Bolivia and government leaders in Washington confirm that the U.S. government did not suspect the MNR of communist affiliation despite concerns about communism's potential to undermine the MNR government.[72] Since Bolivia was an important regional ally, State Department aid helped keep the MNR in power and prevent a theoretical communist takeover.[73]

Yet communism's supposed influence on Bolivia, especially at the University of Cochabamba, disturbed Bauer. He claimed the medical school, constructed in 1936, never should have been built at all because the university had "the reputation of being much more interested in political intrigue than in academic endeavor" and was the "seat of the most aggressive type of Communistic activity in Bolivia." The rector, Urquidi, was a "militant Communist" with a "distinctly hostile" attitude during the survey. According to Bauer, Urquidi "gave us a long lecture about the evil of the United States' imperialistic exploitation of poor Bolivia," and demanded mining profits sent abroad be returned. Yet this was not a unique perspective, as MNR members frequently voiced similar, albeit more tempered, opinions.[74] Bauer was most troubled that the rector was elected by a two-thirds vote from an *asamblea universitaria* composed of an equal number of faculty and student representatives. The rector presided over a *consejo universitario* involving a smaller number of deans and directors with an equal number of student representatives.[75] Based on this process, Bauer claimed "the students seem to take much greater part in the administrative policies of the School than either the faculty or the Dean," including students from Chile, Brazil, and Peru allegedly "expelled from their own universities for Communistic activities." Without providing additional evidence, Bauer asserted it was "quite obvious that not only the Rector but also a fair percentage of the faculty and most of the student body here are militant Communists," including the dean, "although he seems to be somewhat less bellicose than the Rector."[76]

As Bauer wrote in his report, Urquidi "emphasized to the students repeatedly that taking part in national politics is their first duty, and their scientific pursuits second. To this the students seem to respond readily, as shown by the percentage of failures in the scholastic work."[77] In this way, Bauer equated academic underachievement with political engagement, and blamed Urquidi. Why was Bauer so convinced that leftist political ideology could undermine scientific merit? The answer lies in a complex constellation of cultural and political changes both within and outside of the United States.

First, the RF started questioning its international role as a public health champion after World War II. For instance, U.S. occupying authorities in Germany welcomed RF assistance in rebuilding German scientific and medical research, but the foundation was hesitant to resume the program. In part, this hesitation derived from RF discomfort with the link between medical research and Nazi policies made public by the Nuremberg Trials, which detailed the extent of medical experiments on Nazi prisoners.[78] For this reason, RF staffers questioned German scientists' morals and ethics. Reflecting the foundation's lack of enthusiasm for the project, Bauer himself "reluctantly" participated in surveys of German universities in the U.S. zone in 1947 to identify the potential for building a public health school. He concluded the project would require brand-new infrastructure and a fellowship program to adequately train German faculty under U.S. and British supervision. This assessment ultimately prevented the project's development.[79]

Second, Bauer's ideas about the proper use of scientific knowledge were rooted in fears about student and scientific activism in the United States dating back to the 1930s.[80] Amid anticommunist fervor and McCarthyism's growing hold on the country, U.S. politicians manipulated national-security scares and fears of communist subversion to boost budgetary support for the House Un-American Activities Committee.[81] Prominent scientists with leftist or even liberal leanings, such as J. Robert Oppenheimer and Edward Condon, were subject to federal scrutiny and characterized as a "security risk" based on their international connections and criticism of nuclear ambitions. High-profile trials taught U.S. scientists a valuable lesson during the early Cold War: keep their personal political views separate from their science to maintain their professional authority and government funding.[82] If these respected scientists and researchers were accused of espionage or disloyalty and closely scrutinized in this suspicious climate, surely leftists' presence in universities in a nation undergoing a revolutionary transformation, like Bolivia, signaled alarm for U.S. philanthropies.

Third, philanthropic foundations themselves came under scrutiny in this period. In August 1951, Georgia Democratic representative Eugene Cox questioned whether tax-exempt foundations' activities conflicted with U.S. national security concerns. In April 1952 Cox convened a special committee to investigate foundations' potential funding of "un-American activities." The RF was just one of this investigation's targets, which also included the Ford Foundation and the Carnegie Institution, but Cox's specific concerns about the RF derived from grants it provided to Chinese universities and organizations associated with communist doctrine in the 1940s.[83] At the committee's request, each institution replied to a questionnaire about its organization, finances, and programs, to which the RF provided "an extensive reply" of more than one hundred pages.[84] The RF's president, Dean Rusk, testified before the congressional committee on December 8 and 9, 1952, to discuss award decisions, arguing that philanthropic organizations helped extend the frontiers of human knowledge to benefit humankind.[85] In answering the questionnaire and preparing Rusk's testimony, top-level RF staff compiled extensive documentation about its activities abroad, including information pertaining to Bauer's 1945 visit to Poland, his 1946 travels in Czechoslovakia, Yugoslavia, Poland, and Romania, and his 1948 survey of public health in Hungary. The RF gathered this information right around the time Bauer left for his Bolivia trip, so he was likely keenly aware of the need to distance the foundation from any communist association.[86]

The Cox investigations in November and December found little evidence that communists had infiltrated tax-exempt foundations but nevertheless created a climate in which foundation activities were scrutinized. One of the committee's members, B. Carroll Reece—a Republican representative from Tennessee—called for further investigation, claiming the committee lacked sufficient time to carry out its probe, even though he was only present at three of the twenty-eight meetings.[87] As Reece wrote in 1957, more scrutiny was necessary to uncover an insidious conspiracy whereby foundations' irresponsible spending allowed socialism to pervade the United States.[88] Reece's committee conducted additional hearings in May, June, and July 1954.

While critics of Reece's committee suggested it was an attempt by a minority political ideology to hijack the political system, philanthropic foundations like the RF understood they were under considerable pressure to prove they were not funding "un-American activities."[89] For instance, Rusk devoted a significant portion of his "President's Review" in the RF's 1953 annual report to discussing the Cox and Reece investigations, noting, "The Foundation refrains as a matter of policy from making grants to known Communists. This rests upon two elements, the clearly expressed public policies of the United States, within which we operate, and the increasing assaults by Communism upon science and scholarship which would lead us, on intellectual grounds alone, to withhold support."[90] These public investigations sent a loud and clear message to the philanthropic community: communism and science were incompatible.[91]

Finally, as the Cold War gained momentum in the United States, "the foundation's officers found themselves having to choose between retaining a credible posture abroad [in Europe], where fears of communism among scientists were far more muted, and retaining trust and support at home, where concerns about scientists' loyalty and security grew increasingly strident." As in Germany and other European countries, RF concerns about political subversion, security breaches, and economic sabotage affected financial assistance to scientific institutions in Bolivia and elsewhere in Latin America. This "politicization of awards" led to the position that rigorous scientific inquiry could be undermined or tainted by political ideologies: in other words, "a Communist could not be a man of science." Communist affiliations became "unacceptable, both at a personal and an institutional level," and resulted in the denial of awards to numerous scientists in Europe.[92] This exclusionary rationale shaped RF attitudes toward Bolivia—the foundation did not want to be associated with controversial topics like Nazi experimentation or affiliated with radical politics in a revolutionary society.

Although this context helps explain Bauer's misunderstanding of communism's place in Bolivian society, his disdain for the Cochabamba medical school went far beyond its faculty's and students' political involvement. For instance, he wrote that the Hospital Viedma, where University of Cochabamba medical students gained practical experience, was "badly managed" since "the wards on the whole are dirty and no attempt seems to be made to give the institution the aspect of orderly cleanliness." He described the operating rooms as disorganized and was appalled that professors assisted procedures in their street clothes, which he felt served as a "poor example for future doctors to follow." However, as Bauer noted in his report, the Ministry of Public Health was financially and administratively responsible for the Hospital Viedma, so its mismanagement reflected poorly on the national government, not the University of Cochabamba or its medical school per se.[93] Given the financial strain caused by the recent revolution, the Health Ministry's material shortcomings were understandable.

Bauer also claimed that most of the hospital's patients were terminally ill, which "adds to [its] general depressive atmosphere." His evidence for this assertion was the hospital's high mortality rate, "shown by the fact that there is at least one autopsy per day, and often more. Consequently there is a profusion of material for pathological studies."[94] While he suggested the hospital was bad for Bolivians but good for medical students, he based this assertion on sketchy evidence. First, he did not account for the fact that Viedma had a well-known tuberculosis wing that housed patients suffering from what was the fourth-largest cause of death in Bolivia between 1950 and 1953. Other infectious diseases—influenza, malaria, enteritis, and dysentery—also beleaguered Cochabambinos.[95] Additionally, the bodies of people who died in their homes could be brought to the hospital for autopsies, which, based on Bauer's deductions, would make the hospital's mortality rate seem artificially high. He further elaborated, "The fact that the patients are generally admitted in the terminal stages of their illness, where the fatal outcome is almost certain, would seem to give the students a rather poor demonstration of the effectiveness of modern healing art."[96] Bauer seemed to think terminally ill Bolivians had a greater impact on developing medical students than either the hospital's maternity ward or children's care center, which were Viedma's other specialties.[97] Bauer made it clear that he felt that the University of Cochabamba's medical school was not only a potential communist threat but a bad RF investment.

Bauer's vitriolic assessment of Cochabamba's medical school stood in stark contrast to his praise for Sucre's medical school, which he noted was "regarded highly, not only in Bolivia but also in the neighboring countries" for its "high standards and excellent methods of teaching." As evidence, he cited the school's competitive admissions procedures, including personal interviews and rigorous examinations, leading to fewer students failing than in either La Paz or Cochabamba. He described the facilities as "excellent," buildings as "well equipped," and research and teaching staff as "first-rate," with only its clinical instruction facilities being "rather poor" (noting again that the Health Ministry ran the Hospital Santa Bárbara, not the medical school). Most importantly, Bauer described Sucre's rector, Dr. Guillermo Francovich, as an individual with leftist tendencies but who had "never been accused of being a communist"—unlike Urquidi.[98] Bauer implied that Francovich was a better administrator because he was not a communist.

Overall, Bauer lauded Sucre's medical school, its faculty, and its curriculum. However, he noted that the Hospital Santa Bárbara, the region's primary teaching hospital, was "antiquated and unsatisfactory in every respect"—it was more than three hundred years old with earthquake damage that had only received "makeshift repairs," making it a "delapidated [*sic*] institution and ill-suited for teaching purposes." He noted that the Ministry of Health had plans to replace the Hospital Santa Bárbara with a new, five-hundred-bed general hospital and a new medical faculty building. After these renovations, Bauer concluded, "the Medical School of the University of Sucre will be in an excellent position to compare favorably with any similar institution in the southern hemisphere. It will have the advantage of being in a small town and rather isolated from the turbulent politics of La Paz and Cochabamba, where the university students generally take active part in the frequent revolutions and other disturbances." However, he recommended only that a representative should "keep in touch" with the University of Sucre on the chance that a small amount of foundation assistance "would accomplish something of lasting value."[99] Given the excellence of all areas except clinical instruction, it seems that funding for renovating the Hospital Santa Bárbara would have improved the university's regional stature and provided a tangible example of success for the RF's medical-education initiative. Yet the RF's annual reports indicate that no grant-in-aid for such a project was ever forthcoming.

Although Bauer's distaste for the University of Cochabamba's political activities likely colored his assessment of its facilities and instruction, Cochabamba's and Sucre's respective histories may have also shaped his perceptions. Since the nineteenth century, Sucre was reputed as the "intellectual center of the nation." It was the Conservative stronghold in the 1890s until declining global silver prices shifted political power in favor of the Liberals, who led a revolt in 1899 and moved the national capital from Sucre to La Paz.[100] In contrast, the department of Cochabamba has a long history of political activity and mobilization in favor of Indigenous land rights. The town of Ucureña was the site of the first rural uprisings and land occupations following the 1952 revolution and the place where the MNR announced the 1953 Agrarian Reform decree. Ucureña and the Cochabamba region were the symbolic center of the agrarian revolution from the 1930s to the 1950s.[101] Given the RF's reticence regarding politically volatile situations, this history of political activism could certainly have colored Bauer's assessment of the medical school's potential.

Bauer's general conclusions suggested that a university's level of political activity determined the quality of the education. In sum, only the University of Sucre made a good impression, based on a combination of strict entrance examinations, high quality of instruction, and subdued politics. The University of La Paz struggled due to its location in the nation's capital, where "politics always seem to be in turmoil," evidenced, he held, by the fact that university students installed machine guns on the building's roof during the recent revolution. Bauer also claimed that students tended to be leftists whereas the faculty were conservative, creating an unhealthy academic atmosphere. For example, students denounced several faculty members and administrators, including the university rector, for funneling money to exiles in Chile and Argentina to buy arms for a counterrevolution. However, he noted, "while the political atmosphere in the University of La Paz is bad, in the University of Cochabamba it is much worse." Not only did he consider Cochabamba's medical school "more of a joke than an institution of higher learning," he also claimed the entire university functioned as a communist hub. At its center was the infamous Urquidi, who Bauer alleged made an average of fifteen public speeches a year advocating communism and avowing "the duty and responsibility of the university to take part in national politics." As Bauer concluded, prospects for RF cooperation were "not very promising at present."[102]

Bauer's claims reflected prevailing political attitudes in the United States at the time regarding communism's potential to undermine scientific objectivity. His assessment also had lasting consequences regarding the ability of Bolivian medical schools to attract RF financial assistance. The foundation's Division of Medicine and Public Health (DMPH, the IHD's successor) continued to refer to Bolivian medical education as "backward," as Bauer did in his report. In correspondence regarding South American medical schools in 1956, one staffer noted, "I hesitate to mention Bolivia which must be one of the most backward countries in the world as far as medical education is concerned." This same staffer identified the University of San Marcos in Peru, not the medical school in Sucre, as "the best medical school" in the Andean countries.[103] In 1956 the DMPH decided, "It would be advisable for the RF to concentrate its efforts in Brazil, Chile, and Colombia for the present and to encourage the utilization of schools in these countries by students from the less favorably equipped ones," referring specifically to Bolivia, Ecuador, and Peru.[104] While the RF did not provide funding to Bolivian universities in the 1950s, the DMPH did furnish grants-in-aid to other medical schools in Latin America that were located in what the RF president had identified as "strategic places" in 1951.[105] This support went to institutions in Brazil, Chile, and Colombia, as well as Mexico and Puerto Rico.[106] The DMPH did continue to support Bolivia's Division of Rural Endemic Diseases through grants-in-aid after the IHD closed its Bolivia field office in 1951–1952.[107] This program, concerned with the control of transmissible diseases such as yellow fever, malaria, hookworm, and typhus, had been developed under RF supervision during the 1940s and was transferred to the Ministry of Public Health in 1952. The DMPH also provided individual grants to Bolivian doctors associated with the Division of Rural Endemic Diseases and the Health Ministry, although both operational and individual support appears to have concluded by 1953.[108]

When Bauer argued that the RF should avoid involvement with Bolivian medical schools, he did not solely blame the institutions' limited facilities, antiquated curriculum, or substandard equipment. He also articulated a cultural explanation rooted in Bolivia's majority Indigenous population, prominence of Indigenous languages, and lack of mandatory Spanish-only education. Most importantly, he highlighted political instability and student activism as the main obstacles to forging a productive relationship, thereby suggesting that student activism correlated with neglect of academic volition and lower institutional standards. Specifically, he presented a skewed vision of communism's sway in Bolivian universities, which resulted in serious financial consequences for the institutions in question. For this reason, the survey's repeated emphasis on communist influence shows how Cold War ideological dogmatism and diplomatic concerns directly affected RF funding for Bolivian medical schools. No one represented the RF viewpoint that rigorous academic standards and leftist politics were incompatible more than the University of Cochabamba's rector, Dr. Arturo Urquidi.

The U.S. State Department and the Politics of Foreign Aid

Paradoxically, Bauer's recommendations diverged from State Department policy in the early 1950s, which justified supporting the MNR, mostly in the form of food assistance and economic stabilization, out of fear of communist inroads. In 1957 the U.S. Operations Missions (USOM), a State Department agency supervised by the International Cooperation Administration (a precursor to USAID), undertook a survey similar to Bauer's of La Paz's medical school to assess the possibility of developing a cooperative program.[109] The USOM's Dr. Benjamin Horning, who conducted the survey, came to many of the same conclusions about medical education at the University of La Paz as Bauer in 1952. He claimed the faculty received only a "token salary," the building was inadequate without laboratories or refrigeration for cadavers, and the curriculum too antiquated to address Bolivia's public health needs. While the hospital's director, Dr. Jorge Ergueta, lacked training in hospital administration, he struck Horning as capable and efficient. Horning also described the majority of young faculty as impressive, dedicated, and willing to reorganize the medical school. As he concluded, "Bolivia has a splendid group of medical educators and leaders. They are struggling against almost insurmountable difficulties to improve medical education and to provide able leadership to public health and medical care programs." Yet although Horning came to the same conclusions as Bauer, he made the opposite recommendation: USOM should develop a cooperative program with Bolivian medical schools. He saw collaboration as the best method to modernize medical instruction, support the medical faculty, and address Bolivia's public health needs.[110]

That RF and State Department interests did not align is a conundrum. The RF might have helped promote U.S. ideas of scientific modernity by funding Bolivian medical institutions to undercut local political movements' influence. Yet it did exactly the opposite, and used political activism as an excuse to refrain from funding Bolivian medical schools. The RF looked at the La Paz medical school (and the Cochabamba school) and deemed its students and faculty too politically radical for foundation assistance. The USOM, meanwhile, saw the same school as an opportunity for investment that could help "resist 'the totalitarian aggression' of communism that thrived on conditions of want and privation in disadvantaged nations," as the Congressional Foreign Relations Committee phrased it.[111] What explains this discrepancy?

First, conditions within Bolivia had changed dramatically between 1952 and 1957. In the early 1950s, conditions favoring the rise of communism, such as economic exploitation and land monopolization, certainly existed in Bolivia. However, communist parties were unable to gain the workers' and campesinos' support because the MNR effectively responded to popular pressures and enacted policies that undermined communism's appeal, including nationalization of the mining industry and land redistribution.[112] MNR reforms garnered workers' and peasants' support during the early 1950s but also co-opted their political activism.[113] Furthermore, these programs helped the MNR control Bolivia's powerful labor movement—which was a key Eisenhower administration objective—by ensuring that redistribution was a state-driven initiative instead of a union platform.[114]

However, by the late 1950s the MNR was heading a "revolution in retreat."[115] As the MNR tried to consolidate power, its leaders became increasingly conservative, and leftists like the PCB openly denounced MNR policies. Economic instability grew throughout the 1950s, and rampant inflation and wage controls hit the working class especially hard. Diplomatic memos during this time suggest that the State Department was concerned about communism's potential to undermine the MNR government. As tension grew between the MNR's left and moderate factions, U.S. diplomats told the State Department that a communist-inspired ousting of President Hernán Siles Zuazo (1956–1960) was possible. As the embassy counselor wrote on September 28, 1956, "I consider it highly probable that left-wing, possibly Communist-dominated elements

COB [Central Obrera Boliviana] leadership [sic] may be spearheading anti-Siles moves."[116]

Second, Bolivia's MNR, like many nationalist parties during the 1950s and 1960s, manipulated Cold War tensions between the United States and the USSR to acquire greater financial assistance and advance their domestic agenda.[117] For example, President Siles told U.S. ambassador Gerald Drew in 1956 that "he feared [Bolivia's economic problems] would accentuate inflation, inspire Communist and radical elements to redouble efforts to take power and cause pressure to come upon the present regime to go left. . . . He said that if foreign assistance, obviously from the United States, was not forthcoming, the inflationary process would bring about the downfall of the present liberal, democratic regime *inevitably* to be followed by a Communist Government."[118] MNR officials astutely played on U.S. fears of a potential communist threat to negotiate sustained financial aid for economic stabilization, food assistance, education, and public health programs, the latter representing roughly 3.5 percent of total USAID expenditures in Bolivia between 1954 and 1964.[119] State Department funding for medical education was just one program to foster economic development, court political loyalty to the United States, and undermine the potential communist threat.

The State Department's USOM ultimately came to a different conclusion about funding Bolivian medical education in 1957 than did Bauer in 1952. Despite persistent problems such as lack of resources and an overburdened faculty, USOM recommended that the State Department develop a cooperative relationship with medical schools. This decision reflects Bolivia's changing political and economic conditions and evolving U.S.-Bolivian relations. Whereas the U.S. government was not terribly concerned about communism in Bolivia in the early 1950s, by the middle of the decade U.S. diplomats feared its potential subversive impact. Bolivian officials also skillfully stoked these anxieties to negotiate financial assistance for its domestic agenda. U.S. aid was therefore a means to protect a strategic ally in the region, showing that discussions about scientific and technological assistance became ideological during the Cold War.

Although the RF is often considered an extension of U.S. foreign policy, this case highlights contrasting approaches. Ultimately, both the RF's and State Department's decisions were reactions to the presence of actual and exaggerated communist activity in Bolivia at the time. Foundation officials decided against cooperating with Bolivian institutions even remotely associated with communism because the RF was under investigation for supposedly financing un-American activities abroad. Conversely, the U.S. government engaged these institutions hoping that financial assistance would undermine communism's influence. State Department aid to developing countries was designed to depoliticize activist movements. Even though these programs generated disagreement in the United States between liberals, who supported the MNR as modernizers and excused the party's authoritarian tendencies, and conservatives, who decried revolutionary "despotism," they constituted an important part of U.S. foreign policy in Latin America, especially after the 1954 coup in Guatemala and the Cuban Revolution's success in 1959.[120] Whereas the RF disparaged Bolivian medical schools so as not to be seen as supporting communism, the State Department promised funding for social programs to keep Bolivia safely within the U.S. sphere of influence and undercut communism's potential appeal.

Disagreements about medical education show that scientific knowledge and philanthropic aid became politicized during the Cold War. When RF officials and U.S. diplomats debated the efficacy of Bolivia's medical education system, they were really discussing the pervasiveness of communist ideology in Bolivian society. Discussions about Bolivian medical education's effectiveness were a pretext for the RF and State Department to investigate communism's influence on Bolivian politics, a concern both parties shared, albeit for different reasons.

Medical Education and the Strategic Value of Science

The RF's and State Department's divergent approaches to Bolivian medical education represent varying conceptions of science's strategic value. For the State Department, Bolivia's strategic value lay in its geopolitical position. Aid for social programs was one means by which the State Department ensured the MNR government's stability so that it could continue to hold communism at bay. Conversely, for philanthropies, as Paul Weindling has noted, a "new ethos of Cold War science in which strategic value took priority" emerged after World War II, resulting in an emphasis on scientific research that produced knowledge valuable for navigating and winning the Cold War.[121] This new ethos, where the RF weighed the merit of scientific research against its political value, resulted in what John Krige has called the "politicization of awards"—that is, political and ideological considerations gradually came to factor prominently into funding decisions, and the RF flatly refused support to any scientist or researcher even remotely associated with communism, regardless of the quality of their work or institutional affiliation.[122] This case demonstrates that U.S. philanthropies' concerns about communism extended beyond

North American and European scientists and institutions and also shaped RF funding decisions in Latin America.

The portrayal of the strategic value of science is clear in the RF's annual reports from the 1940s and 1950s. Reports from the end of the 1940s detail the change in priorities from public health to professional development, research, and medical education, which also coincided with the IHD's closing. Additionally, these reports reflect the Cold War's impact on the organization's funding decisions. For example, in the "President's Review" in the 1949 annual report, titled "The Changing Scene," President Chester Barnard identified that "the Iron Curtain now dividing the world into two parts" would be one of the most important influences on RF policy and activities in the 1950s.[123] His report details a shift away from public health and disease control programs and a prioritization of ecology, genetics, and agricultural research. It also highlights a few RF pet projects that came to dominate the Division of Medicine and Public Health's reports for the 1950s: tropical-virus research on yellow fever in Brazil and agricultural research in Mexico and Colombia.[124]

A clear pattern emerges from these reports, demonstrating that, after the IHD's closing in 1951, the RF chose to focus its resources on a few priority countries—Mexico, Brazil, Colombia, and to some extent Argentina and Chile. These "strategic countries," as Barnard termed them in 1951, were places where important campaigns were carried out and from which knowledge could be derived that was valuable for waging and winning the Cold War. One example of these endeavors was a biomedical research program on tropical viruses in Brazil, resulting in knowledge about how to manage infectious diseases in tropical environments.[125] Another example is the Mexican Agricultural Program, touted as one of the RF's "highlights of the year" in 1949.[126] This program, which received ongoing plaudits from the RF leadership throughout the 1950s, was expanded to Colombia for further investigation about how to increase yields and improve nutrition in order to reduce poverty—one of the characteristics of Latin American society that U.S. policymakers thought made communism an attractive political philosophy. Colombian agricultural projects after 1951 included the development of rust-resistant wheat, high-yield varieties of corn, cereals, and legumes, and seed banks.[127] Finally, the RF specifically identified Peru's Institute of Andean Biology as a center for high altitude research, which Barnard mentioned could produce new information for innovation in aviation. He further averred that high altitude physiology would produce valuable knowledge about how humans could adapt to new and difficult conditions, such as prolonged exposure to the elements or the pressures of high altitude living.[128] Throughout the 1950s these programs and countries were celebrated in the RF annual reports, while public health programs and marginal countries, like Bolivia, were quietly removed from the conversation. Bolivia's last specific mention in these reports was in 1952, the year Bauer completed his report on Bolivian medical education.

Bolivia was a peripheral country for the RF not solely as a consequence of the country's size or the "backwardness" of its medical schools, but also because it was considered neither a potential site of strategic knowledge production nor a leader in developing effective public health models. The supposed prevalence of communism in Bolivian universities was an added strike against the country's suitability for RF funding under a Cold War mentality. Barnard wrote in the 1951 annual report that the foundation's "experience in fostering research and learning had made us believe that only the free mind can do really productive work in intellectual fields . . . and that the man or woman who has an ideological ax to grind is conspicuously less successful as a contributor of knowledge than one who is free of such a restriction."[129] Urquidi, in Bauer's diagnosis, was a communist (and therefore ideological) and clearly had an ax to grind against the United States. Therefore, in the RF's view, Bolivia was a place that was incapable of producing knowledge useful for winning the Cold War.

Notes

1 J. H. Bauer, "A Survey of Medical Education in Bolivia," Lima, Peru (September 1952), 52–53, Rockefeller Archive Center, Sleepy Hollow, NY (RAC), record group 1.2, series 300A, box 2A, folder 6B.

2 Bauer, "Survey of Medical Education in Bolivia," 23, 25.

3 Marcos Cueto, "Rockefeller Foundation's Medical Policy"; Zulawski, Unequal Cures.

4 Balcázar, Historia de la Medicina.

5 See Marcos Cueto, "Visions of Science and Development"; Cottam, Images and Intervention; Joseph, LeGrand, and Salvatore, Close Encounters of Empire; Thomas O'Brien, Making the Americas; Birn, Marriage of Convenience.

6 See Krige, American Hegemony, 118. On U.S. anticommunism during the 1950s, see Blasier, Hovering Giant; Rabe, Eisenhower and Latin America.

7 Whitehead, "Bolivian National Revolution"; Patch, "Bolivia." See also Dunkerley, Rebellion in the Veins.

8 John, Bolivia's Radical Tradition; Poppino, International Communism in Latin America; Rothwell, Transpacific Revolutionaries.

9 Malloy, Bolivia.

10 John, Bolivia's Radical Tradition, 126, 163, 176–80.

11 Cited in John, *Bolivia's Radical Tradition*, 88–89. See also Alexander, *Communism in Latin America*; Lora, *History of the Bolivian Labour Movement*; Alexander and Parker, *History of Organized Labor in Bolivia*.

12 Dorn, *Truman Administration and Bolivia*.

13 Siles Zuazo declared that the National Revolution and the labor movement would not be "at the mercy of the POR's and PCB's incessant agitation" and positioned the MNR between the "right's constant coup attempts" and the POR's and PCB's "anarchistic union tactics." Hernán Siles Zuazo, Presidente Constitucional de la República de Bolivia, "Cuatro Años de Gobierno," Mensaje al Honorable Congreso Nacional, August 6, 1960, 46–47.

14 See Marcos Cueto, "Rockefeller Foundation's Medical Policy"; Birn, *Marriage of Convenience*; Marcos Cueto, *Cold War, Deadly Fevers*; Zulawski, *Unequal Cures*.

15 Marcos Cueto, "Introduction," x–xi; Birn, "Revolution, the Scatological Way." See also Palmer, *Launching Global Health*.

16 Quevedo et al., *Café y Gusanos, Mosquitos y Petróleo*.

17 Balcázar, *Historia de la Medicina en Bolivia*; Farley, *To Cast Out Disease*.

18 See Zulawski, *Unequal Cures*; Gotkowitz, *Revolution for Our Rights*; Gotkowitz, "Commemorating the Heroínas."

19 Birn, *Marriage of Convenience*, 176–233.

20 Marcos Cueto, "Rockefeller Foundation's Medical Policy," 127–34.

21 Rockefeller Foundation, *Annual Report, 1952*, 25–27.

22 Abel, "External Philanthropy and Domestic Change in Colombian Health Care," 365–67.

23 See Pistorius, *Scientists, Plants, and Politics*; Fitzgerald, "Exporting American Agriculture"; Cotter, "Rockefeller Foundation's Mexican Agricultural Project."

24 Marcos Cueto, "Rockefeller Foundation's Medical Policy," 138.

25 Zulawski, *Unequal Cures*, 115.

26 Marcos Cueto, "Visions of Science and Development."

27 Marcos Cueto, "Rockefeller Foundation's Medical Policy," 140. See also Fosdick, *Story of the Rockefeller Foundation*, 93–122.

28 Solomon and Krementsov, "Giving and Taking across Borders."

29 Those funded included Polish hygienist Ludwik Rajchman (head of the League of Nations Health Organization), Croatian public health leader Andrija Štampar (a socialist who observed Maoist forces in 1930s China after he was forced into exile from Yugoslavia), and esteemed Johns Hopkins professor Henry Sigerist of Switzerland (who carried out a comprehensive review of Soviet social security and health services in the 1930s). See Birn and Brown, "Making of Health Internationalists."

30 Krige, *American Hegemony*, 118.

31 See Hunt, *Ideology and U.S. Foreign Policy*; LaFeber, *Inevitable Revolutions*; Schlesinger and Kinzer, *Bitter Fruit*.

32 Víctor Paz Estenssoro, "Fundamentos Científicos de la Revolución Nacional," quoted in John, *Bolivia's Radical Tradition*, 124.

33 See Siekmeier, "Trailblazer Diplomat"; Siekmeier, *Bolivian Revolution and the United States*.

34 Wilkie, *Bolivian Revolution and U.S. Aid since 1952*.

35 See Lehman, "Revolutions and Attributions."

36 See Latham, *Right Kind of Revolution*.

37 Dwight Eisenhower cited in Lehman, "Revolutions and Attributions," 208; "Bolivia: Chaos in the Clouds," 27.

38 Siekmeier, "Most Generous Assistance."

39 See National Archives and Records Administration online guide to Federal Records of U.S. Foreign Assistance Agencies, 1948–1961 (record group 469), http://www.archives.gov/research/guide-fed-records/groups/469.html.

40 U.S. Agency for International Development (USAID), *Economic and Program Statistics, Bolivia* 9 (1968): 37–38, 41, cited in Wilkie, *Bolivian Revolution and U.S. Aid*, 10.

41 See Geidel, "Sowing Death in Our Women's Wombs"; Geidel, *Peace Corps Fantasies*; Field, "Ideology as Strategy." For further discussion of the Peace Corps's impact in 1960s Bolivia, see Nelson, "Birth Rights."

42 Bauer, "Survey of Medical Education in Bolivia," 23, 53.

43 See the introduction to Virreira Sánchez, *Bibliografía del Doctor Arturo Urquidi Morales*.

44 Rivera Cusicanqui, *Oppressed but Not Defeated*.

45 Urquidi Morales, *Feudalismo en América*. See also Agosto Guzmán's assessment of this book, "Juicio Crítico a la Obra 'El Feudalismo en América y la Reforma Agraria Boliviana,'" in Virreira Sánchez, *Bibliografía del Doctor Arturo Urquidi Morales*, 81–83.

46 Quoted in "Valioso Juicio Periodístico sobre un Discurso del Rector de la Universidad," *El País*, March 31, 1950, in Virreira Sánchez, *Bibliografía del Doctor Arturo Urquidi Morales*, 193.

47 Urquidi Morales, *Labor Universitaria*, 115–27.

48 Blanes, "Bolivia, El Papel de la Universidad," 64.

49 Fernando Díez de Medina, "Cochabamba: la Revelación de un Mundo Nuevo," *Tribuna*, November 26, 1951, in Virreira Sánchez, *Bibliografía del Doctor Arturo Urquidi Morales*, 181.

50 "Discurso del Doctor Arturo Urquidi," in Virreira Sánchez, *Bibliografía del Doctor Arturo Urquidi Morales*, 206. Urquidi, a Communist, according to Bauer, fought for intellectual freedom and institutional autonomy at roughly the same time that professors in the University of California system were forced to sign loyalty oaths. See the University of California Loyalty Oath Controversy Material, 1949–1952, Bancroft Library, UC Berkeley; Innis, "Lessons from the Controversy over the Loyalty Oath"; Brickman, "Medical McCarthyism."

51 Virreira Sánchez, *Bibliografía del Doctor Arturo Urquidi Morales*, 82, 202.

52 Jorge Domínguez and Mitchell, "Roads Not Taken."

53 "Discurso del Presidente de la República, Dr. Víctor Paz Estenssoro," in Urquidi Morales, *Labor Universitaria*, 469–70; Urquidi Morales, "¿Revoluciones Universitarias? Manifiesto al Pueblo de Cochabamba," in Urquidi Morales, *Labor Universitaria*, 129–58.

54 Urquidi Morales, "¿Revoluciones Universitarias?," in Urquidi Morales, *Labor Universitaria*, 131–33, 155.

55 "Discurso del Doctor Arturo Urquidi," in Virreira Sánchez, *Bibliografía del Doctor Arturo Urquidi Morales*, 211.

56 "Discurso del Doctor Arturo Urquidi," in Virreira Sánchez, *Bibliografía del Doctor Arturo Urquidi Morales*, 209, 221–22.

57 "Discurso del Doctor Arturo Urquidi," in Virreira Sánchez, *Bibliografía del Doctor Arturo Urquidi Morales*, 209.

58 Raúl Prebisch first made these ideas famous in *The Economic Development of Latin America and Its Principal Problems*. See also Stein and Stein, *Colonial Heritage of Latin America*; Galeano, *Open Veins of Latin America*; Cardoso and Faletto, *Dependency and Development in Latin America*.

59 The reassessment of the role of universities during moments of political and social upheaval was not unique to either Bolivia or the 1950s. See, for example, Soto Laveaga, "Bringing the Revolution to Medical Schools."

60 Rothwell, *Transpacific Revolutionaries*, 132–33; John, *Bolivia's Radical Tradition*, 56–59, 74.

61 Balcázar, *Historia de la Medicina en Bolivia*, 630.

62 Bauer, "Survey of Medical Education in Bolivia," 7–8; Zulawski, *Unequal Cures*, 26.

63 Bauer, "Survey of Medical Education in Bolivia," 10–11, 18–19, 26–27, 29.

64 Bauer, "Survey of Medical Education in Bolivia," 9–10.

65 Balcázar, *Historia de la Medicina en Bolivia,* 649–51.

66 Johannes H. Bauer, officer diary, 156, RAC, record group 12, box 29. Special thanks to Tom Rosenbaum for sending me these files.

67 Bauer, "Survey of Medical Education in Bolivia," 5.

68 Luykx, *Citizen Factory*.

69 Bauer, "Survey of Medical Education in Bolivia," 4.

70 U.S. officials' overstatement of communism's prevalence in Latin America among labor unions, student movements, and leftist leaders, particularly after Cuba's 1959 revolution, was certainly not unique to Bolivia. See Schlesinger and Kinzer, *Bitter Fruit*; and Schoultz, *Beneath the United States*.

71 Siekmeier also makes this claim in *Bolivian Revolution and the United States*, 5, 61–64.

72 For additional examples, see U.S. Department of State, *Foreign Relations of the United States* (FRUS).

73 John, *Bolivia's Radical Tradition*, 121; Klein, *Bolivia*, 233.

74 Quotes from Bauer diary, 159. For MNR leaders' opinions on this subject, see Alexander, *Bolivian National Revolution*, 133, 256.

75 This was true of all medical schools in Bolivia. See Bauer, "Survey of Medical Education in Bolivia," 9.

76 Bauer, "Survey of Medical Education in Bolivia," 23, 25, 26. On the alleged risks communism posed to students, see Hochman and Paiva's chapter in this volume.

77 Bauer, "Survey of Medical Education in Bolivia," 53.

78 Weindling, "Out of the Ghetto."

79 Farley, *To Cast Out Disease*, 271.

80 Kuznick, *Beyond the Laboratory*; Cohen, *When the Old Left Was Young*; Lear, "American Medical Support for Spanish Democracy."

81 Jessica Wang, "Science, Security, and the Cold War."

82 Brickman, "Medical McCarthyism."

83 U.S. Congress, *Tax-Exempt Foundations*, 505, 542–49.

84 Quotation from Rockefeller Foundation, *Annual Report, 1952*, 11.

85 Rusk's testimony can be found in U.S. Congress, *Tax-Exempt Foundations*, 475–505, 507–55, 647–48.

86 RAC, Cox and Reece Investigations (1952–1954), Series 1—Digest Files, Subseries 1—Individuals, box 18, folder 399 (528—Bauer, J. H., 1945–1948). Special thanks to Tom Rosenbaum for sending me these files.

87 Macdonald and Sutton, *Ford Foundation*, 28–31.

88 Reece, "Tax-Exempt Subversion," 57.

89 Gideonse, "Congressional Committee's Investigation of the Foundations."

90 Rockefeller Foundation, *Annual Report, 1953*, 27.

91 On the role of U.S. congressional hearings in the Cold War, see also Soto Laveaga's chapter in this volume.

92 Krige, *American Hegemony*, 117–18, 129, 151.

93 Krige, *American Hegemony*, 29–30.

94 Krige, *American Hegemony*, 30.

95 Pan American Sanitary Bureau, XIV Pan American Sanitary Conference, VI Meeting Regional Committee, Santiago, Chile, 1954, "Summary of Reports of the Member States, 1950–1953," September 10, 1954, 19, RAC, record group 2.1954, series 200, box 21, folder 148.

96 Bauer, "Survey of Medical Education in Bolivia," 31.

97 Mendizábal Lozano, *Historia de la Salud Pública en Bolivia*, 142.

98 Bauer, "Survey of Medical Education in Bolivia," 33–35, 38–40.

99 Bauer, "Survey of Medical Education in Bolivia," 40, 42, 52–54.

100 Klein, *Bolivia*, 155, 161–63.

101 Gotkowitz, *Revolution for Our Rights*. See also Alexander, *Bolivian National Revolution*, 64; Malloy, *Bolivia*, 198–207.

102 Bauer, "Survey of Medical Education in Bolivia," 13, 52–54.

103 Correspondence between John Bugher (director of medical education and public health), John Weir (associate director of medical education and public health), and John Janney (staff member, Medical Education and Public Health Division), November 1956; quotation from Janney to Weir, November 22, 1956, RAC, record group 2.1956, series 300, box 56, folder 368.

104 Correspondence between Bugher and Janney, November 29, 1956, RAC, record group 1.1, series 303, box 1, folder 6.

105 Rockefeller Foundation, *Annual Report, 1951*, 26–27.

106 See Rockefeller Foundation *Annual Reports, 1954–1959*.

107 Approved grant-in-aid request for ten thousand dollars for the Division of Rural Endemic Diseases, October 26, 1951, RAC, record group 2.1956, series 300, box 56, folder 368; Rockefeller Foundation, *Annual Report, 1951*, 205.

108 Rockefeller Foundation, *Annual Report, 1951*, 211; Rockefeller Foundation, *Annual Report, 1952*, 96.

109 For more information on these programs, see Wilkie, *Bolivian Revolution and U.S. Aid since 1952*; Alexander, *Bolivian National Revolution*.

110 Dr. Benjamin Horning, medical education consultant, to Dr. Harald Frederiksen, director of the Health, Welfare, and Housing Field Party of the Institute of Inter-American Affairs, United States Operations Mission to Bolivia, April 16, 1957, National Archives and Records Administration, Washington, DC, record group 469, box 9, 1957.

111 Marcos Cueto, "International Health, the Early Cold War and Latin America," 27–28.

112 Alexander, *Communism in Latin America*, 212.

113 Rivera Cusicanqui, *Oppressed but Not Defeated*, 59.

114 See Lehman, *Bolivia and the United States*.

115 Dunkerley, *Rebellion in the Veins*, 83–119.

116 Telegram from the counselor of the embassy in Bolivia (Gilmore) to the U.S. Department of State, September 28, 1956, in *FRUS*, 65.

117 Latham, *Right Kind of Revolution*; Lehman, *Bolivia and the United States*, chapters 4, 5. The MNR sought aid from the Soviet Union in the late 1950s in hopes that appealing to the Eastern Bloc could leverage more assistance from the United States. See Siekmeier, *Bolivian Revolution and the United States*, 79.

118 Dispatch from Ambassador Drew in Bolivia to the U.S. Department of State, January 27, 1956, in *FRUS*, 533; my emphasis.

119 USAID, *Economic and Program Statistics*, 41, cited in Blasier, "United States and the Revolution," 79.

120 On international aid as foreign policy, see Siekmeier, "Most Generous Assistance"; Field, *From Development to Dictatorship*.

121 Weindling, "Out of the Ghetto," 211–12.

122 Krige, *American Hegemony*, 118, 151.

123 Rockefeller Foundation, *Annual Report, 1949*, 5.

124 Rockefeller Foundation, *Annual Report, 1951*, 63–68. There is also information about the interest in yellow fever research in *Annual Report, 1948*, 77.

125 Rockefeller Foundation, *Annual Report, 1951*; Barnard quotation on 26–27.

126 Rockefeller Foundation, *Annual Report, 1949*, 26.

127 Rockefeller Foundation, *Annual Report, 1951*, 41.

128 Rockefeller Foundation, *Annual Report, 1949*, 60–63.

129 Rockefeller Foundation, *Annual Report, 1951*, 10.

3

Cold War Mexico in a Time of "Wonder Drugs"

GABRIELA SOTO LAVEAGA

En la periferia la guerra no fue tan fría.

[On the periphery, the war was
not so cold.]

—Lorenzo Meyer, in Daniela Spenser,
Espejos de la Guerra Fría

"Gentlemen, I can assure you that the drawing is not of a missile," claimed a
Soviet professor before an entranced London audience of more than two thousand physicians who had come to hear him speak.[1] Professor L. F. Larionov had
traveled from the Institute of Experimental Pathology and Cancer Therapy
in Moscow to reveal his "self-guided medicine" against cancer. Thunderous
applause greeted the news that the medication, strangely rocket-shaped, targeted affected tissue while preserving healthy cells that surrounded a tumor. A
possible cure for ever-elusive and deadly cancers seemed a certain reality in the
fall of 1958. Not surprisingly for many champions of science and technology,
the pill came in the shape of Soviet technological innovation: a space rocket.

Within a few months, the Mexican embassy in Moscow began receiving telegrams and letters from desperate Mexicans seeking "the auto-guided
treatment" for relatives wasting away from malignant tumors. Some had
heard of Professor Larionov, "the wise Soviet," through the press, others via
acquaintances who had acquired the medication through circuitous means.[2]
This was not the first time that Mexicans were writing to request medication
from the Moscow-based embassy, but this time letter writers seemed to agree
that only with the "critical" aid of Soviet medication could their loved ones
potentially survive. Diplomatic correspondence reveals that in the 1950s the
Mexican ambassador in Moscow often sent experimental "not yet approved

for commercial use" Soviet medication to ailing patients in Mexico and, in at least one instance, to the frantic Mexican ambassador in Havana.[3] The letters, written by the ambassador or his staff in Moscow and overflowing with explicit translated instructions on dosages and secondary effects—that is, "the rapid drop of leucocytes in the blood after taking Dopan indicates that the dosage was not sufficient"—were certainly not the typical correspondence one finds in diplomatic files.[4] Increasing faith in Soviet pharmaceuticals could not cure, however, "the inhumanity of our [Mexican] bureaucracy," which often filed away anxious requests for medications while those ailing, as in the case of the patient in Havana, died days before the medication arrived.[5] The embassy's glacial pace in addressing demands for Soviet medications may also indicate that requests for pharmaceuticals, though not plentiful, were common. In fact, the increased interest in Soviet pharmaceuticals and demand for Soviet cures—in particular for cancer, glaucoma, and polio—seemed to parallel growing tensions between Mexican and U.S. pharmaceutical companies at the time. These embassy letters also suggest that the demand for Soviet pharmaceuticals was part of a complex circuit of exchange in the context of the Cold War. Moreover, the circulation of Soviet medications crystallizes how diplomacy and technological diffusion were intertwined at that time.[6]

Pharmaceutical "wars" were not unusual during that era. Around the globe, national pharmaceutical industries became sites of the "early skirmish" for global control in the Cold War. For example, India, described as a "Cold War hot spot" between expanding American and Soviet pharmaceutical industries, was a key site for these geopolitical struggles.[7] According to historian Jeremy Greene, Merck Sharpe & Dohme International (later known as Merck) fervently pressured India to stop accepting Soviet financing for its burgeoning pharmaceutical industry. The decision in favor of U.S. companies was, allegedly, swayed by the Indian public's hopes of obtaining the coveted American antihypertensive drug, Diuril, in exchange.[8]

This success in South Asia was described as an early battle against "the coming Russian drive on the other front—the war against disease."[9] An increasing number of studies have shown how Cold War rhetoric influenced notions of disease and invigorated health campaigns in key geopolitical regions. Most recently, scholars have used the history of experimentation to propose new geographies based on pharmaceutical capital and marketing power.[10] Though Latin America was not immune to pharmaceutical industry dealings, the region is rarely the focus of historical discussions on the pharmaceutical struggles of the Cold War.

The aims of this chapter are twofold. First, I revisit my earlier work on the case of steroid hormone production in Mexico, resituate it—explicitly—as part of a larger Cold War dialogue over pharmaceutical control, and examine the meaning of this shifted lens.[11] Second, I explore the claims made by U.S. policy-makers about the perceived threat of losing Latin America, especially Mexico, to the Soviet Union in the pharmaceutical battle. By exploring evidence of pharmaceutical trade (or lack thereof) between Russia and Mexico in the 1950s and 1960s, we can better understand how the claims of communist infiltration of the medications market in Latin America often served as a facade for capitalist expansion of the American pharmaceutical industry into the region. Moreover, an examination of the Mexican desire for Soviet pharmaceuticals challenges dominant Cold War narratives that tend to dismiss Russian medical and scientific influence as secondary in the region. By examining demand for Soviet pharmaceuticals on the same plane as that for American pharmaceuticals, we expand the meaning of the quest for "modernity" in a politically divided world. For, as Sujit Sivasundaram reminds us when examining global histories of science, "to be modern in a global age of knowledge, by the twentieth century, meant using science and technology to intervene in problems of hunger, disease, and development."[12]

Washington's Challenge to Mexican Steroid Production

The mid-twentieth century offered a seemingly unending display of medical marvels emerging from both sides of the Cold War. For example, on July 5, 1956, a short medical film transfixed members of a U.S. Senate subcommittee. Made by the National Institutes of Health, the movie showed "the miraculous effect obtained by a particular hormone, a cortical hormone."[13] It likely contained the now-famous clips of once-paralyzed men and women walking, jumping, and almost skipping after only a few daily doses of cortisone. What most clearly made an impact on viewers was how patients reverted to their previous near-invalid states as soon as the cortisone injections ceased. It was obvious that steroid hormones were indeed "wonder drugs," but with limited powers. Although not a cure, steroids could alleviate the symptoms of some troubling ailments, such as "mankind's most crippling disease," rheumatoid arthritis. They also purportedly gave superhuman powers to athletes, and by the early 1950s, they were being used in animal husbandry to produce more beef at less expense.[14] Despite these many uses, a parade of scientists and pharmaceutical executives testified during the subcommittee hearings that, disturbingly, the United States was unable to get a steady, reliable flow of steroids because the raw material needed to produce commercial quantities of—in this instance—cortisone came from Mexican wild yams. In fact, Senate hearings were taking place that summer to study the antitrust actions of a Mexico City company, Syntex Laboratories, that controlled much of the world's steroid trade. Syntex was the first firm to synthesize commercial quantities of progesterone from *dioscoreas*, commonly referred to as yams, found in southern Mexico. Locally called *barbasco*, these wild yams contain diosgenin, the chemical precursor for the mass production of synthetic steroid hormones.

As I detailed in *Jungle Laboratories*, in 1954, a mere ten years after its founding, Syntex—with 3,000 workers, including 150 chemists and technicians, and reported annual sales of $5 million—was the largest steroid-producing company in the world. But starting in the early 1950s, smaller companies within Mexico began to sell diosgenin to European cartels, thus undercutting Syntex's profits. In 1951, at the behest of Syntex, the Mexican government raised tariffs on the export of barbasco-derived products and later limited forestry permits for harvesting barbasco.[15] In response, several foreign company owners, among them famed African American chemist Percy Julian, demanded an explanation from the Mexican government for its apparent collusion with Syntex (which had not been denied any forestry permits).

During the U.S. Senate's 1956 "Wonder Drugs" hearings, the president of Syntex denied any wrongdoing, but Julian insisted that his earlier attempts to build a company in Mexico had failed because "the [forestry] permit was denied at every turn," mainly due to "the objection of the Syntex Co."[16] In addition, Syntex, as the world's leading supplier of synthetic steroids, was considering establishing a state-owned company to regulate the barbasco trade—thus potentially placing the United States, its leading buyer, in a vulnerable and dependent position relative to a Third World nation.[17] Furthermore, Syntex announced the synthesis of cortisone *and* the first viable oral contraceptive, enabling Mexico to continue to dominate the steroid industry.[18] This was no minor feat. Mexico had lagged behind Europe and the United States in pharmaceutical development until after World War II. In the 1940s, the Mexican government, through the Alien Property Act, seized all German laboratories and pharmaceutical houses and the licensing agreements that came with them. It appeared that, thanks to steroids, Mexico might become a leading pharmaceutical contender in a Western hemisphere market then dominated by the United States. But the situation swiftly changed as the "spectre of steroids" became linked to potential Soviet superiority.[19] While focusing on Mexico, the summer hearings in Washington, D.C., were also part of a larger conversation fueled by Cold War anxieties that the Soviets could and would use "their medical personnel, know-how, technologies, and drugs to capture support of people in underdeveloped countries."[20] Indeed, the possibility of a Soviet-style, state-run steroid industry that could appeal to and perhaps be emulated by Third World nations served as one of the leading rationales for U.S. scrutiny of Mexican steroid producers.

In a world divided by the allegiances demanded by the Cold War, steroid hormones fueled anxieties by threatening to tilt the axis in favor of East or West.[21] The inability of U.S. markets to ensure a steady supply of raw material caused much unease both in Washington and on Wall Street. This unease was conveyed in the popular press, such as in a *Fortune Magazine* article explaining that much sought-after cortisone was "in tragically short supply," a situation made worse because the Mexican company Syntex had "already pulled off a stunning raid on the U.S. sex-hormone industry." The article pointed out that by 1951 "about half of all sex hormones sold in the U.S." came from Mexico.[22] Not only was America's health at stake; so too, politicians argued, were cherished American business practices.[23] Only through a robust economy, the article reminded readers, could the United States be "outstandingly the most powerful country in the world."[24] As if to drive the point home, another article in the same issue extolled "Russia's Industrial Expansion."[25] The timing of the interest in Syntex, Mexican barbasco, and its steroid derivatives coincided with both increased scrutiny of the U.S. pharmaceutical industry's price-fixing of medications and the pharmaceutical companies' use of Cold War rhetoric to defend that practice. Some scholars have suggested that the competition for pharmaceutical domination was comparable in importance to the launching of Sputnik, which ignited the Space Race, and was no less aggressive in its goals.[26]

In the case of Mexico and steroids, the Cold War framing was more indirect but no less significant in how it affected business ventures, allegiances, and even the development of science and medicine in the country. Attempts by the Mexican government to protect the steroid trade, mainly through tariffs, were reinterpreted in U.S. congressional hearings as direct attacks on American capitalism.[27]

As early as 1941, the United States had sought a way to control steroid production. That year U.S. espionage "picked up the exciting rumor that the Luftwaffe was using adrenal extracts, which permitted German pilots to fly at great altitudes without suffering oxygen deficiency and without fatigue."[28] The rumor was not far-fetched, for at the time amphetamines were part of the "daily diet" of American GIs. Indeed, army scientists and physicians had documented unbelievable acts of "heroism" performed while under the influence of "speed."[29] Though the Luftwaffe rumor turned out to be false, the U.S. National Defense Research Council immediately began to fund research on steroids. During the Cold War, concerns over steroids rose again when rumors began to circulate that Eastern Bloc athletes were using steroids to compete in the peaceful but politically potent East–West battleground of the Olympic Games.[30] It seemed that if the United States wanted to win the pharmaceutical war, it would have to pay close attention not only to steroids but to the pharmaceutical industry across the world.

In 1955, seven companies were processing barbasco in Mexico; only one, Beisa, was a subsidiary of a transnational corporation.[31] A few years later the main Mexican laboratories had U.S. and European owners. Two principal changes occurred over the ensuing five years to edge out Mexican control of the trade. First, tinged with Cold War rhetoric about national security, debates and U.S. Senate hearings on price-fixing of pharmaceuticals spilled over the border. Second, the Mexican government's attempts to regulate the barbasco trade became the backdrop for Mexico's steroid hormone industry to embrace the "freedom" of capitalism instead of the "regressive" alternative of government restrictions. The attitude was best summarized by the president of American Ciba Pharmaceuticals when speaking of steroid production: "We do not feel it consistent either with our company's interests or with our general concept of freedom of trade and commerce to be subjected to a supply market which would be restricted as to its competitiveness."[32] Foreign pharmaceutical executives' negative attitude toward Syntex was rooted in the company's rapid success and the Mexican government's seeming preference for a national company over foreign pharmaceutical companies.

On May 13, 1955, the Mexican government's official legal register, *Diario Oficial*, published a decree that raised the tariffs on all "tubers, roots, stalks, and parts of plant extracts for manufacture of pharmaceutical products, natural or synthetic hormones, etc."[33] Syntex, as a Mexican company, received priority in the granting of permits and a reduction in prohibitive taxes. Critics argued that this undermined the very core of (American) capitalism. Yet at the same time, U.S. pharmaceutical firms were under investigation for the high prices of medications that, some argued, placed the United States at a global disadvantage because U.S. medications could not compete against lower-cost Soviet counterparts.

Despite these concerns about the prohibitive costs of U.S. pharmaceuticals, Latin American consumption of U.S. drugs and medical supplies went from $18 million to $119 million between 1942 and 1953.[34] As historian Marcos Cueto has argued, this created a growing dependence on a U.S.-style of medicine that focused increasingly on managing chronic diseases instead of infectious ones.[35] Pharmaceuticals also became a pivotal component in the unfolding Cold War via U.S. support to the World Health Organization's disease campaigns. As such, U.S. foreign aid (in the guise of pharmaceuticals) also subsidized U.S. business interests. Industry leaders in turn convincingly deployed Cold War rhetoric to defend their price-fixing schemes into the late 1950s and early 1960s.[36] For example, in the summer of 1959, the president of Merck & Co., John T. Connor, remarking on the power of pharmaceutical companies, stated, "Now that we are forced to take stock, we find that our industry has grown into a significant national asset, these daily contributions to the war against disease are well known . . . but [its] potential contributions to the world struggle against Communism are only beginning to become apparent."[37]

By this time, in an attempt to preserve a for-profit business model in the face of proposed regulation of drug pricing and marketing strategies, the major U.S. drug houses joined together to protest these policies, drawing on the fear of encroaching communism. As the chairman of the Pharmaceutical Manufacturers Association stated, "Probably through no other industry can the superiority of our American competitive system be demonstrated so impressively." In the midst of the Cold War, the pharmaceutical industry showcased itself as "a model of American free enterprise and sought, through the development" of ever more medications as well as donations of pharmaceutical supplies to the Third World, to stanch the spread of communism.[38] The heads of the pharmaceutical industry took the position that any attempts to challenge the industry's free-market ethos threatened the United States in the fight against communism, thereby bringing the menace of socialized medicine closer to U.S. shores.[39]

The Wonder Drugs hearings, led by Senator Estes Kefauver, sought to address the challenges involved in the U.S. pharmaceutical industry's production of four key drugs: antibiotics, oral anti-diabetes medication, tranquilizers, and, most crucially, corticosteroids. In addition to the concerns expressed above with regard to steroids, witnesses before the Senate hearings expressed a growing fear that the U.S. pharmaceutical industry could not produce enough of the medication to treat its own population. As one witness grimly told Senate subcommittee members, "The total number of victims [of rheumatic diseases in the United States] is greater than the combined populations of Chicago and Los Angeles, and of those ten million sufferers . . . one million are permanently disabled."[40] Physicians presented a list of at least forty different diseases that could be treated with steroids, and they explained that, given the rising number of Americans suffering from arthritis, controlling the production of synthetic steroid hormones was of vital clinical importance, and even a matter of national security.

In 1955, in a letter presented as evidence to the U.S. Senate hearings, John L. Davenport, executive vice president of Charles Pfizer & Co., stated that Pfizer was familiar with the Mexican steroid processing plant in Mexico City because in the previous two years it had "actively participated in the modernization of this plant and in the installation of the latest equipment."[41] It is unclear what Pfizer's investment entailed, but it led the company to regard the new Syntex installation "as at least as modern and efficient as any other existing plant anywhere in the world for the manufacture of hormone products." Indeed, American companies, it appeared, were competing against each other to gain a foothold in the lucrative steroid trade.

These actions ultimately contributed to Mexico's loss of control of the steroid hormone industry in 1956, when American interests purchased Syntex and relocated its headquarters to Palo Alto, California. The impact of this move significantly diminished Mexico's ability to maintain a successful, domestic pharmaceutical industry. By 1960, Mexico's small, independent pharmaceutical companies had disappeared, and all of the entities processing barbasco had become subsidiaries of larger corporations. Even more telling, none were Mexican.

From American Pharmaceutical Friendships to the Moscow-Mexico Nexus: Fellows and Fellowship

Notwithstanding U.S. pharmaceutical companies' overwhelming financial interest in displacing and overtaking Mexican hormone production, they also recognized that the pharmaceutical sector had a role to play in forging ties with potential U.S. allies. Moreover, there were ways other than technical support or installing a plant in a country to ensure political allegiances. For example, in a 1953 memo, Antonie T. Knoppers, the director of Merck's international division, questioned why thirty-four postdoctoral fellowships his company sponsored (nearly 40 percent of the total) were granted that year to scientists from Great Britain compared to seven grantees from Mexico and only one from Uruguay.[42] He added an illustrative quote paraphrasing the Bible, "Those who are well have no need for a physician, but those who are sick do," to explain why giving postgraduate training funding to so many British citizens had "little value." Moreover, he argued, British scientists "are excellently trained and have fully equipped laboratories of high standing." Knoppers proposed, instead, to select "75% of the fellowships from semi-developed countries" because a few of these scientists are "real gems." But beyond this, he stressed:

> With such a choice one would really foster science, as such fellows will improve laboratories, and introduce and adopt new methods when they return to their countries; further, these people will be more valuable as good-will contacts for the USA, from a scientific and a more general point of view (during my visits in foreign countries, I experienced many proofs of this attitude), and in the third place, these "fellows" are of vital value to the Intl. Division of Merck & Co., Inc. as points of contact.[43]

The underlying argument about the importance of securing U.S.-friendly "points of contact" in the Mexican scientific community played directly into the Cold War rhetoric. After all, becoming a scientist in Mexico required funding that was often not easy to obtain. Understandably, aspiring Mexican scientists welcomed financial backing and opportunities to study abroad—many of which, as we shall see, came from the Soviets.[44]

In 1957, a few years after Merck's fellowship program, the Mexican government again attempted to regulate the sale of the increasingly lucrative steroid hormone. The pharmaceutical war was expanding to the training of scholars through strategic fellowships and grants. The heads of several American pharmaceutical companies had previously written to the U.S. Senate to complain that this ill-advised protectionist stance would deeply hurt the pharmaceutical industry's business model and affect the spread of American goals around the globe. To make clear which type of model was favored, a senior vice president of Merck & Co. stated, "As to the matter of government regulation, we recognize in principle the sovereign right of any government to regulate its industry in a manner required to best serve the interests of its people. In our own country, we believe that this has been accomplished, barring the unusual necessities of wartime, without undue restriction on the principle of free enterprise, which we as a people have embraced and zealously guard." In case his message was not clear enough, a bit later in the letter, he underscored, "We believe, however, that local industry can best grow in an atmosphere of freedom from unnecessary regulation, and with full opportunity for free and open competition in price and service with other local firms in the same industry."[45]

In other words, only those practices that did not directly affect American pharmaceutical interests could be deemed free and necessary. If Mexico were to continue being a valued recipient of grants, fellowships, equipment and, above all, medications, these "unnecessary regulations" would have to be rethought. Along with its aggressive challenge to Mexico's independent steroid industry, the United States was also sending a message about its conditional willingness to include Mexicans or any foreigners in a large-scale training program. Put differently, there was willingness to help train Mexicans in U.S. laboratories but not to accept an independent, successful Mexican pharmaceutical competitor.

For example, the U.S. "Health for Peace" bill, or Senate Joint Resolution 41, proposed the creation of an international medical research initiative. The bill passed the Senate with strong support (sixty-three to seventeen votes) on May 20, 1959, but was blocked in the House later that summer. The bill proposed an international research effort modeled on the National Institutes of Health for the "training of promising scholars in other lands."[46] As a doctor in support of the bill was quoted as saying, "In many countries, such as Italy, the amount of research support available is so small that men of great skill and intellect are compelled to carry on only token research concerning problems which are selected because they do not require manpower, equipment, or modern research facilities."[47] Despite Senate support, congressional representatives voted to block the bill and effectively killed federal programs to fund the training of foreign researchers. U.S. government support for training foreign scientists was subsumed under the Fulbright program (which did not emphasize the sciences), although private philanthropies, such as the Rockefeller, Carnegie, and Kellogg Foundations, continued to offer thousands of fellowships throughout the Cold War period.[48]

The Soviet government, meanwhile, took a decidedly different stance on training of Mexican and other Third World scientific professionals. As the Mexican Embassy in Moscow enthusiastically commented, the Soviet Union had launched a vigorous program to attract foreign students and fund their studies either through direct government sponsorship or through a series of accords with forty-seven countries. In 1959 there were fourteen thousand foreign students studying in Soviet institutions.[49] While many of these students were focusing on the arts and humanities, even more were specializing in "electricity, petroleum, machinery construction, geography, hydraulics, medicine, economy, etc." Remarkably, "90% of these students are from the Middle East, India, South Asia, or Africa, in other words from nearly every developing nation." Though Latin America was not explicitly mentioned, that year Mexico had thirty-one scholars in the USSR specializing in fields from petrochemicals to ballet. As the Mexican diplomat noted, the Soviet Union was "the only country in the world that currently offers such an important number of scholarships and in such favorable conditions for the recipients." The embassy attaché's concluding remarks would certainly have chilled many

American hearts: "Within a few years many of the professionals—and possibly even politicians—who will be charged with leading the public in developing countries will be the product of a solid scientific formation acquired in the Soviet Union."[50] To put it differently, at roughly the same time that the United States had rejected dedicating funds to train foreign scientists, and while it had aggressively pursued ways to curtail Mexico's growing steroid industry, Mexico and the Soviet Union were venturing into agreements that ultimately led to technological exchanges and study-abroad programs.

In addition, the Soviet Union was keen on publicly displaying the strong cultural and historical affinities between Mexico and Russia. For instance, in April 1959, two associations—the Society for the Diffusion of Political and Scientific Knowledge and the Soviet Association for Friendship and Cultural Collaboration with the Countries of Latin America—organized a series of talks on Mexican revolutionary hero Emiliano Zapata to commemorate the forty-year anniversary of his death.[51] In his report of the events, a Mexican Embassy employee gushed that "it is not often that the opportunity arises for a foreigner to speak to a Soviet audience in praise of a Revolution that is not the 1917 Russian Revolution (or the Chinese, or of the democratic populations, which appear to be the only ones that are officially recognized as historical)." A rapt audience of nearly eight hundred Muscovites, among them "members of the Academy of Science and the Institute of History, journalists, writers, students, etc.," listened as the talk illustrated the common struggles against *latifundistas* (large rural landholders) in the two countries. As one speaker explained, though Zapata had no formal training, and despite difficulties in communications, when the revolutionary icon found out that "an insurrection had exploded in czarist Russia, he, as an example of his extraordinary political savvy, pledged his solidarity with the October Revolution." In closing statements, the representative of the Mexican Embassy underlined that "little moves a Mexican as much as an homage to la Patria," and he assured the audience that the Mexican nation viewed the Soviet Union with great satisfaction.[52]

Half a year later, the Soviets again delighted Mexicans, now on their home turf, when the touring Pyatnitsky Choir executed a perfect rendition of *Las Golondrinas* at the Auditorio Nacional. An audience of more than ten thousand was captivated "by the perfect pronunciation of Spanish" by the Russian choir singing traditional Mexican songs. For nearly six weeks, the choir toured Mexico and was welcomed on stages "magnificently constructed, others that were totally inadequate and rapidly improvised, in sports fields, in stadiums, movie theaters, bull-fight rings." The quality of the venue, however, did not matter: as the popular newspaper *Últimas Noticias* reported, listening to the

Soviet choir was deeply "impressive and we were all filled by a feeling of deep tenderness and love for humanity."[53] As beguiling to Mexicans as were Russian voices singing Mexican folk songs, the display of Soviet medical advances, of which the choir was an incidental component, was even more engrossing.

Evidence of this is a series of newspaper clippings and translated articles about Soviet scientific developments sent to the Ministry of Foreign Relations in Mexico City by its embassy staff in Moscow.[54] Though the diseases and interventions covered in these exchanges varied, it is clear, as recounted in an article on cancer, that Mexicans found it worthwhile to monitor the USSR's ambitions and relentless technological and medical progress, in order to learn from Soviet successes.

But Mexicans were no strangers to Soviet scientific progress. Mexico City's Auditorio Nacional was also the site of the November 1959 three-week "Soviet Exposition in Mexico." One of its organizers, vice president of the Soviet Chamber of Commerce Dmitri Borisenko, enthused in an interview that those who attended the exposition would be treated to "models of artificial satellites . . . launched into the Cosmos by Soviet scientists and [visitors] can learn how in our country the atom is made to work for peace." In addition to the expected exhibits about space travel, Mexicans would be able to see work by jewelers, late-model cars, models of "maternity houses, preschools, color pictures of our nation's clinics, where hundreds of thousands of Soviet citizens can rest and be treated."[55] The medical exhibit showcased medical advances such as "thoracic surgery, diagnosis and treatment of cancer," and other medical wonders. The importance of this exhibit and the value of Latin America for the Soviet Union was succinctly spelled out in an article in *Pravda*: "Spring has Arrived in Latin America." The "spring" of the title referred, of course, to the presence of the Soviet Union. As the author of the article intoned, "some leaders want to sow the seeds of doubt about the Soviet people's sincerity in foreign relations" with Latin America, but as was becoming apparent, "it is more difficult every day to cultivate discord and enemies on Latin American soil . . . because peace and friendship is what is growing."[56]

As a 1959 article explained, the Soviet government "is devoting special attention to the struggle against cancer," and funds would be funneled to building "new oncological institutes in Moscow and Leningrad and to enlist alongside medical men, chemists, physicists and biologists in work on the problem of cancer."[57] Next to these articles, in the same folder, was a letter giddily describing "the great honor of the letter writer" to send copies of a Soviet newspaper showing images of the moon captured during that nation's third successful rocket launch.[58] The implication was clear: with Soviet manpower focusing on deadly diseases, the prospects of success in conquering cancer might well be realized by the first country to launch a rocket. Indeed, the Soviet Information Bureau underscored such promise in declaring that "the launching of a ballistic rocket with scientific equipment and test animals into high-altitude is another great success for Soviet science."[59] Even as U.S. politicians showed little interest in funding the training of foreign scientists, the Soviet Union insistently conveyed the opposite message, not just in terms of training but also in their willingness to broaden the availability of their pharmaceuticals and their benefits in Latin America.

It is not surprising, then, that Professor Larionov's treatment against cancer, with its unique rocket shape, would cause such a frenzied response in Mexico. Of all possible medical therapeutics, none inspired as much hope as alleged pharmaceutical cures for cancer. Requests for cancer drugs were common into the 1970s, as attested by a 1971 letter from a self-described "52-year old, physically strong, professor with a family history of cancers." The professor herself had been diagnosed with breast cancer and sought the Soviet medication Forafur, "which had positive results in 70% of all breast cancers."[60] Like all such earlier missives, the professor's lengthy and clinically detailed letter ended with the plea "to please send the treatment, with instructions, and cost" because this Soviet medication "is our last hope." Though the medication was sent on an Air France flight just days after receipt of her request, the professor died before the pills arrived in Mexico.

News that there was a potential Soviet cure for the physical havoc caused by polio also elicited responses from several Mexicans. Most notable, for its hopeful tone, was one penned by Alfonso Martínez Domínguez, who was clearly a personal friend of the ambassador, begging for any information on this breakthrough for his young son. The worried father attached a newspaper clipping extolling Soviet science and revealing that "in some instances [the medication] restored motor function in patients struck by paralysis." In July 1959 the embassy's response to Martínez Domínguez explained that Galantamina was an experimental medication that required direct approval from Moscow's Ministry of Public Health and that there had been no response from this ministry. In early September, two months after his request, Martínez Domínguez was sent a dosage of medication via airmail. Earlier that summer he had been sent a report that explained how Soviet Galantamina worked by "increasing the skeletal structure's sensibility."[61] Archival material did not reveal if the much-awaited medication had any effect on his son's illness.

Mexico was not the only Latin American country where requests for new Soviet pharmaceutical cures originated, but it seemed to be an important point of contact. For example, a brief news report that Soviet researchers had found a cure for glaucoma, Fosarbin, prompted a request from the Mexican Embassy in Caracas on behalf of a three-year-old Venezuelan boy who was quickly losing his sight.[62] The letter writer ended with the plaintive plea to "help me with this act of charity." An embassy employee responded that Fosarbin was known "on that side of the world" as the commonly available drug pilocarpine and, though he would be happy to send the Soviet sample, it would probably be best for the letter writer to obtain the medication locally.[63]

While most letters attached the newspaper or magazine articles that referred to promising and tried Soviet pharmaceuticals, others mentioned scientific venues, for example, "a chemistry conference in Lima, Peru," where attendees had learned of Soviet research on antibiotics that revealed a possible link to cancer cures.[64] The latter illustrates the concerted efforts by the Soviet Union to publicize their medical advances and also to make this information available to nonexperts who would, emotionally, pin their hopes for cures on the Soviet Union's progress.

Mexicans' staunch belief in the superiority of Soviet medicine is perhaps best illustrated in the figure of muralist Diego Rivera. In 1956, shortly after receiving a cancer diagnosis, Rivera traveled to Moscow for cobalt treatment at Botkin Hospital. At that time, such treatment was not available in Mexico. Rivera had previously visited Moscow in 1927 as part of a delegation of Mexican "peasants and workers" invited to celebrate the ten-year anniversary of the October Revolution.[65] Rivera's biographers agree that the parades, shows of military might, and worker processions deeply influenced his work and expanded his vision beyond the "confines of Mexican nationalism."[66] The trip also seemed to elicit Rivera's awe at Soviet advances. A recent Mexico City exhibition showcasing Rivera's time in Moscow displayed photographs of "innovative architectural projects, factories, metalworking plants, petroleum fields, technological advances, schools, theater, and general life and Russian culture" that had been given to Rivera and which he had preserved.[67] His post-Moscow murals and sketches bear the influence of his time there. When he returned to Moscow nearly thirty years later, his sketches again appeared heavily influenced by his surroundings, yet this time doctors and nurses, as seen from a sick man's bed, took the place of parades and factories.

After his four-month treatment, Rivera returned to Mexico, where he died in 1957. Ironically, before his cancer diagnosis and trip to the Soviet Union the Mexican government had requested that he paint a mural about the eventual triumph of humanity over cancer. The finished mural, *Apology of the Future Triumph of Medical Science over Cancer*, ultimately painted not by Rivera but by David Alfaro Siqueiros, alluded to the multiple cancers that can attack humankind, including political injustice and social inequality.[68] Front and center in the mural is a Theraton 60 with treatment table, purveying cobalt treatment against cancer.

Attempts to influence medical knowledge were not unidirectional, as the Mexican Embassy in Moscow files reveal. For example, in July 1967 the director of the Mexican Institute for Social Security (IMSS), Ignacio Morones Prieto, received a memo tagged as "very urgent, sent by messenger." Originating in Mexico's London Embassy, the memo demanded immediate action. In contrast to the urgent tone of the message, however, the request seemed trivial: 35mm color photographs of murals. Three specific murals formed part of the detailed list: Diego Rivera's mural for the Hospital de la Raza, the exterior patio ones for the Hospital de Jesús, and the newest ones for the recently inaugurated Centro Médico. In addition, murals from "other IMSS institutions from throughout the nation" could be included.[69] The pressing request came from a Dr. Francisco Guerra, a historian of medicine and Mexican researcher in Britain's Wellcome Trust library. Dr. Guerra needed the slides for a paper, "Anthropological Bases for Welfare Assistance in Hispanic America," which he would present a few weeks later as part of a course for hospital administrators organized by the World Health Organization in Moscow. The images were vital, the London attaché claimed, because they clearly showed the advances in medical assistance provided by the state in both urban and rural areas in Mexico. Moreover, it was, presumably, an important opportunity to showcase Mexico's hospitals to the world, which likely contributed to the request receiving "ample support" from Mexico's ambassador in London. While Mexicans were certainly proud of their compatriot's artistic talent, they also sought to highlight their own medical assets. The letter, filed in the Soviet Bloc files of Mexico's Ministry of Foreign Relations archives, raises other, potentially more intriguing issues that go beyond pharmaceutical influence and instead focus on health care models as modes of influence. An example is IMSS, founded in 1943, which provided comprehensive social security measures, including state-run health care services, retirement pensions, and other benefits for industrial workers. More than twenty years later, at the height of the Cold War, when the above request was made, Mexican scholars sought to showcase their own model of health care delivery as a powerful national approach that transcended the ideological divide.

Concluding Thoughts

In the late 1950s, the global monopoly on hormone production was not held by either of the superpowers—both of which hoped to harness steroids' medical potential—but rather by an unlikely country, Mexico. Yet some U.S. politicians believed that as a "less developed" nation, Mexico and its supply of cortisone could come under the sway of expanding Soviet influence and its model of state production. The Mexican government's attempts to regulate the barbasco trade heightened that fear, and U.S. pharmaceutical companies refused to sit idly by waiting to see what would transpire. Following the Wonder Drugs hearings, some industry representatives still sounded relatively confident in the pharmaceutical advantage the United States held over the USSR. John Connor, president of Merck, for example, noted in 1960 that "the United States has now drawn so far ahead in pharmaceutical research that it will take the Soviets more than ten years and more than a billion dollars to close the gap."[70] Yet as discussed above, most pharmaceutical executives at the Wonder Drugs hearings resorted to (rhetorical) arguments about the repercussions of Soviet inroads in this sector, while deflecting attention from domestic allegations of their companies' price-fixing. Thus, although the threat of communism had not been the initial catalyst for pharmaceutical houses to demand greater U.S. control of the lucrative Mexican synthetic steroid industry, such a threat resonated in pharmaceutical executives' testimony in the 1956 hearings. Later events seemed to confirm the industrialists' alarm. For U.S. policymakers, Sputnik's 1957 launch was proof that the Soviet Union could surpass the United States in technology and innovation, and that it could also use prescription drugs "to win the hearts and minds of the third world."[71] Even before Sputnik, pharmaceutical companies manipulated this fear and, in the case of the Wonder Drug hearings, translated it into the need for complete control of Mexico's domestic steroid hormone industry as a defensive action against communism.

Through intensive publicity campaigns, tours to Latin American countries, fellowships to Soviet centers of higher learning, and a vibrant exchange program, the Soviet Union seemed intent on educating Mexico and other Latin American countries about the Soviet production of, allegedly, better medications. As the many letters sent to the Mexican Embassy in Moscow demonstrate, the battle over how Mexicans would procure medication included personal appeals far removed from the strategic geopolitics of the Cold War or the industrial logic of corporate acquisitions and, instead, centered squarely on trying to save the lives of loved ones by reaching out to apparent allies with resources. The success of Soviet overtures in Latin America is apparent not just in Mexican missives requesting Soviet medication, but in the fact that individual Mexicans bypassed the United States and went directly to Moscow to seek medical treatment. Even as the decision to seek treatment in either the United States or Mexico was personal (for those who had the means to decide), these choices also had significant public reverberations, as in the case of Diego Rivera.

While some "ordinary" Mexicans charted a pragmatic and hopeful path, the stance of the Mexican state was more complicated, requiring caution and daring amid U.S. and Soviet efforts both to dominate global pharmaceutical innovation and production and to curry strategic allies in the Third World. The Soviet Union was geographically distant, but not alien in its societal aspirations, and it appeared well-disposed to help Mexican trainees, appreciate Mexican culture, and share medical innovations. On the other hand, despite its proximity, the United States—especially given the 1950s hearings to curtail Mexican pharmaceutical independence (targeting steroids in particular)—appeared less accommodating. Ultimately, in the Cold War struggle over pharmaceutical production, it is clear that Mexico acquired a brief but pivotal position on the world stage thanks to its control of a coveted natural resource, barbasco, and its favoring of a local company, Syntex. Under these circumstances, Mexico was able to play off the rivalry of the two world powers, putting one on the defensive and encouraging overtures from the other, and, at least for a time, forge its own path.

Notes

A version of this chapter was originally presented as part of a 2010 workshop on the Cold War in Latin America organized by Anne-Emanuelle Birn and Raúl Necochea López at the University of Toronto. I am grateful to both of them for their incisive comments, suggestions, and invitation to submit this chapter. An earlier version of this chapter was published in Spanish: "Medicamentos Milagrosos: Embajadas y Enfermedades en el México de la Guerra Fría," in *Aproximaciones a lo Local y lo Global: América Latina en la Historia de la Ciencia Contemporánea*, edited by Gisela Mateos and Edna Suárez-Díaz (Mexico City: UNAM, 2016), 243–67. I am also grateful to Angélica Márquez-Osuna for her timely research assistance.

1   Siméon J. André, "Médicament-Boussole contre le Cancer," *Constellation*, no. 125 (September 1958), translated article found in Secretaría de Relaciones Exteriores de México, Fondo Embajada de México en la URSS (SRE), folder 16, file 12.

2   André, "Médicament-Boussole contre le Cancer."

3   Gilberto Bosques, Mexican Ambassador in Cuba, to Mexican Embassy in Moscow (telegram), SRE, folder 16, file 12. The requests, which started in 1957, can also be found in SRE, folder 12, file 5. On similar international requests for a putative cure for cancer developed in the Soviet Union, see Krementsov, *Cure*.

4   Several examples of dosage explanations are found in SRE, folder 16, file 12, but a rather illustrative one is labeled "Certificado por el Comité Farmacológico del Consejo Científico del Ministerio de Salubridad de la U.R.S.S., Instrucciones."

5   Gilberto Bosques to Ernesto Madero, Mexican Embassy in Moscow, SRE, folder 16, file 12.

6   More than a decade ago, James A. Secord pointed out the importance of asking about science as a form of communication and about the patterns of circulation of knowledge. See Secord, "Knowledge in Transit." More recently, Marcos Cueto's analysis of the dynamics of the global circulation of science illustrates how the flow of "scientific practices, materials, and of institutional norms" is asymmetric. Examining the case of Mexican physiology during the Cold War, he shows how this asymmetrical circulation of knowledge also provided opportunities for the expansion and growth of scientific institutions and training of researchers. See Marcos Cueto, "Asymmetrical Network." Rather than addressing the "circulation of knowledge," Edna Suárez-Díaz explores the notion of travel and how knowledge moves across national borders, particularly the U.S.-Mexican border. In analyzing Rubén Lisker's research on the genetic hematological traits of Mexican Indigenous populations during the Cold War period, she shows how Lisker, as a member of an international circuit of researchers, became part of a new generation of experts who contributed to Mexico's dual modernization-nationalist impetus. See Suárez-Díaz, "Indigenous Populations in Mexico."

7   Greene, *Prescribing by Numbers*, 45. The pharmaceutical industry as a key element for geopolitical struggles is also analyzed by Timothy Barney. He argues that the scientific fields of medicine and geography were connected during the Cold War through development projects such as the Atlas of Disease, a joint initiative of the U.S. Armed Forces, the American Geographical Society, and international pharmaceutical corporations. In the classification of Third World nations during the Cold War, diseases became "markers" of boundaries between the North and South. The map represented the distribution of diseases throughout the world, in effect isolating the areas where some diseases, such as cholera, were more prevalent. Barney illustrates how Pfizer's interest in these maps was part of a new form of colonization in which sickness represented a risk to international security. See Barney, "Diagnosing the Third World."

8   Greene, *Prescribing by Numbers*, 45; Greene, "Releasing the Flood Waters."

9   Greene, *Prescribing by Numbers*, 45.

10 See Tobbell, *Pills, Power, and Policy*; Rasmussen, *On Speed*; Greene, *Prescribing by Numbers*. For Mexico, see especially Marcos Cueto, *Cold War, Deadly Fevers* (on the pharmaceuticals needed for malaria eradication); Birn, *Marriage of Convenience*; Petryna, *When Experiments Travel*; Graboyes, *Experiment Must Continue*.

11   Applying this new lens was prompted by the editors of this volume. See Soto
     Laveaga, *Jungle Laboratories*.

12   Sivasundaram, "Sciences and the Global," 156. For a historiographical analysis of
     local-global approaches in the history of medicine and health in Latin America,
     see Espinosa, "Globalizing the History of Disease"; Birn and Necochea López,
     "Footprints on the Future."

13   "Hearings before the Subcommittee on Patents, Trademarks, and Copyrights of
     the Committee on the Judiciary," U.S. Senate, 84th Cong., 2nd sess.; "Removal of
     Obstacles to the Production of Essential Materials from the Cheapest Source for
     the Manufacture of Cortisone and Other Hormones," July 5–6, 1956, located in UC
     Santa Barbara library, p. 93 (hereafter cited as "Wonder Drugs"). The film is also
     mentioned in different testimony on page III ("as was shown in that excellent film
     yesterday . . .").

14   "Wonder Drugs," 116.

15   "Wonder Drugs," 52.

16   "Wonder Drugs," 83.

17   "Wonder Drugs," 121; Soto Laveaga, *Jungle Laboratories*.

18   Soto Laveaga, *Jungle Laboratories*; Marks, *Sexual Chemistry*.

19   Beamish and Ritchie, "Spectre of Steroids."

20   Tobbell, *Pills, Power, and Policy*, 95. Another case reflecting similar Cold War anxi-
     eties in the field of nuclear technologies is analyzed by Gisela Mateos and Edna
     Suárez-Díaz, "Atoms for Peace." This was a training and technical-assistance
     campaign propagated by the Eisenhower administration in Latin America to
     keep countries from using nuclear technology for military purposes. Mateos and
     Suárez-Díaz, "We Are Not a Rich Country."

21   Beamish and Ritchie, "Spectre of Steroids."

22   "Cortisone Shortage," 83.

23   "Mexican Hormones," 86–90, 161–62, 166.

24   "MacArthur and National Purpose," 71.

25   "Russia's Industrial Expansion," 106–7.

26   Greene, *Prescribing by Numbers*, 46. See also Tobbell, "Who's Winning the Human
     Race?"; Tobbell, *Pills, Power, and Policy*.

27   On the role of U.S. congressional hearings in the Cold War, see also Pacino's
     chapter in this volume.

28   "Cortisone Shortage," 85.

29   Rasmussen, *On Speed*.

30   Beamish and Ritchie, "Spectre of Steroids."

31   The six that were not subsidiaries were: General Mills (1956), Ogden Corporation
     (1956), Syntex (1958, when it became a private company again), G. D. Searle and
     Company (1958), American Home Products (1959), and Smith, Kline, and French
     (1961). See Gereffi, *Pharmaceutical Industry and Dependency in the Third World*. The
     European companies that established themselves in Mexico were the same ones
     that in the 1930s and 1940s had controlled the global steroid hormone industry,

among them Schering AG in Mexico in 1963 (German), Organon in 1969 (Dutch), and Ciba Geigy in 1970 (Swiss).

32 CIBA president T. F. Davies Haines in "Wonder Drugs," 65.

33 A translated version of the decree can be found in "Wonder Drugs," 58.

34 Marcos Cueto, *Cold War, Deadly Fevers*, 29.

35 Marcos Cueto, *Cold War, Deadly Fevers*, 61.

36 Tobbell, "Who's Winning the Human Race?"

37 Cited in Tobbell, "Who's Winning the Human Race?," 430.

38 Tobbell, "Who's Winning the Human Race?," 433.

39 Tobbell, "Who's Winning the Human Race?"

40 "Wonder Drugs," 5.

41 "Wonder Drugs," 71.

42 I am deeply grateful to Dominique Tobbell for generously sharing with me this memo found during her time in the Merck Archives. Merck Archives Bush 73/1748, Whitehouse Station, NJ.

43 Merck Archives Bush 73/1748.

44 Fortes and Adler Lomnitz, *Becoming a Scientist in Mexico*. On Soviet internationalism in Latin America and Russia, see Rupprecht, *Soviet Internationalism after Stalin*. On the nuances of medical cooperation sans the United States, see also Anderson's chapter in this volume.

45 "Wonder Drugs," 68.

46 Gardner, "Progress Report on the 'Health for Peace' Bill."

47 Gardner, "Progress Report on the 'Health for Peace' Bill," 145.

48 Tournès and Scott-Smith, *Global Exchanges*.

49 "Estudiantes Extranjeros en la Unión Soviética, April 9, 1959," SRE, folder 14, file 4.

50 "Estudiantes Extranjeros en la Unión Soviética, April 9, 1959," SRE folder 14, file 4. A vibrant academic exchange was also taking place between Mexico and Moscow. For example, a Mexican "expert from each area"—anthropology, history, sociology, and law—"was sent for a total of three weeks" to the Soviet Union so that educational systems, including the USSR's "open university," could be better understood and, it was hoped, so that a validation (*reconocimiento*) of degrees between the two countries could occur.

51 "Homenaje a Zapata, 9 de abril, 1959," SRE, folder 14, file 4.

52 "Carta de Ernesto Madero a Secretario de Relaciones Exteriores," April 13, 1959, SRE.

53 Translation of "Cultura Soviética," "Admiración y Cariño de los Mexicanos," November 19, 1959, SRE.

54 SRE, folder 14, file 4

55 SRE, "La Mujer Soviética," no. 10, 1959.

56 SRE, folder 17, file 2, visita de Mikoyan.

57 "Daily Review of Soviet Press Published by Soviet Information Bureau—Cancer and the Battle against It," June 11, 1959, SRE, folder 14, file 5.

58 "Asunto: Tercer Cohete Cósmico Soviético," October 27, 1959, SRE, folder 14, file 5.

59 "Daily Review of Soviet Press Published by Soviet Information Bureau—Great Success of Science." July 7, 1959, SRE, folder 14, file 5.

60 SRE, folder 69, file 5, 1971.

61 SRE, folder 18, file 1.

62 SRE, folder 18, file 1, January 26, 1959.

63 SRE, folder 69, file 5, Certificado October 4, 1971.

64 But Soviet expertise was not limited to pharmaceuticals. There is indication that some Mexicans were traveling to Moscow for surgeries—as in the case of a woman who had sought out Soviet surgeons at Moscow's Center for Ears, Nose and Throat. SRE, folder 69, file 5, October 27, 1971.

65 Richardson, "Dilemmas of a Communist Artist"; special exhibit, *Diego Rivera y la Experiencia en la URSS*, Museo Casa Estudio Diego Rivera y Frida Kahlo and Museo Mural Diego Rivera, January–April 2018. The exhibit was covered by various press reports and blogs, including Alex González, "Diego Rivera en la Unión Soviética."

66 Richardson, "Dilemmas of a Communist Artist."

67 *Diego Rivera y la Experiencia en la URSS.*

68 López Orozco, Ramírez Sánchez, and Cruz Porchini, "Siqueiros y la Victoria de la Medicina sobre el Cáncer," 75, 77.

69 SRE, folder 49, file 9; Soto Laveaga, "Building the Nation of the Future."

70 John Connor, "Drug Profits," cited in Greene, *Prescribing by Numbers*, 46.

71 Tobbell, "Who's Winning the Human Race?," 440.

Part II

**Health Experts/
Expertise and
Contested Ideologies**

4

The Puerto Rico Family Life Study and the Cold War Politics of Fertility Surveys

RAÚL NECOCHEA LÓPEZ

In the mid-1940s the University of Puerto Rico's Center for Social Research launched the Puerto Rico Family Life Study. Its goal was to document popular attitudes about reproduction, and to use such knowledge to persuade people to favor smaller families. It was the prototype for many fertility surveys carried out worldwide over the next three decades. These "KAP studies" (known by this acronym because they aimed to uncover *k*nowledge, *a*ttitudes, and *p*ractices about reproduction and sexuality) took place in scores of countries across Latin America, South and Southeast Asia, Africa, and the Middle East that the United States was courting as allies during the Cold War.[1] In the late 1940s, U.S. demographers and politicians worried about rapid population growth's potential to fuel poverty and social discontent, thereby enabling communist inroads. The Cold War accelerated this change in experts' views of fertility, from considering it a private matter determined by sociocultural dynamics to a public matter of strategic import. KAP studies pointedly responded to this change: those funding and directing the surveys believed that population limitation ought to be a component of policies to modernize "underdeveloped" nations along Western lines and steer their populations away from communism.[2]

Years before the Cold War, the U.S. government had already made its Puerto Rican colony a testing ground for the hypothesis that capitalist industrial development could create prosperity even in the most "backward" places of the globe.[3] Because rapid population growth could counter the benefits of economic reforms, mid-twentieth-century U.S. authorities in Puerto Rico came to view family planning services, and greater understanding of how laypeople might use them, as necessary complements to economic measures.[4] The Cold War heightened the interest of the United

States in replicating the Puerto Rican experiment regionally in order to sway other Latin American states grappling with how to align themselves in the East–West divide. As Governor Luis Muñoz Marín put it in 1953, Puerto Rico could "create a better understanding among Latin Americans of the sincerity and devotion of the United States to the principles of respect for human freedom."[5]

The Family Life Study (FLS) built on existing clinical initiatives, namely the Asociación Pro Salud Maternal e Infantil, a birth control advocacy and services organization established in 1936, and the legalization of sterilization surgery in 1937. However, the aim of the FLS was not clinical per se, but rather to foster changes in popular attitudes regarding family size. Its main report, *The Family and Population Control*, published in 1959 after a decade and a half of intensive research, argued that Puerto Ricans' unfavorable views of fertility limitation could be modified, provided family planning programs made their services more consonant with Puerto Rican values. *The Family and Population Control* made broad generalizations about how a lack of communication about sexuality between partners, the "sexual modesty" of Puerto Rican married women, and their "respect" for their husbands' desires, were traits that stood in the way of contraceptive use by married couples. To change this, family planning must become "a central and explicit feature of government policy," paralleling "the island's successful program of economic development." Were the government able to "reach couples early in their marital histories with an authoritative message concerning family planning, it is probable that knowledge and motivation could be crystallized at a point in the family cycle more strategic for fertility."[6]

Seen from a Puerto Rican perspective, however, the FLS was more than a pioneering social engineering intervention in a colony. Outlining a pattern discernable throughout Latin America during the Cold War's middle years, the FLS was a key site of contestation and accommodation regarding family planning between local and foreign actors. The range of positions in Puerto Rico appears all the more remarkable given the near-complete U.S. political control over the island. As important as U.S. funds and technical expertise were to the FLS, the project's direction was determined by the crucial yet underrated participation of a trio of actors: local political patrons who created a space for it within academic institutions; native fieldworkers paradoxically expected to grow into researchers while remaining subordinate assistants; and academic critics who pointed out the flaws and biases in the research. Seeing the FLS through the eyes of these different actors, we can take stock of the enthusiasm and controversy surrounding the early production of knowledge about family planning in Latin America, as well as of the Cold War exigencies that made novel social science research possible.

Puerto Rican Politics and the Patronage of Fertility Surveys

The local patronage of the FLS owed much to the 1940s rise of the Partido Popular Democrático (PPD, Popular Democratic Party), which increased the role of the University of Puerto Rico (UPR) as a producer of knowledge to serve the government's modernization agenda, which, in turn, included the limitation of population growth from the earliest stage of the Cold War.[7] The 1940s began with a reconfigured map of political forces, owing to changes within and outside Puerto Rico—which had been under U.S. control since 1898, following centuries of Spanish colonialism—that nonetheless kept the island well within the sphere of U.S. colonial domination. The declining price of sugar (Puerto Rico's main source of income), the Great Depression, and the mobilization of impoverished workers had weakened the Puerto Rican Senate's ruling coalition between the Partido Socialista (Socialist Party), which spoke for the Federación Libre de los Trabajadores (Free Workers' Federation), and the Partido Republicano (Republican Party), representing sugar producers.[8]

Workers demanding salary increases looked for new leadership in the 1930s, but most took little notice of the Partido Comunista Puertorriqueño (PCP, Puerto Rican Communist Party), established in 1934 with help from the Communist International (Comintern).[9] Much more attractive was a broad and motley coalition that included agricultural workers, the petty bourgeoisie, and former Communists disaffected with the PCP. This coalition gave rise to a nationalist, pro-independence movement that blamed U.S. corporate interests and colonial rule for the island's poverty. The Partido Nacionalista (PN, Nationalist Party) served as the movement's political arm, and Pedro Albizu Campos as its leader. The PN coordinated hundreds of strikes in the early 1930s, with Albizu a visible agitator. Violent clashes with the police landed Albizu in U.S. jails for a decade. Tensions reached a high point with the Ponce Massacre, in which the police killed twenty pro-PN demonstrators and wounded hundreds of others in February 1937. In the aftermath, Puerto Rican police escalated harassment and persecution of activists opposed to U.S. control of the island.[10] Uncompromising and diminished, the PN ceased to be a viable political option for Puerto Ricans dissatisfied with the status quo in the late 1930s.

The PPD, founded by Senator Luis Muñoz Marín in 1938, benefited from this political vacuum. It called for a program of economic modernization based on the financial interests of sectors other than sugar production while capitalizing on U.S. strategic designs on Puerto Rico as a military and commercial outpost. As Emilio Pantojas-García has argued, PPD leaders did not wish to challenge U.S. dominance. Instead, they portrayed themselves as technocrats free of ties to the foundering sugar economy and as honest brokers for the different factions vying for representation.[11] Muñoz Marín's charisma and tireless campaigning earned the PPD a Senate majority in the 1940 election, and the Senate presidency for Muñoz Marín himself.

The rise of the PPD in the 1940s also rested on external factors, particularly the 1941 appointment as governor of Rexford Tugwell, one of the architects of Franklin Roosevelt's New Deal, and a short-term windfall of World War II–related U.S. expenditures in military infrastructure building. A Columbia-trained economist, Tugwell had joined Roosevelt's "Brain Trust" of advisers in 1932. He had visited Puerto Rico as assistant secretary of agriculture in 1934, a visit that led to government proposals addressing the long-term economic reconstruction of the island after the Depression, involving state-directed land reform and diversification of agricultural production. But back in mainland United States, opposition to Tugwell's ambitious plans for state-led planning of suburban communities provoked accusations of communism in Congress and his resignation in 1936.[12] Five years later, Tugwell returned to the Roosevelt administration, as governor of Puerto Rico, eager to showcase the merits of the expert-driven reformism that had been frustrated in the United States.

During his tenure as governor (1941–1946), Tugwell collaborated with the PPD to set up a planning board to guide economic development as well as promote light manufacturing of goods such as glass, paper, and rum. The modest agrarian and industrialization reforms Tugwell implemented eased social tensions without imperiling the status of sugar as Puerto Rico's leading export. In addition, the construction of U.S. military bases and roads in this period generated new jobs, while two federally funded programs, the Puerto Rico Emergency Relief Administration and the Puerto Rico Reconstruction Administration, bankrolled social welfare projects that benefited many of the poorest Puerto Ricans.[13]

With the onset of the Cold War, foreign direct investment (FDI), especially directed to the production and export of raw materials, grew in importance for U.S. strategic interests. Coupled with technical cooperation and military "assistance," FDI became a defining development policy of the United States in the Third World under Harry Truman.[14] Given these circumstances, both Tugwell and Muñoz Marín began to envision U.S. capital investment, instead of redistributive policies or local industrialization plans, as the most viable way to turn Puerto Rico into a prosperous showcase for liberal democracy. The victory of Muñoz Marín in the gubernatorial election of 1948 paved the way for Operación Manos a la Obra (Operation Bootstrap), a landmark economic policy that defined the public sector's primary role as that of supporting investment in whatever area U.S. capitalists deemed promising.[15]

In this climate, Muñoz Marín was not inclined to press for altering the colonial status of Puerto Rico. As the first person elected, rather than appointed, to the post of governor, he represented a nod by the United States to greater Puerto Rican self-government, but he ended up disappointing those who expected a stauncher defense of Puerto Rican sovereignty. Instead, Muñoz Marín and the PPD promoted the establishment of the Estado Libre Asociado (ELA, the Puerto Rican Commonwealth) as a new model of local governance with greater self-rule powers yet still under the control of the U.S. Congress, which could annul or amend bills passed by local legislators. Despite occupying a subordinate place relative to U.S. congressional power, the PPD's position in Puerto Rico was strong, particularly after the defeat of its leading opponents in the PN. As a bulwark of U.S. Cold War development policies, the PPD was an essential partner in all aspects of Puerto Rican life, including the fields of education and research.

A crucial player in this regard was the UPR. Established in San Juan in 1903, the UPR was the island's largest and most prestigious higher education institution. In the early 1940s, its administrators called for significant changes in the university's structure and operations that had to be negotiated with the rising PPD. The university reform law of 1942, for example, shielded the UPR from excessive legislative oversight. On the other hand, the reform also called for sanctions against student-activists (particularly those in the PN). Just as importantly, the reform led to the creation of the School of Public Administration and the Centro de Investigaciones Sociales (CIS, Center for Social Research) in 1944. The latter's purpose was to produce policy-relevant research that government authorities could use. With a mandate to "avoid [both] the immediate practical utility often desired by government agencies, and the purely general scientific interest often displayed by scholars," the CIS rose to become the most influential social science research center in Puerto Rico through the 1950s.[16] The FLS was one of its leading projects.

The Political Context of the Family Life Study

Between 1945 and 1955, the CIS zeroed in on four research areas: "population growth," "industrialization," "distribution of economic benefits," and "social

structure patterns," each unapologetically tied to the Puerto Rican government's priorities. The research areas comprised projects directed by prestigious scholars recruited in the United States, including Lloyd Reynolds (Yale),
John Kenneth Galbraith (Harvard), and Melvin Tumin (Princeton). As the CIS
put it, "when competent observers, university people, and officers of the Government show persistent interest and concern" in certain areas, these should
be considered as research targets.[17]

The study of fertility knowledge, attitudes, and practices at the CIS started
in 1946 with a pilot project codirected by Clarence Senior, the CIS director, and
demographers Kingsley Davis and Frank Notestein of the Princeton University Office of Population Research. The pilot, conducted by José Janer, chief
of Puerto Rico's Department of Health, and sociologist Paul Hatt, also from
the Princeton University Office of Population Research, was meant to be a
first step in a larger project to ascertain how Puerto Rico's population could
be made to decrease so as not to slow down industrialization.[18] Over the next
fourteen years, social research on fertility grew into one of the pillars of the
CIS. By the mid-1950s, projects dealing with population growth, including the
FLS, consumed almost half (US$199,000) of the CIS's budget, nearly as much
as projects dealing with aspects of industrialization (US$206,000), the most
expensive category of research projects.[19]

Although the CIS's financial standing was solid, in the first decade of operations its administrators complained of a dearth of qualified Puerto Rican researchers.[20] University chancellor Jaime Benítez, a PPD appointee, supported
hiring U.S. experts to make up for this. In fact, Benítez welcomed the outsider perspectives of the CIS's U.S. personnel, comparing them to the revealing
analyses of U.S. life produced at distinct moments by foreign observers such as
Gunnar Myrdal and Alexis de Tocqueville.[21] Echoing the PPD's economic and
political alignment with the United States, Benítez portrayed Puerto Rico as
defined by and contributing to Western culture. As such, there was no place
at the UPR for political or intellectual positions that made "the West" into an
adversary of Puerto Rico. Benítez was not referring to the insignificant forces
of communism, but rather to those of nationalism, vigorous at the UPR despite
the PPD's popularity outside the university.[22]

To nationalist critics, however, Benítez's observations, and the higher
salaries of U.S. researchers at the CIS relative to those of Puerto Ricans in the
Faculty of Social Sciences, were evidence of his contempt for native culture
and talent. This unease grew amid the unfolding Cold War, with the election
of Luis Muñoz Marín as governor, the implementation of Operación Manos a
la Obra, and the rising prestige of the CIS. All of these factors exacerbated the

university community's apprehension over the UPR turning into an enclave of Western scholars, much like Puerto Rico had become an enclave of U.S. capital. As former dean of the Faculty of Social Sciences Antonio Colorado carped, "Ours must not be just another university in the world, but the university of Puerto Rico and for Puerto Rico."[23]

Nationalist resentment boiled over again in 1948, when an unrepentant Pedro Albizu was released from prison and returned home to continue advocating for independence. Supporters at the UPR, such as political science professor Marcos Ramírez, sympathized with Albizu's fiery, pro-Catholic, and Hispanophile rhetoric about Puerto Rican uniqueness, which they considered "intimately tied to the preservation of our culture."[24] Students petitioned to have Albizu address them at the university theater. After being turned down, the students began a strike of several months. Albizu's return also triggered a new wave of violence, including the attempted assassinations by Puerto Rican nationalists of Governor Luis Muñoz Marín and President Harry Truman in 1950, and a shooting attack inside the U.S. Congress in 1954. In response to this militancy, the government brought back its policy of imprisonment, harassment, censorship, and surveillance against nationalists. Albizu and his closest collaborators were once again incarcerated, and scores of UPR students and faculty were respectively expelled and fired.[25]

The repression of nationalism eliminated a strong rival of the PPD and diminished student activism at the UPR significantly by 1952. As a sign of how serene the 1950s had become, Benítez even defended his students and staff from charges of communism brought on by members of the Puerto Rican Senate looking to grandstand at the height of McCarthy's red-baiting campaign. His defense of the integrity of the university community had not been as vigorous in the tumultuous late 1940s.[26] More significantly, as we have seen, it was nationalist, rather than communist, agitation that UPR and PPD authorities considered threatening. The resulting tensions and accommodation between FLS workers played out at different levels.

The Project in Practice

Notwithstanding the turbulence of the late 1940s, I have found no traces of CIS researchers' claiming to be affected by the conflict between the PPD and nationalist activists at the UPR. In 1949, with Paul Hatt's pilot complete, Clarence Senior's successor at the helm of the CIS, Millard Hansen, began to lay the groundwork for a more ambitious population study. Using UPR funds and contributions from the Rockefeller Foundation, the Milbank Fund, and the

Population Council, Hansen recruited University of North Carolina sociologist Reuben Hill as director of the Puerto Rico FLS, which encompassed two subprojects.[27] The first dealt with child-rearing practices in a rural area, led by anthropologist David Landy of Harvard. The second, which commanded a greater share of Hill's attention, was a survey-based study of fertility attitudes in rural and urban areas led by sociologist Joseph Mayone Stycos of Columbia.[28]

Hill and Stycos's plan was to begin with a survey of child-rearing styles, sex roles, courtship patterns, the nature of consensual unions, and attitudes and practices related to marriage, fertility decision-making, and birth control. The survey's sample would be expanded from seventy-two to twelve hundred respondents in a second phase to refine hypotheses developed in the first phase. The work involved the design of questionnaires, the deployment of surveyors to data-collection sites throughout Puerto Rico, the centralized aggregation and analysis of field data, and its ultimate preparation and presentation in the form of tables and bullet points that Puerto Rican decision-makers could use. The FLS was to conclude with an experimental stage in which different forms of intervention would be tested to determine how best to popularize the small family ideal, per the CIS's policy-shaping imperative.[29] Among the tactics used in the experimental phase was widespread distribution of informational pamphlets on birth control and the Emko spermicidal foam by volunteers in rural areas.[30]

At the time he took on responsibility for the survey, Joseph Stycos already had experience in fertility research at the CIS. In 1947, he worked for Paul Hatt and José Janer in Puerto Rico, supervising the Princeton project's local fieldworkers. Stycos's early experiences are telling of his encounter with a university community that was deeply ambivalent about U.S. participation in the island's political and economic life. Governor Tugwell had interpreted this ambivalence as an expression of a dysfunctional pride that "prevent[ed] the public acknowledgment of inferiority of any kind." In a similar vein, Stycos viewed the concerns of Puerto Ricans as emerging from an "irrational desire to keep from being absorbed" by U.S. culture.[31] Neither acknowledged how the stagnation of the local light manufacturing drive in favor of FDI, and the longstanding humiliation of having an appointed governor rather than an elected one, fueled resentment. Yet, as seen earlier, these had been key factors driving nationalist fervor since the 1930s.

Following his involvement with the Princeton study, Stycos had enrolled in the PhD program at Columbia University. As a graduate student, he worked in several of the advertising and public opinion projects of Columbia's Bureau of Applied Social Research (BASR) under Kingsley Davis.[32] Once appointed to the FLS, Stycos's first challenge was turning the educated Puerto Ricans he had known previously into reliable information-gathering fieldworkers. Between 1951 and 1957, he worked with forty-four of them, all but five of whom were women.[33] Not surprisingly, following the purge of nationalist activists from the UPR, these fieldworkers professed strong PPD leanings.[34]

Importantly, it was the CIS, not Stycos directly, that hired the fieldworkers. Once hired, they became part of a pool of research assistants that the CIS then deployed as needed for the multiple projects the principal investigators directed. Thus, both the native research assistants and the principal investigators depended on the UPR's patronage, although the financial and career advancement opportunities for these two groups differed markedly. Project directors tended to be prestigious scholars from the United States with lucrative multiyear contracts. They included Hill and early-career experts, such as Stycos and Landy, whose work might result in interesting publications that would make them more attractive in U.S. academic and policymaking circles. Subsequent work opportunities for research assistants, meanwhile, were overwhelmingly in Puerto Rico, in local civil service and allied health fields. Nonetheless, the CIS portrayed research assistance as an apprenticeship that "provides valuable training, which prepares these younger scholars to use their improved competence in graduate study, in research and teaching, or in government services."[35]

Rather ethnocentrically, Stycos viewed his staff's high morale not as a sign of their satisfaction with steady, interesting employment alongside politically like-minded people, but as a result of their "loyalty to the *jefe* [boss]"; he characterized the assistants as belonging to "folk cultures" that put their "faith in a personality rather than a cause."[36] To be sure, research assistants did appreciate Stycos's cordial demeanor and his commitment to preparing them to conduct fertility surveys. Stycos allocated three weeks to the fieldworkers' training, which comprised background readings and lectures about the FLS, interviewing tips, and mock interviews. It was particularly difficult to motivate fieldworkers to broach the sexuality-laden subjects, which they at first deemed indelicate and distasteful.[37]

The three-week training fell vastly short of the minimum demanded by researchers engaged in similar studies in the United States; sexologist Alfred Kinsey, for example, mentored his interviewers for a whole year. It also failed to acquaint research assistants with the broad social scientific literature Columbia's BASR routinely provided its trainees.[38] The research patrons' expectations of cost minimization and rapid delivery of policy recommendations determined the quick pace of quantitative data gathering, to the detriment of the training of local subordinates. This turned the day-to-day work into some-thing akin to guerrilla sociology: lightly equipped but motivated fieldworkers deployed by the project's leaders to visit locales for short bursts of questioning, followed by swift retreats to prevent any backlash against the interview topic. Former fieldworker Angelina Saavedra recalled how she eluded confrontation with a man who was fuming after learning of the scabrous questions she had posed to his wife. Similarly, repeat canvassing of La Perla in San Juan was not possible because of the entire neighborhood's negative disposition toward the questionnaire. Word-of-mouth communication turned it into a topic of local censure after a single day of interviewing.[39]

The treatment of local personnel as ad-hoc subordinates contradicted the CIS's formal mission to mentor research assistants as scientific apprentices. As Stycos saw it, though, "the task of the interviewer is to receive the information from the respondent and to transmit it for analysis. For this function, the in-formation has to be complete, accurate and not influenced by the interviewer himself."[40] In practice, then, the FLS treated research assistants as little more than conduits of "objective data" between the field and the research direc-tors. Hill and Stycos's purported scientific objectivity struck some observers as misguided. Anthropologist Julian Steward, another CIS researcher direct-ing a multisited ethnography of the island, noted skeptically that "one cannot enter a home as a stranger and straight off inquire into sex life, family rela-tions, or attitudes toward local authorities."[41] Quantifying responses without analyzing the context in which they were elicited also raised eyebrows. Even FLS assistant director David Landy complained that Hill's "faith in numbers" led him to "often mistake them for the social facts of life."[42] The neutrality in human interactions to which Hill and Stycos aspired seemed to these crit-ics self-delusional, though understandable in a context that favored making rapid policy-relevant recommendations based on quantitative data. After all, as Chancellor Benítez explained, the ultimate goal of this research was to pro-duce "skillfully-devised methods of suggestion and propaganda to modify aspi-rations and behavior in the manner of commercial enterprises."[43]

Local social scientists' critiques of the FLS irritated its directors more than those made by fellow U.S. social scientists at the CIS. David Landy came to detest Puerto Rican colleagues' pugnacious attempts to engage U.S. research-ers in debate, "their noisy and transparent attempts to out-American the Americanos." He preferred the "open frankness" of rural Puerto Ricans to the "stuffy, synthetic and half-bright people that clutter up the university."[44] The young anthropologist Sidney Mintz, then a member of Julian Steward's team, believed that the deep knowledge of the lives of the poor acquired by foreigners like himself aroused the envy of his UPR colleagues.[45] It is possible that envy played a role, though the tensions probably also encompassed a sense of unfairness. After all, the CIS lavished resources on multiyear contracts for foreign investigators, while excluding local scientists except as research assistants.

To Puerto Rican social scientists, the CIS created hierarchies in the research establishment in service of the Cold War aims of capitalist industrialization and population limitation. The PPD was complicit. Puerto Rican intellectuals such as Luis Nieves Falcón, Eduardo Seda Bonilla, and Charles Rosario reacted to their belief that a PPD-sanctioned form of colonialism had extended to the social sciences, one that dictated the questions worth asking while neglecting others that also mattered.[46] Rather than personal attacks on U.S. researchers or a rejection of the risks of rapid population growth, the critiques expressed exasperation with the PPD's narrow, Cold War–bound emphasis on small families as a lever of prosperity and security, to the detriment of policy research on education programs, women's employment, or migration, for example.

Regarding migration, most notably, the CIS squandered the opportunity to be at the forefront of a dramatic change in Puerto Rican society. The decade during which the bulk of the FLS took place also witnessed the onset of mass migration of Puerto Ricans to the U.S. mainland, profoundly affecting the size and composition of the island's population for years to come. After a significant jump to 2.2 million inhabitants from 1.8 million between 1940 and 1950, Puerto Rico's population grew to only 2.3 million by 1960, not thanks to the increased popularity of birth control, but to the out-migration of some 470,000 people between 1950 and 1960.[47] The FLS did not seek to address the factors that led to such large-scale migration, notwithstanding its indirect impact on the birth rate.

Puerto Rican intellectuals did not just take aim at the CIS's biases and its political patrons, but also at fellow Puerto Ricans working at the organization. University of Puerto Rico sociologist Carlos Buitrago, for example, acknowledged the creativity of CIS research assistants, but lambasted them for favoring social activities, such as fieldwork and conference presentations, over the honing of scholarly "aptitudes for lonesome reflection." Along the same lines, René Marqués referred to them as "docile" social scientists, adept at following directions, "but often in need of a different expert—a foreigner usually—when the time for analysis, interpretation, and conclusion-drawing came."[48] To be fair, the research assistant role, as encountered in practice at the CIS, did little to strengthen individual analytical skills, connect research assistants to other related research outside the CIS, or award them the academic credentials that could further their professional autonomy outside the confines of the CIS. In short, as an anonymous writer claimed, the CIS "had not made any serious effort to create a corps of Puerto Rican researchers."[49] As a result, no CIS research assistants became the scholars the CIS envisioned in the early 1950s, although former FLS fieldworkers Doris Díaz, Nilsa Torres, and Angelina Saavedra did conduct independent research beyond their CIS employment.[50]

For Stycos, on the other hand, Puerto Rican research assistants fulfilled his needs exactly, and he unabashedly promoted the role of fieldworkers in his employ as mere conduits of data between the field and himself in subsequent fertility surveys he directed in Jamaica, Haiti, and Peru. His Puerto Rican sojourn convinced him that governments and educational institutions must devote energies to developing a motivated pool of part-time workers who could be repeatedly summoned for whatever projects social scientists might have in mind.[51] Proper training and job security were certainly issues to be resolved, but "most important of all is to give the interviewer a sense of his professional status; to alter the traditional concept of the interviewer as an enumerator who fills in blanks on a questionnaire, to that of the junior social scientist who conscientiously strives to secure reliable and valid information as the crucial first stage of a scientific project."[52] Fertility surveys in Cold War Puerto Rico, in other words, did more than pull social science into the politically fraught sphere of population policymaking. As detailed in the next section, they also inspired the need for a new subordinate workforce in the Third World.

The FLS from the Bottom Up: An Asymmetric Cold War Partnership

Despite the aforementioned shortcomings, many of the "junior social scientists" were pleased with the work conditions and learning experiences the FLS offered. For instance, as Angelina Saavedra proudly noted, the CIS "was a school for me." Others used the experience as a stepping stone in their careers. Nilda Anaya went on to become a health promoter, while Sila Nazario followed up with other research and administration posts in the public sector, and even became a state senator for San Juan in 1969.[53] It is important to see their satisfaction in its Cold War context. The UPR in the 1950s, financially strong, recently purged of nationalist malcontents, and bent on highlighting its similarities to the industrialized capitalist United States, sponsored U.S. researchers aligned with the PPD's industrialization agenda. This situation also effected a new dynamic at the CIS: the identification of a number of educated locals with suitable interpersonal skills, who were then turned into an inexpensively trained class of research subordinates that could serve as interlocutors able to mediate between research patrons' thirst for quantifiable data and the wariness of people asked to bare details about their sexual and reproductive lives.

But FLS research assistants also challenged their subordinate positions in several ways. To begin with, they found that the research-assistant-as-conduit model was at odds not only with the CIS's formal mission toward its trainees and with the views of other CIS researchers, but also with the field's practical demands. Stycos and Hill insisted that research assistants stick to the script provided, emphasizing their affiliation with the prestigious UPR, to create an authoritative distance from which to compel complete and accurate answers to questions.[54] However, in practice, fieldworkers often sought to diminish social distances in order to make respondents comfortable. This occurred most often when fieldworkers confronted the squalor in which some of their interviewees lived. Moved by pity and a paternalistic sense of responsibility for the poor in rural areas, fieldworkers brought clothes for children or advocated on behalf of interviewees at health posts, for example. Reciprocally, interviewers accepted food, horse rides, and even invitations to Christmas pig roasts as tokens of gratitude for their visits.[55]

Another way in which FLS research assistants asserted themselves within the project was through their devising of original tactics to broach the delicate subjects of sexuality and contraception with interviewees. Research assistants reported enjoying the challenge of getting others to bare details of their intimate lives, by asking questions in roundabout ways, seeming empathic, cajoling answers from unwilling respondents, and praising their looks, homes, and children. One particularly successful fieldworker concluded that "every person can talk freely to anybody whom he believes to be serious and trustful in character, and especially who have proved to be friendly [to] him."[56] Yet a third way in which research assistants challenged the FLS's definition of their role can be gleaned from interviews and the few reports they filed in addition to the questionnaires they completed while in the field. What little exists shows that research assistants' interests in the FLS extended beyond family planning. One interviewer, for example, recorded a man's disapproval of U.S. beauty contests that objectified women's bodies. Another was shocked by the twelve-year-old daughter of an interviewee, who verbally assailed her mother for leaving her husband for a new man. Yet a third noted a link the woman made between her poverty and family size preference ("If I were rich I would have many [children]"), contravening the FLS's assumption that wealth correlated with a desire for fewer offspring.[57] And a fourth reacted with astonishment and amused contempt to her discovery of rural men's sexual liaisons with tropical fruits. These observations make it clear that the surveyors charged with zeroing in on the social barriers to contraceptive use were also drawn to other aspects of the lives of their countrymen and women—such as domestic strife, material deprivation, and disapproval of U.S. customs—that the official FLS documentation omitted from its cultural diagnostics and policy advice. The latter focused narrowly on birth control popularization, sidestepping the broader conflicts and social issues that surveyors observed but had little leeway to explore further.

Whatever Hill and Stycos may have intended, then, FLS research assistants saw themselves, and acted as, far more than data conduits. As other scholars have found, Cold War–bound social scientific projects sponsored by the United States elsewhere in Latin America treated the transmission of scientific knowledge, along with values of individualism and self-reliance, as markers of modernity.[58] The Puerto Rican evidence indicates that this process influenced not only the subjects of research, but also, more immediately, the subordinate personnel who carried out portions of the research. Though very little is known about these workers, they are pivotal actors, given that they were on the front lines of the birth control movement throughout the Third World. Rather than mere reporters of data, they developed identities on the ground as keen observers of their own societies. It is important to remember, however, that the benign paternalism that the CIS research assistants displayed toward their fellow citizens was laced with racialized prejudices about people in rural areas of the island, colloquially known as *jíbaros*, as more ignorant and more resistant to embracing birth control than lighter-skinned, urban Puerto Ricans. Both U.S. and Puerto Rican CIS personnel shared these beliefs about the demographic makeup of the island. This did not bother Stycos in the least, who was chiefly concerned with the data-gathering skills of his assistants. In fact, he was pleasantly surprised by the performance of these fieldworkers and praised their "unanticipated excellence" to Millard Hansen.[59]

While the FLS highlighted racial and cultural cleavages among Puerto Ricans, it simultaneously reinforced among U.S. social scientists the image of the non-U.S. researcher as a professional sidekick, crafty but naive, and lacking initiative. Others seemed to embrace such an exploitative image, with little thought to the deleterious effect this had on the cultivation of Latin American talent. For example, Immanuel Wallerstein, of Columbia's BASR, came to believe that U.S. scientists had a duty to train local researchers, to "turn out not scholars but workmanlike applied social researchers who could design a study, utilize the necessary research tools, know basic methodology and some statistics, [and] be able to supervise a field staff."[60] In his opinion, Third World governments would more readily accept policy recommendations from U.S.

social scientists if locals were involved in the research, regardless of the token conditions of their participation. U.S. Cold War leadership of the anticommunist bloc encouraged U.S. scholars to enlist not only Western European research partners but also Third World players, even as it made the latter's questions, needs, and critiques subservient to those advanced by U.S. experts. Ultimately, then, such partnerships were markedly asymmetrical. Ironically, Wallerstein's best-known intellectual contribution of the 1970s, World Systems Theory, offered a trenchant critique of powerful nations' exploitation of peripheral ones.[61]

The Cold War–inspired asymmetric research partnership model of the FLS, of course, could not have been put in place without the collaboration of Puerto Ricans themselves. Puerto Rican academic authorities ignored local critics of the CIS and tacitly approved of the limited mentoring offered to local research assistants because it made for more rapid and less expensive data collection and a more expedient formulation of policy recommendations. As a result, the FLS strengthened U.S. social scientists' ethnocentric biases about their superior technical and leadership skills, which Latin Americans understandably found odious. As KAP surveys became more popular in the Americas in the 1960s and 1970s, the codependence of U.S. and local researchers increased, as did the frictions between them. In 1963, a frustrated Stycos mocked these "jobless intellectuals" who felt survey work was beneath them, who added their own interpretations to the data collected (instead of simply recording it), and who "argued verbosely about grand theoretical points in the social sciences."[62] According to the asymmetric partnership model he favored, it was the U.S. researchers' prerogative to interpret findings, understand theoretical implications, and pursue policy recommendations, regardless of their ignorance of local history, culture, and politics, and of their unacknowledged dependence on Latin American research patrons in government circles.

Like other social science projects during the Cold War, the Puerto Rico FLS reveals a particular flavor of research patronage.[63] Authorities of the PPD and U.S. government officers bent on demonstrating the salutary effect of capitalist development and population limitation created a place for the FLS within the University of Puerto Rico. But while the FLS yielded its intended policy-shaping insights, it also led to subtle and overt contestations of the asymmetric research partnership model the FLS exemplified, both on the part of nationalist academic critics at the UPR and of the CIS's own research assistants. Because of the extent to which it implicated both sets of local researchers, the FLS directs our attention to the relations between U.S. and Latin American personnel in a rapidly changing university, instead of solely to the relations between researchers and their patrons. For the CIS research assistants, their relationship to the FLS was mainly one of subordination, despite the opportunities they had to shape the day-to-day data collection and the pride and pleasure they derived from their jobs. For the Puerto Rican social scientists shunned by the CIS because of their doubts about the PPD's agenda and their sympathy toward nationalism, the relationship to the FLS was mainly antagonistic and in need of radical redress. By the late 1960s, as I show in the next section, this group finally got the upper hand. Thus, although squarely inspired by U.S. Cold War needs, the FLS produced local struggles and adaptation that were not simply functions of the conflict between capitalism and communism in mid-twentieth-century Latin America.

The FLS's Denouement and Its Legacy for Population Research

The FLS nearly ended in disaster when university authorities, under pressure from PPD leaders, threatened to censor the project's final report in 1958. The university had done this only once before, shortly before the start of the FLS, in the case of an ethnography written by CIS scholar Morris Siegel. His study of the town of Lajas was critical of the poverty-worsening effects of PPD projects, the failure of English instruction in schools, the petty corruption of PPD officers, and the colonial control of the United States over the island. University chancellor Benítez requested opinions from eminent colleagues. Demographer Kingsley Davis of Columbia, dean of the Faculty of Social Sciences Antonio Colorado, and Governor Luis Muñoz Marín had misgivings about both the study's antiestablishment stance and the generalizability of its conclusions. As a result, the book was disavowed and did not appear in print until 2005.[64]

University patrons also asserted their censorship prerogative over the FLS. The CIS director, Millard Hansen, told FLS director Reuben Hill preemptively that "the University and I wish to impose a restriction on publication of results except those the University determines will be in the best interest of the University and the People of Puerto Rico" and not cause "injury to the Island."[65] Yet during the final stages of the production of the FLS's main report, *The Family and Population Control*, government officials learned of Hill's proposal to expand and diversify publicity about birth control services, which drew attention to the sensitive issue of the PPD's population limitation agenda. Governor Muñoz Marín instructed secretary of health Guillermo Arbona to remind Hill that, were the administration to follow such recommendations, "the opposition would feel challenged to do something, and according to [the governor's] experience, a vocal minority can squelch a program." Arbona explained that the scientists had "overstepped [their] bounds," exposing the government to a political attack. Reuben Hill, on his next visit to Puerto Rico, succeeded in lowering the tension and secured the publication of the book.[66]

Rather audaciously, *The Family and Population Control* nonetheless got away with accusing state maternal health clinics of a "clear intention of 'playing down' the birth control aspect," which made them "quite unsuccessful in making families systematic, regular, and efficient in their use of contraceptives."[67] It is a sign of the administration's Cold War–driven worries about population growth that *The Family and Population Control* did not suffer the same fate Siegel's book did. Still, in order to distance itself from future potential scandals, the CIS began to phase out population as a field of research following the completion of the FLS.[68] As the fate of Siegel's and Hill's texts shows, local political patrons played a key role determining the suitability of CIS work. Specifically, to please its sponsors, the FLS had to contribute to the crafting of family planning policies that would hasten Puerto Rico's capitalist development. This imperative, however, limited scholarly attention to the identification of cultural barriers to contraceptive use, rather than inspiring new ideas to improve women's health or correct gendered wage disparities, which could also lower fertility.[69]

The FLS's narrow emphasis on the promotion of birth control as a lever of rapid industrialization, its overreliance on governmental policies as tools to transform popular attitudes, and its tendency to pigeonhole Latin American workers as professionally inferior, reverberated far beyond Puerto Rico. Approximately four hundred KAP studies had been carried out worldwide by the early 1970s, at national and subnational levels, though not all as sophisticated as the FLS.[70] By this time U.S. social scientists began to question the remarkable uniformity of KAP studies' recommendations. Despite the diversity of human and geographic terrains covered, most studies urged the same tactics: governmental action to lower cultural barriers to contraceptive use, to persuade individuals of the benefits of lower fertility, and to stress the economic and health disadvantages of large families.[71]

Demographic evidence from Cold War Latin America, however, showed that government policies' impact on popular attitudes toward fertility was not straightforward. For example, the governments of Cuba, Panama, the Dominican Republic, Mexico, and Colombia, all of which adopted family planning policies in the 1960s and early 1970s, reduced their total fertility rates between forty and sixty percent between the mid-1960s and the early 1990s. Yet El Salvador and Guatemala, whose family planning policies date from 1974 and 1975, did not achieve such reductions. Meanwhile, countries such as Chile,

Uruguay, and Argentina reached replacement fertility rates without governmental intervention. Other countries, including Venezuela, Brazil, Costa Rica, and Peru, also reduced their fertility rates by more than thirty-five percent, either without policies or with policies implemented only in the 1980s.[72] Clearly, and contrary to what CIS researchers in the 1950s and population experts in the 1970s argued, governmental involvement was not the sole factor driving fertility changes.[73]

A more significant challenge to KAP research arose from developing nations themselves. The UN-sponsored World Conference on Population held in Bucharest in 1974 provided a venue for Third World critics to converge. At the end of it, representatives from 136 states (all except the Vatican) agreed to a World Population Plan of Action championed by Francophone sub-Saharan African countries, Algeria, Argentina, China, Albania, Romania, Cuba, and Peru. Third World countries ran against and defeated the U.S. proposal to establish demographic growth quotas and instead demanded respect for national sovereignty in population policymaking. More radically, Third World representatives moved away from defining rapid population growth as their leading problem, and instead claimed that "alien and colonial domination, foreign occupation, wars of aggression, racial discrimination, apartheid and neo-colonialism in all its forms, continue to be among the greatest obstacles to the full emancipation and progress of the developing countries and all the people involved."[74] From this perspective, underdevelopment caused rapid population growth, rather than the other way around. In addition, Third World representatives maintained, contraceptive-based population policies were shortsighted, racist, and colonialist technical fixes that failed to address developing nations' main concerns, although none of the signatories of the World Population Plan of Action denied the existence of popular demand for family planning, nor the social problems exacerbated by rapid demographic growth. Third World nations' insistence that population problems derived from social and economic ones, and that development was, therefore, necessary to tackle population problems effectively, contrasted sharply with the priorities of KAP research: producing knowledge about people's attitudes toward contraception to come up with more effective population-limitation strategies.

In Puerto Rico, nationalist critiques of KAP surveys encompassed a related assessment of the PPD's influence in determining the direction of social science research. In the early 1960s, the CIS had started to shift its focus to new areas beyond those deemed most relevant to the PPD's early policymaking priorities, including education, political sociology, and psychiatry. Though still dominated by U.S. researchers, the CIS's contingent of local scholars grew. No longer defining itself in terms of its service to the government, the CIS now did so as "a community of scholars with a common interest in Puerto Rican society."[75] Yet, the center's debt to Puerto Ricans was not settled, in the opinion of Luis Nieves Falcón, who became CIS director in 1970, after the PPD was voted out of office in 1968. As one of the sharpest critics of Millard Hansen's tenure, Nieves Falcón repudiated the work the CIS sponsored in the 1940s and 1950s, and looked to Brazil, Peru, and Venezuela as models for a more integral and sustained promotion of local talent and research.[76]

Méndez and Quintero see 1968 as a turning point in the history of local social science, when Puerto Ricans ceased being "mere objects of research" and became "observers and investigators of [their] own processes."[77] However, while Puerto Rican social scientists certainly became more involved as lead researchers after Nieves Falcón took the helm of the CIS, changes were already underway in the early 1960s. More importantly, long before that, Puerto Ricans had been heavily involved in determining the course of health policy research from their leadership positions in the university's administration, from the trenches of research assistance, and from their critical intellectual platforms. Their actions were framed by the U.S. priorities of limiting population growth, promoting capitalist development, and curbing nationalist agitation. These Cold War imperatives essentially made Puerto Rican actors subservient to U.S. social and geopolitical exigencies, but they do not erase the variegated ways in which local research patrons, assistants, and intellectuals shaped fertility research alongside and even contesting U.S. experts.

Notes

1   Stycos, *Human Fertility in Latin America*; Population Council, *Manual for Surveys of Fertility and Family Planning*, 4.
2   Davis, "Latin America's Multiplying Peoples"; Janer, Arbona, and McKenzie-Pollock, "Place of Demography." See also Szreter, "Idea of Demographic Transition"; Dörnemann and Huhle, "Population Problems."
3   Lapp, "Rise and Fall of Puerto Rico"; Goldstein, "Attributes of Sovereignty"; Elisa González, "Nurturing the Citizens of the Future"; Rostow, *Stages of Economic Growth*. The same attitude echoed among Indian elites preparing for independence. See Nair, "Construction of a 'Population Problem.'"
4   Lopez, *Matters of Choice*; Ramírez de Arellano and Seipp, *Colonialism, Catholicism, and Contraception*; Laura Briggs, *Reproducing Empire*.

5   Luis Muñoz Marín, "Puerto Rico since Columbus, 19 November 1953," 2, University of Minnesota Archives, Family Study Center Collection (FSC), box 10, folder Fertility Control in Underdeveloped Areas—The Case of Puerto Rico.

6   Hill, Stycos, and Back, *Family and Population Control*, 331, 339, 364, 366, 381, 388.

7   Méndez, *Las Ciencias Sociales*; Duany, "¿Modernizar la Nación o Nacionalizar la Modernidad?"; Duncan and Richardson, *Social Research in Puerto Rico*; Quintero Rivera, "La Ideología Populista."

8   Competition from the Philippines and Hawaii lowered sugar prices beginning in the mid-1920s, a trend exacerbated by the onset of the Great Depression in 1929. See Pantojas-García, "Puerto Rican Populism Revisited." Through the Jones Act, the U.S. Congress established the Senate of Puerto Rico in 1917 as a popularly elected body with local legislative jurisdiction. Emphasizing U.S. political dominance over the island, the Jones Act also reserved the U.S. Congress's right to annul or amend bills passed by the Puerto Rican Senate and required that the U.S. president, with the advice and consent of the Puerto Rican Senate, appoint the directors of the local departments of the interior, agriculture, health, and treasury. The two remaining local department heads, the attorney general and the commissioner of education, would be named solely by the U.S. president. See U.S. House of Representatives, History, Art, and Archives, "Puerto Rico." On Puerto Rican labor history, see Silvestrini, *Trabajadores Puertorriqueños*; Quintero Rivera, *Liderato Local*.

9   The PCP's failure to attract popular support led to its demise in 1944. See Pujals, "Perla en el Caribe Soviético."

10   Ferrao, *Pedro Albizu Campos*; Fernandez, *Macheteros*; Bosque-Perez and Colón Morera, *Puerto Rico under Colonial Rule*.

11   Pantojas-García, "Puerto Rican Populism Revisited." See also Ayala and Bernabe, *Puerto Rico in the American Century*; Pantojas-García, *Development Strategies as Ideology*.

12   See Sternsher, *Rexford Tugwell*, chapter 24.

13   Goodsell, *Administration of a Revolution*.

14   See Ekbladh, *Great American Mission*.

15   Zapata, *De Independentista a Autonomista*; Dietz, *Economic History of Puerto Rico*.

16   "The Family in Puerto Rico Research Project," 5, FSC, box 15, folder Progress Reports, University of Puerto Rico Project.

17   "Informe Anual del CIS, 1956–57," 4, University of Puerto Rico Archive (UPR Archive), Informes Anuales, box C-48.

18   Hatt, *Backgrounds of Human Fertility*.

19   "Informe Anual del CIS, 1954–55," UPR Archive, Informes Anuales, box C-48.

20   "Informe Anual del CIS, 1954–55," UPR Archive, Informes Anuales, box C-48.

21   "Informe de conferencia de Jaime Benítez con el Gobernador," November 23, 1954, Luis Muñoz Marín Archive (LMM), box 8, series 17, subseries 7, folder 5b.

22   See Benítez, *Junto a la Torre*, especially "La Universidad y sus Símbolos." On the university as a nexus of Cold War conflicts, see also Pacino's chapter in this volume.

23 Antonio Colorado, "¿Autonomía Universitaria o Absolutismo Rectoral?," February 13, 1955, UPR Archive, series 73, Organización y Sus Funciones, box A-1; Efraín Sanchez Hidalgo to Consejo Universitario, December 27, 1957, and Ismael Rodríguez Bou to Rector Jaime Benítez, December 26, 1952, LMM, box 8, series 17, subseries 7, folders 5f, 5a.

24 Marcos A. Ramírez, "La Universidad, La Colonia, y la Independencia," March 1, 1948, UPR Archive, recopilación especial 1 "Reforma Universitaria 1942–1962," box 1–2, folder "Reforma Universitaria, Años 1942–1948."

25 Acosta, *La Mordaza*. For a timely critique of the revealing place of Puerto Rican nationalism in the history of colonialism, see the essays in *Radical History Review* 128 (2017), edited by Margaret Power and Andor Skotnes.

26 "Elementos Subversivos en la UPR," April 5, 1951, UPR Archive, Correspondencia del Rector 1949–1955, box 330.

27 Millard Hansen to Reuben Hill, June 17, 1951, FSC, box 15, folder Progress Reports, University of Puerto Rico Project. On Hill's specialty, the sociology of the family, see his biographical file at the University of Minnesota Archives, Reuben Hill Papers (RHP).

28 Landy, *Tropical Childhood*. Landy never coauthored with Hill. In contrast, Stycos and Hill coauthored several articles as well as a book, *The Family and Population Control* (with Kurt Back). See the CV in Cornell University, J. Mayone Stycos Papers, (JMS), box 13, folder 1. See Millard Hansen to Reuben Hill, June 17, 1951, and Millard Hansen to David Landy, n.d., FSC, box 15, folder Progress Reports, University of Puerto Rico Project.

29 "Stages in a Long-Term Project in Family Life," FSC, box 15, folder Progress Reports, University of Puerto Rico Project. See also Stycos and Hill, "Prospects of Birth Control."

30 Paniagua, Vaillant, and Gamble, "Field Trial of a Contraceptive Foam."

31 "Puerto Rican Strength," 64–65, JMS, box 11, folder 16; Tugwell, *Stricken Land*, 8.

32 Kingsley Davis to Reuben Hill, June 25, 1951, FSC, box 15, folder Progress Reports, University of Puerto Rico Project.

33 See CIS annual reports, 1951–1957, in UPR Archive, Informes Anuales, box C-48.

34 Telephone interview with former CIS research assistant Teté Fabregás, June 16, 2011.

35 "Informe Anual del CIS, 1950–51," UPR Archive, Informes Anuales, box C-48.

36 Stycos, *Family and Fertility in Puerto Rico*, 278.

37 Stycos, "Further Observations"; Stycos, "Interviewer Training in Another Culture."

38 Kinsey, Pomeroy, and Martin, *Sexual Behavior in the Human Male*; "Training Guide on the Techniques of Qualitative Interviews, 1948," box 155, Columbia University, Records of the Bureau of Applied Social Research, 1944–1976.

39 Telephone interview with Angelina Saavedra, San Juan, Puerto Rico, May 16, 2011.

40 Kurt Back and J. M. Stycos, "The Survey under Unusual Conditions, 1959," 34, JMS, box 11, folder 18.

41 Steward et al., *People of Puerto Rico*, 22.

42 David Landy to Reuben Hill, December 8, 1951, April 7, 1952, FSC, box 10, folder Family Life Project (Prospectus).

43 Jaime Benítez, "La Iniciación Universitaria y las Ciencias Sociales, 1952," 48, 53. LMM, box 13, series 17, subseries 7, folder 41.

44 David Landy to Reuben Hill, April 7, 1952, FSC, box 10, folder Family Life Project (Prospectus).

45 Mintz, "People of Puerto Rico Half a Century Later."

46 Luis Nieves Falcón, "Implicaciones Sociales de la Expansión Cuantitativa en el Sistema de Instrucción de Puerto Rico durante el Periodo de 1940 a 1960," November 5, 1963, LMM, box 10, series 17, subseries 7, folder 20; Seda Bonilla, *Interacción Social y Personalidad*; Maldonado Denis, *Puerto Rico*; Seda Bonilla, *Requiem por una Cultura*.

47 Vázquez Calzada, *Población de Puerto Rico*.

48 Buitrago, "Investigación Social," 101; René Marqués, *Puertorriqueño Dócil*, 41.

49 Anonymous letter to the governor, "Sobre la UPR y el Rector, 1955," 84, LMM, box 9, series 17, subseries 7, folder 15.

50 "Informe Anual del CIS, 1951–52," UPR Archive, Informes Anuales, box C-48; Cáceres et al., *Violencia Nuestra de Cada Día*; Saavedra, *Espiritismo como una Religión*.

51 "The Sample Survey: Its Uses and Problems," 1955, 39, JMS, box 11, folder 18.

52 Stycos, "Further Observations," 77.

53 Telephone interview with Saavedra; telephone interview with Nilda Anaya, Silver Spring, June 20, 2011; "Notas," 36.

54 Such assumptions about the dynamics of interviewing are telling about the state of U.S. sociology in the mid–twentieth century. See Burawoy, "Extended Case Method."

55 See telephone interviews with Fabregás, Socorro Martínez, Saavedra, Anaya.

56 BEGLI, "My Experience as Interviewer in the Family Life Project," 12, RHP, box 41, folder Puerto Rico Study.

57 The full names of these surveyors were not included in the archival source. BEGLI, "Report of interview x-3, February 11, 1952," p. 20; ES, "Report of interview X-3M, February 14, 1952"; MES, "Report of interviews with X-6, February 11–12, 1952," RHP, box 41, folder Puerto Rico Study.

58 See Necochea López, *History of Family Planning in Twentieth-Century Peru*, chapter 4; Pribilsky, "Developing Selves."

59 Joseph Stycos to Millard Hansen, January 14, 1952, RHP, box 41, folder Puerto Rico Study.

60 Immanuel Wallerstein to Bernard Berelson on Special Training Program for Social Researchers from Underdeveloped Areas, 1961, Records of the Bureau of Applied Social Research, 1944–1976, box 106, folder 262.

61 The three volumes of Wallerstein's *The Modern World-System* were published between 1974 and 1989. See Wallerstein, *World-Systems Analysis*.

62 "Encuestas para Ciencias Sociales a Base de Muestreo en las Zonas Subdesarrolladas," CELADE, 1963, 10, JMS, box 11, folder 6.

63 Solovey, "Project Camelot."

64 Siegel, *Pueblo Puertorriqueño*. For a history of the work's censorship, see Jorge Duany's introduction.

65 Millard Hansen to Reuben Hill, June 17, 1951, FSC, box 15, folder Progress Reports, University of Puerto Rico Project.

66 Kurt Back to Reuben Hill, December 4, 1957, Reuben Hill to Kurt Back, January 14, 1958, FSC, box 3, folder Kurt Back 1957–1958.

67 Hill, Stycos, and Back, *Family and Population Control*, 350, 370, 376, 385.

68 "Informe Anual del CIS, 1957–58," UPR Archive, Informes Anuales, box C-48.

69 See Necochea López, *History of Family Planning in Twentieth-Century Peru*, chapter 5.

70 Cleland, "Critique of KAP Studies."

71 Demeny, "Social Science and Population Policy."

72 Aramburú, "Is Population Policy Necessary?"

73 On the importance of community buy-in for family planning programs, for example, see Pieper Mooney's chapter in this volume.

74 Mauldin et al., "Report on Bucharest."

75 "Informe Anual del Centro de Investigaciones Sociales, Enero–Junio 1962," UPR Archive, Informes Anuales, box C-48.

76 Nieves Falcón, "Puerto Rico."

77 Méndez, *Ciencias Sociales*, 101. See also Quintero Rivera, "Luis Nieves Falcón."

5

Parasitology and Communism

Public Health and Politics in Samuel Barnsley Pessoa's Brazil

GILBERTO HOCHMAN AND
CARLOS HENRIQUE ASSUNÇÃO PAIVA

On February 28, 1975, a house in the middle-class neighborhood of Morumbi in São Paulo was surrounded, invaded, and searched without a warrant by agents of the military dictatorship that had governed Brazil since April 1, 1964. The objective of the operation was to look for evidence of subversive activities and to arrest physician, scientist, and professor Samuel Barnsley Pessoa (1898–1976). The agents found neither Dr. Pessoa nor any evidence of his alleged antigovernment activities. They returned the next day and were informed that Pessoa was expected back in São Paulo within twenty-four hours. His son then received a telephone call from "Captain Ubirajara," the code name of a police officer who years later would be identified as one of the most brutal torturers of the military regime. Ubirajara ordered that Dr. Pessoa present himself immediately to the Department of Information Operations (DOI) at the Center for Internal Defense Operations (CODI). The DOI-CODI was the Brazilian Army's repressive antiguerrilla unit, whose headquarters in São Paulo served as a detention, torture, and assassination center in the 1970s. It was not the first time that Samuel Pessoa suffered intimidation tactics by the police. These had been frequent since the late 1940s; after all, the parasitologist and his wife, Jovina Rocha Álvares Pessoa, had been active members of the clandestine Brazilian Communist Party (PCB).[1]

Ironically, while the DOI-CODI was looking for him, Samuel Pessoa was attending an event in his honor at the XI Congress of the Brazilian Society of Tropical Medicine in Rio de Janeiro. Dr. Pessoa had long been the most renowned parasitologist and public health activist in Brazil, having trained generations of physicians and scientists at the University of São Paulo (USP), where he was professor of medical parasitology from 1931 to 1955, and he maintained connections with the university until his death in 1964. The event in Pessoa's honor was attended by the minister of health and other dignitaries linked to the very same government that had sent its agents to arrest him. It was a government that fired, imprisoned, and forced into exile many of Pessoa's colleagues in the department of parasitology of the School of Medicine of the USP, almost all of whom were his former students and collaborators and who, in one way or another, were also affiliated with the PCB.

This honorary event was to be one of the last tributes Pessoa received in his career. Upon returning to São Paulo with his wife, he presented himself to the military authorities to avoid the indignity of being arrested and handcuffed in his own home. At seventy-seven years of age and in poor health, he was arrested, hooded, subjected to a severe interrogation, and held incommunicado for several days. Samuel Pessoa died eighteen months later, on September 3, 1976.[2] Even though the obituaries were detailed, censorship forced omission of many aspects of his public life and political activity.[3]

The career of Samuel Pessoa illustrates the complex relations between medicine and politics in Brazil in the Cold War era. Rather than a biography of a distinguished scientist, this chapter offers an analysis of his ideas and actions, in particular his understanding of the health problems of rural populations, which was informed by his communist beliefs and activism between the 1940s and 1960s. These ideas and political activities were marked by the decidedly diverse political contexts Pessoa experienced as a physician and professor: from the crisis of the liberal-oligarchic republic in the 1920s through the military regime established in 1964, and covering Getúlio Vargas's initial administrations (1930–1937) and his dictatorship (the "Estado Novo," 1937–1945), as well as the Brazilian democratic period from 1945 to 1964 (including Vargas's 1951–1954 elected government). In the post–World War II period, and for the next three decades, Pessoa's professional trajectory was also shaped by the U.S.-Soviet rivalry in Latin America and the Caribbean, by wars and foreign interventions, revolutions and coups d'état. His career is an embodiment of the Cold War in Brazilian science and public health.

For Pessoa, the practice of social medicine, especially in terms of addressing endemic parasitic diseases in rural Brazil, was inseparable from concrete economic and political transformations, such as agrarian reform and eliminating large, exploitative estates—the *latifúndios*—and, more broadly, from a struggle for socialism. With regard to the latter, he differed from other physicians and health workers, both predecessors and contemporaries, with whom he shared a concern about the need for state intervention to tackle rural diseases.

Samuel Pessoa's political activism was linked to a wide network of intellectuals and communist organizations associated with the PCB and pro–Soviet Union movements, both in Brazil and abroad. The tension between being simultaneously recognized nationally and internationally as the most authoritative voice of Brazilian medicine in the field of rural health, and being persecuted for his political views, characterized his life and work for decades. This inseparability of parasitology and communism in Samuel Pessoa's career makes his trajectory a paradigmatic one for our understanding of the dynamics of Brazilian public health in the context of the Cold War.[4]

Samuel Pessoa's biomedical and public health activities and his struggles for equality and socialism have generated incomplete historical analyses. On one hand, there is considerable biographical work written about him, especially by his many colleagues, research and teaching assistants, and former students.[5] Because Samuel Pessoa and his group were victims of political persecution, notably during the military dictatorship, these sources emphasize the suffering they experienced—particularly removal from professional positions, imprisonment, and exile. The memoirs of militant Communists also mythologize him, for example, as the "physician of the peasants," for his work in rural areas. In the field of public health, Pessoa's nation-building and reformist leanings were associated with the struggle for democracy and health reform in Brazil during the 1970s and 1980s, particularly with the promotion of a national, public, and universal health care system.

On the other hand, the consensus about Samuel Pessoa's contribution to the scientific and public health communities has precluded more systematic scrutiny of his political activism. Some scholars have addressed aspects of Pessoa's scientific work, his political thought, his public health activities at the university, and his relations with the Rockefeller Foundation (RF).[6] Precious little, however, has been written about his communist and antinuclear activism or about the relations between science and left-wing politics in the postwar era.[7] Pessoa is occasionally mentioned as a political activist in studies of the Brazilian left and its intellectuals,[8] but they give short shrift to his scientific work. This chapter aims to integrate discussion of Pessoa's public health work and his politics, especially during the Cold War, but also going back to the 1920s, when Samuel Pessoa became a physician and began his career as a parasitologist.

This chapter is divided into two parts. In the first, we analyze Pessoa's trajectory from his medical school graduation until the end of the Vargas dictatorship, his relations with the RF, his work as a professor of medical parasitology, and his ideas and actions in the field of rural health starting in the 1930s. The objective is to show how his practice of parasitology was linked with communism in the context of the Estado Novo dictatorship and the outbreak of World War II. The second part deals with the 1946–1964 period, as the connections between parasitology and communism in Pessoa's work unfolded in the context of the Cold War. This section addresses Pessoa's ideas and work at the USP and in Brazilian public health, as well as his activities in the "peace movement," and the setbacks he suffered due to his communist activism, including following the civil-military coup of 1964.

From Parasitology to Communism, 1922–1945

Samuel Barnsley Pessoa was born in May 1898 in São Paulo, the son of Leonel Pessoa, a physician from the state of Paraíba, and Anna Barnsley Pessoa, daughter of a couple who migrated to Brazil along with twenty thousand other U.S. southerners after the American Civil War. Pessoa's extended family belonged to Brazil's northeastern political elite and had even produced a president, Epitácio Pessoa (1919–1922), and a Paraíba state governor, João Pessoa, during the First Republic (1889–1930). Samuel Pessoa attended high school at the Colégio Anglo-Brasileiro, where most of the scions of São Paulo state's elites studied, and in 1916 he enrolled at the newly established School of Medicine of São Paulo.[9]

It was precisely at this juncture that the RF's International Health Board (IHB) began providing substantial backing to the School of Medicine of São Paulo, fueling research and the modernization of the curriculum. Most importantly, starting in 1918, the IHB helped found an Institute of Hygiene, which offered public health courses, ran field stations, and was directed until 1922 by American scientists (and RF staff members) Samuel Taylor Darling and Wilson George Smillie.[10] Pessoa studied and worked with both men, launching his long-term ties to the RF.[11]

From 1920 onward, the RF supported the modernization of curriculum in traditional and new disciplines, relying initially on the presence of U.S. instructors, and then on Brazilian scientists who received scholarships to study in the United States, particularly at the Johns Hopkins School of Public Health. The RF recommended reforms, emphasizing laboratory research, limits on the number of students admitted, and the creation of a hospital attached to the School of Medicine, which were implemented during the 1920s by the government of the state of São Paulo. Through the 1940s, the RF continued funding medical researchers working in a range of specialties and institutions in São Paulo.[12]

As of 1916, a significant part of the Brazilian medical and intellectual elite was involved in a political and nationalist campaign for public health reform, with particular emphasis on the diseases of rural populations and medical attention seen as a form of absolution for the circumstances of racialized poverty and ill health.[13] Given this larger environment, the reforms of medical education at São Paulo, and the IHB's agenda, which included combating anemia-inducing hookworm disease, it is no coincidence that the young Samuel Pessoa's 1922 medical thesis focused on the use of chenopodium oil as a hookworm prophylactic.[14] Researchers on the staff of the IHB, among them Smillie, Pessoa's professor, tested chenopodium oil in several Latin American countries, and the two men coauthored various studies on this topic between 1922 and 1925.[15]

Upon graduation, Pessoa was awarded a Rockefeller scholarship to carry out research on rural health and work in health clinics in the interior of São Paulo, maintaining ties with the Institute of Hygiene. Wishing to remain in the region, he turned down a position in Rio de Janeiro with Mark Boyd, a key figure in the RF's malaria studies at the time. On several occasions, Pessoa credited and thanked Smillie for fostering his interest in a career combining parasitology and fieldwork.[16]

Pessoa's prestige grew rapidly during the first decade of his professional career, as he deepened his connection to the RF and simultaneously increased his contact with and concern for Brazil's rural population. Lewis Hackett, the director of the IHB in Brazil, not only praised Pessoa's medical school thesis and requested copies for distribution, but he also expressed the RF's high esteem for the young researcher, indicating that, despite Pessoa's being unable to work on malaria with Boyd, "our posts are always open to you for duty at any time you desire."[17]

In 1925, with malaria's prominence rising on the national and international health agenda, the IHB commissioned Pessoa to conduct epidemiological and field studies on the disease in São Paulo. Two years later, Pessoa traveled to Europe to further his training in malaria, sponsored by the Committee of Hygiene of the League of Nations. He visited malaria research institutions and clinics in Spain, Italy, and Yugoslavia. At the time, physician Andrija Štampar was the leader of public health in Yugoslavia, having created a school of public health in Zagreb and organized the Central Institute of Hygiene in Belgrade, both strongly backed by the RF.[18] Following his visits to these institutions, Pessoa approvingly noted that, after six years of health reforms, Yugoslavia had become "a true school of hygiene."[19] Before returning to Brazil in 1928, Pessoa also pursued advanced courses at the Hamburg Institute of Tropical Medicine and worked at Émile Brumpt's parasitology laboratory at the Paris School of Medicine. Years later, Pessoa attributed his teaching philosophy to his experiences in Germany and France.[20]

From 1922 to 1931, Pessoa published fifty-seven scientific papers, further establishing him as a rising star in his field. In 1931, at thirty-three years of age, he became a tenured professor of parasitology at the School of Medicine of São Paulo; this was one of the most important teaching and medical research positions in Brazil, a chair (*cátedra*) created and occupied by Brumpt during his stay in São Paulo in 1913 and 1914.

Pessoa's appointment to the School of Medicine occurred in a troubled political and economic context. In October 1930, Getúlio Vargas seized control of the government, ousting the liberal-oligarchic regime that had been in power since 1889 and beginning his fifteen-year regime as president. In the early 1930s Brazil was mired in economic crisis, which had worsened since 1929 and severely affected the state of São Paulo's coffee industry, a leading employment sector. Responding to the crisis through political centralization, Vargas in short order created ministries of labor, industry and commerce, and education and health.[21] Vargas's interventionism rankled states such as São Paulo, which were keen to maintain their autonomy. Dissatisfaction with the political and economic direction of the federal government led São Paulo's political and economic elites to rise up in arms between July and October 1932—the so-called Constitutionalist Revolution. Classes were suspended statewide, including at the School of Medicine. Pessoa, who had been granted a Rockefeller Fellowship that year to study in the United States or Europe, had to cancel his plans due to the tense political environment.[22] The civil war ended with the victory of the federal government and the deaths of hundreds of opponents. In the aftermath, the federal government was forced to call elections for a national assembly in 1933, leading to a new constitution in 1934.

Following an attempted leftist uprising against the government in November 1935, Getúlio Vargas imposed authoritarian measures in November 1937. The administration had the support of the military and civilians alike, many of whom were sympathetic to fascism. Alleging a communist threat, the regime issued yet another constitution and intensified centralizing and repressive tendencies, which were relaxed only after 1942 when Brazil severed relations with the Axis powers. The country's shift toward regional defense priorities and support for the U.S.-led war effort was complemented by its entry into World War II on the side of the Allies. While these events were unfolding, Samuel Pessoa devoted himself to teaching medical parasitology, researching endemic rural diseases in the field, and training students in his laboratory. As he traveled throughout the interior of São Paulo, he got to know people whose lives were marked by poverty, malnutrition, and disease. Their misery, as he wrote in 1940, would be etched in his mind for the rest of his days.[23]

Between 1932 and 1941 Pessoa published some seventy works, almost entirely in national journals and with Brazilian coauthors, unlike in his early career, when he was closer to his U.S. mentors and the RF. His status as a "master of parasitology" rose with his training of new researchers and professors, and his support for new medical schools and new chairs of parasitology in state capitals and cities in the interior. It was during this period that his lectures and articles began to stress the notion that "health issues [were] above all social issues."[24] From 1939 to 1942 he led a commission for the study and prophylaxis of American tegumentary leishmaniasis, which was transmitted via sandflies and caused disabling skin lesions. As part of this work he organized health clinics and treated patients in the interior of São Paulo.

In 1940, Pessoa took a significant political step during an address to the graduating class of the USP medical school, when he called for the centralization of health services, the reform of Brazil's concentrated land ownership, and the improvement of health administration and medical training. Given the authoritarian political environment, the speech prompted threats of arrest from Adhemar Pereira de Barros, governor of São Paulo (1938–1941), a physician who had previously been on friendly terms with Pessoa.[25] Barros was particularly annoyed by Pessoa's depiction of the health situation in the state as dramatic and chaotic.[26]

Had Pessoa given his address a title, he claimed, it would have been "On the Need for Rural Physicians in Brazil" or "On the Urgent Need for Medical and Health Assistance to Brazilian Rural Populations."[27] Pessoa painted a dire picture of rural health, especially in the state of São Paulo, which was generally regarded as "Brazil's engine."[28] He entreated graduating medical students to rectify the "greatest sin of the past generation—the abandonment of the rural populations."[29] The speech clearly revealed his commitment to the poor, marking Pessoa's political activism and his private life, as well as his burgeoning stance decrying foreign (especially U.S.) influence on Brazilian culture.[30]

At first glance, the arguments that Samuel Pessoa expressed in 1940 were similar to, and derived from, those of the sanitary movement of the 1910s and 1920s, which denounced the neglect of the health and education of rural populations, and fought for rural sanitation and public health reform.[31] However, there were also striking differences, signaling Pessoa's firm adherence to socialism. The first was his insistence on holding rural landowners and, less explicitly, Brazilian capitalism, instead of only the government, accountable for the living conditions of rural workers, especially in the areas of agricultural expansion.[32] As he put it, "Landowners are generally responsible . . . , to a greater or lesser degree, for health improvement, the status of hygiene on their properties, and the health of their workers."[33] Pessoa recounted the obstacles imposed by landowners to the establishment of health clinics on their properties, particularly dispensaries for the treatment of tegumentary leishmaniasis, claiming that the presence of such dispensaries and of sick persons devalued their land.[34] Pessoa attributed this obstructionism to selfishness and greed, and also to a deeply ingrained disposition to protect products, cattle, and crops over workers. His critique of the Brazilian capitalist mentality also extended to wealthy landowners' resistance to the presence of state health services on their property and lack of interest in any form of outside health assistance, even in partnership with the RF.[35]

That a considerable portion of the rural population was Indigenous and/or Afro-descendant, however, remained outside this equation. Pessoa, like other Brazilian communists of his era, subsumed the context of racial oppression in Brazil's rural expanses to one of class relations. This prioritizing of economic over racial dimensions of rural misery, whether from a leftist or liberal-reformist perspective, marked Brazilian health and social policy throughout the Cold War period, even as some groups of intellectuals contested the idea of Brazil as a "racial democracy" as early as the 1940s.[36]

In Pessoa's opinion, the federal and state governments were also at fault, although he guardedly approved of the reformist tendencies of the Vargas regime. Despite the state of São Paulo's and the federal government's creation of health posts in the state's interior beginning in the late 1910s, health problems, parasitic infections especially, persisted twenty years later. Pessoa had come to realize that health actions alone were no longer sufficient to address rural misery. A crucial element was the introduction of school-based health education to address precarious health in rural areas.

More damning, though expressed in a discreet manner, was Pessoa's assessment of the social policies of the Vargas government. While acknowledging the virtues of extending legal and social security protection to urban workers, Samuel Pessoa considered overlooking the needs of rural workers to be "unconscionable."[37] Because federal social policies did not cover rural populations (and local power mongers kept services out), the rural milieu remained under the control of private and local powers and forgotten by the federal government, contrary to the intentions of the sanitarians of Brazil's First Republic.

In December 1942, Samuel Pessoa became director of public health of the state of São Paulo, a position he would hold until February 1944, when he resigned and returned to the USP. This was his one and only experience in public administration, and it occurred at a particular local, national, and international juncture: São Paulo was headed by a new *interventor* (an appointed governor), Fernando de Souza Costa, after Vargas fired Adhemar de Barros on charges of corruption in June 1941. The country had mobilized for the war effort, having sent troops to Italy and designated locations for U.S. military bases in the Brazilian Northeast, a move by dictator Vargas to assert "national unity" at a time of war. But the contradictions of the Vargas regime were also evident: an authoritarian and repressive government fighting alongside democracies such as the United Kingdom and the United States, as well as their Soviet allies, against Nazi fascist totalitarianism. Emboldened Brazilian dissenters called for the end of repression and censorship, amnesty for political prisoners, the legalization of political parties, free elections, and a democratic constitution. The pressure of these demands engendered greater government tolerance.

As São Paulo state's director of public health, Pessoa tried to implement (parts of) his agenda for addressing rural endemic diseases. He sought to increase the number and efficiency of health centers. He also reorganized the Malaria Prophylaxis Service to enable better coordination with the medical school and with public hospitals and to improve research, treatment, and disease control. Pessoa championed this coordinated model throughout his career.[38]

Pessoa and his wife likely became affiliated with the PCB in the late 1930s or early 1940, given that his speech of 1940 already included some clear anticapitalist content.[39] Some of his articles condemning the scourges afflicting Brazilians were censored in 1944, indicating that, even in the twilight of the Vargas regime, its surveillance and censorship bureaus monitored opponents' declarations and actions.[40] Not all PCB leaders had been arrested following the 1935 uprising, but by 1940 most of the central committee was imprisoned, liquidating the party and leaving it without national officers or structures until 1943. With the changes in the political environment, the PCB sought to reorganize itself in Rio de Janeiro, São Paulo, and Bahia, holding a clandestine national conference in August 1943.[41] During this period a new generation of PCB leaders and activists gained prominence, broadening the social and political influence of the party in Brazilian society. Alongside Pessoa, a significant number of writers, artists, academics, journalists, and intellectuals joined the PCB.[42]

In 1945, the country's pro-democracy climate led to political amnesty, a call for general elections, the legalization of the PCB, and at the end, the overthrow of Vargas by the army in late October of that year. Party leader Luís

Carlos Prestes, in prison since 1936, was released in April 1945 and appointed party secretary-general.

In these years, Samuel Pessoa's intense political activism ran parallel to his academic activities. In 1946 he completed his most important book, *Parasitologia Médica*, a compendium that became mandatory reading in all medical schools in the country, and which continued to be updated and reissued until 1982.[43] In addition, his political career took a decisive turn when he ran for the National Constituent Assembly as a Communist Party candidate for the state of São Paulo in the general election held on December 2, 1945. His political position had become public and well defined.

Communism and Parasitology, 1946–1964

The PCB made a notable political debut in the elections of 1945, the year it was legalized. After decades of banishment and persecution, the party managed to send one senator (Secretary-General Luís Carlos Prestes) and fourteen deputies to the National Assembly, making it the fourth-largest party in that body. Its presidential candidate received nine percent of the national vote. But Samuel Pessoa was not elected.[44] The PCB's fortune would soon turn, however, as the Cold War winds of anticommunism began blowing toward Brazil. The government of President Eurico Dutra (1946–1951), closely aligned with the United States, once again broke off relations with the Soviet Union in October 1947 (relations had been reestablished in April 1945). Accused of serving Soviet interests, the PCB was declared illegal in May 1947 by electoral authorities, and all party parliamentarians were removed from office in January 1948. Anti-PCB repression followed, including the harassment of party-affiliated trade unions and the imprisonment of party members and leaders. Samuel and Jovina Pessoa were both briefly arrested in January 1948. In response to these actions, the PCB, which had until then engaged in a balancing act between its socialist program and its need for legality, adopted a radical platform of clandestine confrontation, which lasted until the late 1950s. From then on, and well into the 1960s, the secret police monitored, alternately suppressing and sometimes tolerating, the actions of Communist individuals, their organizations, and their newspapers. Such tactics had become common under the Estado Novo dictatorship and even continued under the governments that were democratically elected between 1945 and 1964.[45]

Although Samuel Pessoa never ran for office again, he became more outspoken regarding domestic social problems, the need for a national and international anti-imperialist (i.e., anti-American) struggle, and the importance of eliminating nuclear, biological, and chemical weapons. He participated in progressive and nationalistic movements in favor of a state oil monopoly, the release of political prisoners, and the legalization of the PCB, and against the military agreements Brazil made with the United States. As an academic and a scientist, he continued to train physicians and to create and support chairs of parasitology in medical schools in various regions of the country. He also continued to study rural endemic diseases in situ—especially schistosomiasis and leishmaniasis—in his scholarly work, denouncing the role of poverty in propagating these ailments. Pessoa published another 132 scientific articles and opinion papers between 1945 and 1964, in which he linked the science of parasitology with politics in his own distinctive way.

Pessoa's communism, however, did not translate into an uncritical stance toward Soviet science. For example, two of his most illustrious students, the couple Victor and Ruth Nussenzweig, recalled being drawn to parasitology research in the last two years of medical school, around 1950. One of their goals had been to replicate the results of two Soviet investigators, Grigorii Ruskin and Nina Kliueva (also a couple), who reported having successfully treated certain types of tumors with extracts from *Trypanosoma cruzi*.[46] According to the Nussenzweigs, who married in Pessoa's laboratory, Ruskin and Kliueva's findings did not appear scientifically reasonable to Pessoa. Yet he allowed them to use the resources of his laboratory to draw their own conclusions. Decades later, long after the couple had embarked on other lines of investigation, they expressed great appreciation for Pessoa's support for their early career research.[47]

Over the years, the critical elements already present in Pessoa's 1940 speech to the USP medical graduates acquired greater coherence as a socially transformative project. His 1949 book, *Problemas Brasileiros de Higiene Rural*, clarified and expanded the argument of that controversial speech. In it, Pessoa reaffirmed that the *latifúndios*, which concentrated land in few hands and subjected workers to despicable, quasi-feudal labor relations and draconian labor contracts, were the main obstacles to the improvement of living conditions in rural Brazil.[48] In his opinion, "hygienists or sociologists who have been studying our rural phenomenon stress the need for agrarian reform, without which it will be impossible . . . to improve the precarious conditions of existence in rural areas, including nutrition, clothing, housing, health, and education."[49]

The transformation of the agrarian structure was one of the main concerns of communists and intellectuals in the PCB, and implied challenging large landowners in a society that was still predominantly rural. Pessoa listed numerous other obstacles to the improvement of rural health, including the lack of physicians in rural areas, low government funding for health services and epidemiological studies, a paucity of public health professionals, the difficulties faced by poor and illiterate rural populations when interacting with overly bureaucratic health centers, and the ineffectiveness of health education programs for children and adults.[50] Regarding the last of these, he was inspired by Emilio Willems, chair of anthropology at the USP, who saw the conservative culture of rural communities as one of their few defenses against the "growing instability fostered by the capitalist economy."[51] Going against the mainstream of Brazilian and international public health tenets, Pessoa argued that health efforts in rural areas should refrain "from intervening in the *caboclo* cultures as much as possible."[52]

Because of agrarian reform's strong association with the PCB, critics of communism, even from within the field of public health, resisted this approach as a means of improving living conditions in rural areas. At the VII Brazilian Hygiene Congress, held in São Paulo in 1948, progressive physicians, led by Pessoa, urged that "solving the agrarian problem in Brazil" be included among the congress's resolutions. The motion was defeated after a heated challenge from a distinguished health worker and senior official of the Serviço Especial de Saúde Pública, a U.S.-Brazilian health agency created in 1942 that displayed, according to Pessoa, "blatant North American leanings."[53] Pessoa condemned as absurd the arguments of this "pro-American lackey" that latifúndios did not exist in Brazil and that, to the contrary, there was still a large amount of land that could be occupied and distributed to landless peasants.[54]

Through the 1950s, land reform and structural change were Samuel Pessoa's core proposals to improve the deplorable living conditions, and associated parasitic diseases, of rural populations. After Josué de Castro, a physician and nutritionist from the state of Pernambuco, published his powerful analysis *Geografia da Fome* (Geography of Hunger) in 1946, Pessoa turned also to the issue of hunger. Malnutrition was a particularly pressing problem in the Northeast, where Pessoa traveled frequently, often staying for long periods to carry out research, teach, and provide medical care. He believed that emergency government measures would not free "the people of the Northeast from the shackles of their desperate poverty" unless they were accompanied by "programs to alter the economic structures of the region."[55] In this respect, Samuel Pessoa embraced the "national-developmentalist" trend in Brazilian public health, which rose in opposition to the predominant viewpoint in Brazilian and international health that it was possible to address health problems through better administration, technologies, and campaigns against specific diseases. This latter approach generally dismissed the need for structural changes and cultural negotiations. Importantly, it was also the perspective promoted by international health agencies, such as the World Health Organization (WHO) and the U.S. International Cooperation Administration (subsequently USAID), and was prevalent within Brazilian health services and the Ministry of Health.[56]

Samuel Pessoa began to think about the paths to the socialization of medicine in Brazil, as inspired by the British National Health Service and Soviet state medicine.[57] He also became enthusiastic about China's rural health initiatives, as well as Chinese traditional medicine. He openly advocated for the socialization of medicine in rural areas, although he was aware that the conditions for this to take place in Brazil in the early 1950s were lacking. As he often insisted, concrete actions and steps were first needed to transform utopia into reality: agrarian reform, more health professionals and technicians, and a hospital network in the interior of the country. Pessoa also insisted on employment contracts for physicians with wages paid by the state or by businesses, and on the extension of public health policies and programs for rural areas. Moreover, as a physician and Marxist, he argued that in a capitalist society the socialization of medicine should not, and indeed could not, be pursued in isolation, but had to be part of the process of socialization of the means of production and distribution, in an inexorable march toward socialism.[58]

It was also in the early 1950s that Pessoa became involved with a core set of interrelated issues of the Cold War, namely the arms race, the threat of nuclear war, and the use of chemical and biological weapons. By this time, the brief period of cooperation that followed World War II had ended, and the Cold War was firmly entrenched. As of 1948 the PCB had followed directives from the Soviet Union and the Communist Information Bureau (Cominform) to organize a broad peace movement, which could help contain the political and military actions of the United States and mobilize the masses toward socialism.[59] In 1949, the First World Peace Congress was held simultaneously in Paris and Prague, and the World Peace Council was created with direct links to the Communist Party of the USSR, as well as to independent Christian, humanist, and socialist movements.

In March 1950, the committee of the World Congress of Partisans for Peace launched the "Stockholm Appeal," calling for the total prohibition of nuclear weapons. The goal was to collect millions of signatures from many countries, in support of world peace, to be sent to the United Nations. Though banned and persecuted, Brazilian Communists affiliated with the PCB conducted a widespread publicity campaign through their underground newspapers and their professional and trade-union centers, in addition to relying on the mobilization of noncommunist political groups that adhered to the cause of eliminating nuclear weapons. These activists collected an astonishing two million signatures, including from members of the military, the political elite, the Supreme Court, and the Brazilian national soccer team, many of whom were high-profile noncommunists.[60] The signatures of these so-called "fighters for peace" were taken to the Second World Peace Congress, held in Warsaw in November 1950.

Pessoa was an important activist in this peace movement, participating in public demonstrations and meetings, making speeches, giving interviews, and writing articles for journals and newspapers.[61] He also participated in demonstrations for the commutation of the death sentence of the American couple Julius and Ethel Rosenberg, who were convicted of spying for the Soviet Union. Pessoa even became the vice president of the Humanitarian Crusade for the Prohibition of Atomic Weapons and one of the leaders of the Brazilian Movement of Partisans for Peace. The secret police in São Paulo and Rio de Janeiro monitored the activities of the Brazilian Peace Movement, frequently summoning and arresting its militants, and banning their public meetings and demonstrations.[62]

In 1952, Pessoa was directly involved in a central episode of the Cold War, namely the accusation made by the governments of North Korea and China that the United States had used biological weapons in the Korean War. The accusers, supported by the USSR, rejected the U.S.-backed proposal to form a review committee led by either the WHO or the Red Cross. Instead, the World Peace Council—chaired by the French chemist and physicist Frédéric Joliot-Curie, winner of the 1935 Nobel Prize in Chemistry and member of the French Communist Party—appointed the International Scientific Commission for the Investigation of the Facts Concerning Bacterial Warfare in Korea and China (ISC).

In light of his prestige as a scientist and militant Communist, Pessoa was invited by Joliot-Curie and the Chinese Academy of Sciences to participate in this commission in May 1952.[63] The ISC was led by a prominent Cambridge professor, British biochemist and sinologist Joseph Needham, the only ISC member who could speak Mandarin. The ISC included scientists from various other countries, such as Andrea Andreen (Sweden), Jean Malterre (France), Oliviero Olivo (Italy), and Nikolai Zhukov-Verezhnikov, vice president of the Soviet Academy of Medicine. Between June 31 and August 23, 1952, the commission visited sites in North Korea and China, met with Korean and Chinese witnesses and top officials, including Mao Zedong and Kim Il-sung, and interviewed two U.S. pilots held as prisoners of war, who presumably confessed to dropping biological material on Korean and Chinese territory. The commission produced an extensive, 660-page report, published in Beijing in August 1952, which confirmed the "criminal use of biological weapons by U.S. forces."[64]

The United States and its allies vehemently contested the report, deeming it a farce and a propaganda tool, both because of the partiality of the ISC members, which comprised Communists or communist sympathizers, and because of the limits imposed by Korean and Chinese authorities on the work of the commission. A campaign orchestrated by the United States and United Kingdom singled out Joseph Needham for personal and professional attacks. The ISC report was also the subject of hearings before the U.S. House Un-American Activities Committee (HUAC). As a result of the "Second Red Scare" and McCarthyist fearmongering, the supporters and promoters of the ISC report in the United States found themselves named as defendants in sedition and treason lawsuits.[65]

The activities of the commission and its report generated a massive furor at the time, and a debate that continues to this day, particularly after the opening of Soviet archives and access to Chinese documents by historians.[66] Was the ISC report a communist farce, or did it reveal an uncomfortable truth? Whatever the case, Pessoa's involvement elevated him to a prominent position in the anti-imperialist and peace movement in Brazil and abroad. The Communist press in Brazil touted the conclusions of the commission, attacked the United States, and praised Pessoa. "Microbes from Maryland over Korea and China" and "Proof of Microbial War" read some of the headlines in the second half of 1952, with articles including photographs to emphasize the presence of Pessoa among the "wise men who made decisive revelations."[67] Upon his return to Brazil, a massive entourage of colleagues, students, and activists for the peace movement received Pessoa and his wife at the São Paulo airport. According to A Voz Operária, the couple was warmly and euphorically greeted as they stepped off the plane. The newspaper Imprensa Popular highlighted Pessoa's statement upon landing: "I saw the Bacteriological War."[68] Newspapers affiliated with the PCB praised Pessoa for having lived up "to his status as a man of science" by accepting the difficult mission.[69] To fend off the accusations of partiality, the sympathetic press stressed Pessoa's role as a scientist, noting that his participation on the commission was merely "an extension of the meticulous research that he conducts in his laboratory."[70]

Because of his visibility with the ISC, however, Pessoa also became the target of criticism and retaliation.[71] The mainstream media in Rio de Janeiro and São Paulo were decidedly pro-American and anticommunist. One of the leading Brazilian newspapers, *O Correio da Manhã* of Rio de Janeiro, questioned the selection by "Soviet China" of the members of the commission: "These are communist sympathizers or are already known to be pro-Moscow. . . . As for professor Samuel Pessoa, no more needs to be said. A Professor of Parasitology of the University of São Paulo, he has believed in the miracles of communism since 1940."[72] Curiously, a year later the same newspaper sought out Pessoa for an interview about the high incidence of visceral leishmaniasis in children in the state of Ceará; for this purpose, the Communist reverted to his status as scientist, the foremost Brazilian authority on parasitic diseases.[73] Another newspaper in Rio de Janeiro, *O Globo*, sought to discredit Pessoa, stating that, if he was a Communist, he could not be a scientist, and adding that his wife and three children were also Communists![74] Pessoa's participation on the ISC also led to an order to present himself at the offices of the secret police to provide details about his journey.[75]

Shortly after his experience with the ISC, Pessoa participated as the Brazilian delegate at the Congress of the Peoples for Peace, organized by the pro-USSR World Peace Council, held in Vienna in December 1952. Rising international tensions, including the Korean War, nuclear testing, and accusations of the use of chemical and biological weapons, were the background for this meeting, which also gave China, the Soviet Union, and the Communist Parties from various countries the opportunity to mobilize populations and workers in support of a nationalist and anti-imperialist agenda. The PCB intended to use this platform to advance its campaign to block the sending of Brazilian troops to Korea, to reestablish diplomatic relations with the USSR and China, to denounce the military agreements Brazil had made with the United States, and to defend Brazilian culture against the onslaught of North American cultural products, in the form of films, comics, and literature.[76] While the mainstream media completely ignored the Vienna Congress, workers' and Communist newspapers gave the Brazilian mobilization for peace ample coverage and, once again, highlighted Pessoa's participation.[77]

For the RF, which had supported the scientist Samuel Pessoa since the beginning of his research career, the now Communist Samuel Pessoa had overstepped the mark by participating in the ISC, and it became concerned about his political activities. At the time, the U.S. Congress's Cox-Reece commission was investigating tax-exempt philanthropic foundations, which were suspected of financing Communists and subversives, as well as antisegregationists.[78] When the RF came under fire, its president, Dean Rusk, addressed the commission and published a detailed response about all of the philanthropy's activities.[79] For authors such as Tim Mueller, this was one of the moments when "RF definitions on academic freedom—even then not uncontested within the foundation—bordered on fervently anti-Communist, security obsessed discourses."[80]

Although the pressure on the RF decreased after 1954, apprehension and mistrust persisted among some of its staff members. In 1955, for example, Robert Briggs Watson, a malariologist in charge of the foundation's scientific and medical-education programs in South America (1954–1962), wrote that Pessoa "went to China on a 'germ warfare' commission, thus prostituting his undoubted scientific ability as a parasitologist, invalidating it to his political belief." Watson's suspicions extended to Pessoa's students: "P. has been influential for years in training young men not only in parasitology but also in subversive political activities. While P. . . . has now retired, his influence is still very much felt in the country."[81] These comments reveal the lingering concern about the young professors who were members of an alleged "school of parasitology and subversion" led by Samuel Pessoa, who could be receiving, directly or indirectly, funding from the RF.

As Watson's comments indicate, Pessoa retired in 1955. He was made emeritus professor of parasitology at the USP and continued to devote his time to research and teaching, especially in the Brazilian Northeast. He acquired additional awards, titles, and honors in the 1950s, confirming his status as the de facto national leader in parasitology. As Watson feared, Pessoa's combination of activism and research served as a model for his students, many of whom were, not surprisingly, communist sympathizers, given the distinct intellectual environment of parasitology at the USP; their eye-opening rural fieldwork experiences often took place in the company of Samuel Pessoa.[82]

Despite the RF's growing discomfort with Pessoa, the sentiment was not mutual. Pessoa recognized the RF's pivotal role in Brazil even after his political choices and actions led to his distancing from the American philanthropy. When the RF closed its office in São Paulo in 1944, for example, Pessoa gave interviews to newspapers praising the role of the IHB in improving Brazilian public health and in his own training, stating that "the RF's policy of good neighborly relations preceded [U.S. President Franklin D.] Roosevelt's own by many years."[83]

In 1956, the RF was consulted about the possibility of Pessoa's appointment to a position at the School of Medicine of the University of Minas Gerais (in its state capital Belo Horizonte), where the foundation supported various teaching and research activities.[84] Watson reported in June 1956 that the "RF did not approve of P. nor would RF support him," and, furthermore, that this appointment could threaten the funding of the School of Medicine.[85] The correspondence about this case among Watson, Samuel Bugher (the RF's director of medical education and public health), and Dean Rusk, indicating that Pessoa's appointment would not be well received by the RF, reached the Brazilian government indirectly via Brazilians working for the foundation. The correspondents cited the guideline provided in the RF's annual report of 1953, written during the Cox-Reece commission investigations, that "the Foundation refrains as a matter of policy from making grants to known Communists."[86] The dynamics of the Cold War weighed on Pessoa's life, especially due to his deep involvement with international communist organizations; not even his acknowledged scientific credentials could absolve him in the eyes of the RF this time. Pessoa's detractors succeeded. As Watson noted, "P. did not get the appointment."[87]

The RF's veto and the obstacles created by the secret police did not diminish Pessoa's prestige or his political and academic dynamism. In the second half of the 1950s he remained involved in peace organizations, lecturing and publishing on the subject in both medical and lay journals. He also continued to advance the medicopolitical agenda he had promoted since 1940 to conduct research, teach, and establish parasitology chairs and laboratories in medical schools in several states. The same newspapers that in the mid-1950s had criticized his participation in the ISC and accused him of subordinating science to communist ideology later reported approvingly of his initiatives against schistosomiasis and leishmaniasis and the interventions he organized during health crises in the Northeast. *O Correio da Manhã* described a Pessoa who had grown "tired of theories," and who deserved praise for retiring of his own accord, having chosen to live in an area "most afflicted by the evil" of schistosomiasis, where he studied the "greatest ignominy" of Brazil.[88] For the national press, at least, a Communist could sometimes be virtuous and nationalistic, as well as a good scientist, simultaneously.

Epilogue

Samuel Pessoa's retirement in 1955 and his subsequent activities occurred amid significant transformations in Brazilian and international politics. The suicide of Getúlio Vargas in August 1954 caused an enormous political crisis in Brazil, inaugurating a period of unrest and radicalization that would culminate in the 1964 coup. The death of Joseph Stalin in 1953, the revelation of Stalinism's crimes by the Khrushchev Report, and the Soviet invasion of Hungary in 1956 had a major impact on the PCB, even more so than the admission of the persecutions to which Stalin subjected several leaders of the international communist movement.[89] Years of reflection and perplexity followed for Communist intellectuals and militants, along with turmoil for the PCB, which resulted in the loss of many militants and the overhaul of its strategies by the late 1950s.[90]

Throughout these changes, Pessoa remained a member of the PCB, and even paid tribute to Stalin in 1953 as "one of the greatest men of the century." However, he began to show some signs of discomfort with Stalinism after 1956–1957, reflecting the impact of Khrushchev's report. There was a heated internal debate about the report within the PCB, which ended with Secretary-General Prestes's affirmation of the leadership role of the USSR in international communism and the approval of the expulsion from the party of historical leaders considered treasonous toward the cause of the socialist revolution.[91] The report led a growing number of Communist intellectuals, including the famous writer Jorge Amado, to leave the PCB or to distance themselves from it.[92] Pessoa did not join them and never openly criticized the party, but he became a frequent contributor to the prestigious leftist journal *Brasiliense*, directed by the Marxist historian Caio Prado Jr., which circulated between 1955 and 1964 and kept an editorial line independent of the PCB's leadership and orientation. There, Pessoa wrote about his favorite themes: agrarian reform and the relation between poverty, hunger, and rural endemic diseases.[93]

Another indication of his growing distance from the USSR was his enthusiasm for China, especially after a two-month trip in 1958 to attend a congress in Shanghai, followed by a visit to rural health services established to address endemic diseases. Upon his return, Pessoa gave public talks, some at the Sino-Brazilian Cultural Society, and published articles on the Chinese experience in combating rural endemic diseases, especially schistosomiasis.[94] He also wrote about acupuncture, having become acquainted with, and even undergone, acupuncture treatment during his Chinese sojourn. He believed that Brazil had much to learn from the rural health initiatives of the "New China," which became an alternative model to that of the USSR for some Brazilian Communists in the early 1960s.[95] Yet Pessoa never left the PCB, even when it splintered in 1962 with the founding of a new, Maoist-inspired party. In fact, despite the Sino-Soviet split, complete by the mid-1960s, Pessoa maintained his alignment with the Soviet Union.

Important domestic transformations were underway at the time, including the rise of the national-developmentalist ideology, the acceleration of industrialization, the construction of Brasilia (the new capital in central Brazil), and the achievement of a period of democratic stability during Juscelino Kubitschek's administration (1956–1961). Although, as a candidate, Kubitschek had supported a policy of persecution of the PCB, as president, he relented. The party gave up on its strategy of open confrontation in 1958 and embraced a call for structural reforms and a broad class alliance as the path to socialism.[96] Seeking to broaden its bases and become legalized, the party also changed its name to the Brazilian Communist Party in 1961. International developments also had repercussions locally, especially Kubitschek's proposal for a renegotiation of Latin America's development and economic relations with the United States (Operation Pan America), the Cuban Revolution, and the 1961 launch of the Alliance for Progress by U.S. president John F. Kennedy. In the public health field, the Kubitschek administration placed new emphasis on the control and eradication of rural endemic diseases, unifying previously dispersed services within a single department.[97] Although concerned that these policies did not aim to alter discriminatory/oppressive social structures, Pessoa collaborated with the new department.[98]

The late 1950s and early 1960s also witnessed the intensification of agrarian conflicts and the formation of rural trade unions and peasant movements, such as the Peasant Leagues, particularly in the Brazilian Northeast.[99] The demand for land reform was at the core of the political struggle beleaguering the leftist government of João Goulart (1961–1964) and contributed significantly to the civilian-military coup of March 31, 1964. During these dramatic years of rising social conflict in rural areas, Pessoa insisted publicly that the challenges facing Brazilian society were long-standing and profound, requiring agrarian reform and improvement of the health conditions of rural populations. Forty years had elapsed since his first contact with parasites and with rural workers under the auspices of the RF, twenty of which he had spent as a militant Communist forging his interpretation about the relations between parasitism and capitalism.

The U.S.-backed and strongly anticommunist military dictatorship that began in April 1964 quickly began to persecute trade-union leaders, politicians, intellectuals, and scientists who supported progressive positions, expressed any kind of opposition, or had been connected with the deposed government. It was a new phase of the Cold War in Brazil and in Latin America. The repression hit Brazilian universities with a vengeance. The USP School of Medicine was especially singled out, with the Department of Parasitology suffering the most, as it was considered a "red department," gravitating around Emeritus Professor Samuel Pessoa. Between 1964 and 1969, several department members lost their jobs or were forced to retire, were arrested, and were even pushed into exile.[100] Pessoa, his students, and his collaborators were included in the first purge.[101]

The institutional mood at the USP became marred by suspicion. Almost immediately after the coup, Pessoa was subjected to a military police inquiry for his "subversive" activities, a precursor to the brutal and humiliating interrogation and brief detention he would experience a decade later. At sixty-six years of age, disgusted with what he had experienced at the USP, he vowed never again to set foot in the School of Medicine, a promise he kept. During the last decade of his life, he and his wife continued to defend their political beliefs and fight against the authoritarian regime to the extent possible. He signed, for example, various manifestos of intellectuals and artists against censorship and in support of freedom of the press. He and his wife also reportedly gave shelter to people the dictatorship was pursuing, allegedly because of their involvement in the armed struggle against the government.

The scientific and political career of Samuel Barnsley Pessoa illustrates, in all its aspects, the dynamics of the Cold War and its bitter anticommunism in the Brazilian context, particularly in the fields of medicine and public health. Pessoa's scientific training and passion for agrarian reform were marked by both nationalism and communism, as was the case for a generation of intellectuals, doctors, scientists, and teachers in Brazil and in other Latin America countries in the post–World War II period. It was a generation besieged by authoritarian regimes that were backed by the United States from the 1960s into the 1980s.

After his ouster from the USP and until his death, Pessoa held a meager post at the Butantan Institute, a São Paulo state institution specializing in the production of antivenom, where he carried out research on snake parasites. When friends and followers asked about his decision to study snakes after fifty years working on the gravest parasitic diseases afflicting the rural population of Brazil, Pessoa replied that snake parasites did not cause lawsuits or imprisonment, but "people parasites" did.

Notes

Gilberto Hochman is grateful for a grant-in-aid from the Rockefeller Archive Center and for a fellowship from the National Council for Scientific and Technological Development–CNPq.

1   Founded in 1922, the PCB enjoyed only a few brief years of legal existence in the 1920s and again between 1945 and 1947. In 1975 and 1976, having practically exterminated the guerrilla organizations, the government turned to the elimination

of PCB leaders although the party had not waged an armed struggle against the military regime. For a general history of the PCB, see Chilcote, *Partido Comunista Brasileiro*; Rodrigues, "PCB"; Pandolfi, *Camaradas e Companheiros*.

2   The details of Pessoa's arrest are described in the petition filed by his lawyer, Hélio Navarro, on March 4, 1975, to a military tribunal requesting information regarding his whereabouts and the reasons for his detention. Document on loan from the Samuel Barnsley Pessoa family.

3   For example, in *Folha de São Paulo*, September 4, 1976, 19.

4   On the complex overlap between professional biomedical debates and the Cold War, see also Lambe's chapter in this volume. Studies on the history of health during the Cold War in Brazil have concentrated on the North American influence on models of health care, with special emphasis on the Special Public Health Service or the RF's financing of biomedical research. See, for example, Campos, *Políticas Internacionais de Saúde na Era Vargas*. For Rockefeller funding, see Marinho, *Norte-Americanos no Brasil*; Hochman, "From Autonomy to Partial Alignment."

5   Among the most prestigious are Ruth and Victor Nussenzweig, Luiz Hildebrando Pereira da Silva, Maria and Leonidas Deane, Luiz Rey, Michel Rabinovitch, Thomas Maack, and Erney Plessman de Camargo. See also the testimonial essays accompanying the second edition of Pessoa's *Ensaios Médico-Sociais* (1978); "Entrevista da Editoria da Revista Brasileira."

6   Among these, see Czeresnia and Ribeiro, "Conceito de Espaço em Epidemiologia"; Paiva, "Samuel Pessoa"; Mello, "Pensamento Clássico da Saúde Pública Paulista."

7   Andrade, *Físicos, Mésons e Política*.

8   For example, Limongi, "Marxismo, Nacionalismo e Cultura"; Feltrim, "Perseguição da Delegacia de Ordem Política."

9   See Pessoa, *Ensaios Médico-Sociais* (1978), 53–81.

10 Faria, *Saúde e Política*; Santos, "Reforma Sanitária 'Pelo Alto.'"

11 See biographical files of Samuel B. Pessoa for 1922–1932, available at the Rockefeller Archive Center (RAC), Sleepy Hollow, NY.

12 Marinho, *Norte-Americanos no Brasil*.

13 Lima and Hochman, "Condenado pela Raça."

14 Pessoa, "Estudo dos Componentes de Oleo Essencial de Quenopódio."

15 Palmer, "Toward Responsibility in International Health"; Rita Marques, "Filantropia Científica nos Tempos da Romanização." See also Smillie and Pessoa, "Treatment of Hookworm Disease."

16 See, for example, his interview in *O Bisturi, São Paulo* 22, 72 (1955): 5.

17 Lewis Hackett to Samuel Pessoa, May 19, 1922, in *Memorial apresentado pelo Dr. Samuel Barnsley Pessoa à Congregação da Faculdade de Medicina de São Paulo por Ocasião do Concurso da Cátedra de Parasitologia, 1931*. The RAC records show that the RF followed Pessoa's career closely until the 1950s. See RF/RG 10.2 Fellowship Cards, box MNS, Folder Brazil, Pessoa, Samuel B.

18 On public health in Yugoslavia at the time, see Dugac, "Like Yeast in Fermentation."

19 *Diário Nacional de São Paulo*, May 27, 1928, 4.

20 See, for example, Pessoa's 1969 address, "Conferência de Agradecimento ao Título de Professor Honoris Causa da Universidade Federal de Goiás," in *Ensaios Médico-Sociais* (1978), 304–9.

21 Hochman, "Cambio Político y Reformas."

22 Pessoa's file states, "Fellowship rescinded; Unable to take advantage of fship" (October 19, 1931), as well as "[Pessoa] cannot accept fship this year, due to local political situation" (January 21, 1931), RAC, RF/RG 10.2 Fellowship Cards, box MNS, folder Brazil, Pessoa, Samuel B.

23 "Discurso Proferido pelo Prof. Samuel B. Pessoa ao Paraninfar os Doutorandos de 1940," *Separata da Revista de Medicina* 41 (1941): 14, reprinted in Pessoa, *Ensaios Médico-Sociais* (1978), 238–50.

24 Pessoa, "Verminoses na Zona Rural."

25 Adhemar de Barros studied at the same elite high school as Pessoa. The newspaper *Correio Paulistano* reported visits by Pessoa to the Bandeirantes Palace (the state seat of government) before these tensions and cited alumni meetings of the Colégio Anglo-Americano, attended by both Barros and Pessoa. As coincidence would have it, Barros, as governor of São Paulo (1963–1966) during a subsequent military dictatorship, would become the tormentor of Samuel Pessoa and of many USP professors who were dismissed for activities deemed subversive.

26 Paiva, "Samuel Pessoa."

27 Pessoa, "Discurso Proferido," 11.

28 Expression coined by Arthur Neiva, one of the most important physicians and health leaders in São Paulo in the 1910s.

29 Pessoa, "Discurso Proferido," 12.

30 In an interview with the magazine *Piauí* (40 [January 2010]), Pessoa's grandson, the artist Nuno Ramos, recalls that Coca-Cola was banned at his grandfather's house, that the Brazilian translation of the song "Happy Birthday" could be sung only if followed by a Brazilian song, and that only Brazilian plants and trees were grown in the garden. On the imperative to improve health conditions in rural areas, see also Anderson's and Bliss's chapters in this volume.

31 Lima and Hochman, "Condenado pela Raça."

32 Pessoa, "Discurso Proferido," 11. Belisário Penna, leader of the movement for rural health at the end of the 1910s, also accused rural landowners of this, though in a less elaborate manner. See Hochman, *Sanitation of Brazil*, chapter 2.

33 Pessoa, "Discurso Proferido," 13.

34 Pessoa, "Discurso Proferido," 17. Tegumentary leishmaniasis was endemic in the interior of the state of São Paulo.

35 Pessoa, "Discurso Proferido."

36 Lima and Maio, "Ciências Sociais e Educação Sanitária"; Maio, "Projeto Unesco."

37 Pessoa, "Discurso Proferido," 16.

38 "Discurso de Inauguração do Novo Prédio," 6. It was during this period (1942–1944) that Pessoa published the bulk of the articles he would write on malaria.

39 Pessoa's file at the State Department of Political and Social Order (DEOPS) at the Public Archives of Rio de Janeiro, includes an annotation, likely taken from his

biography when he ran for federal congressman in 1945: "In 1940 he made a famous speech, of a populist and socialist slant, due to which he became a victim of persecution. From that time onwards, he became closer to the PCB." This is the most telling evidence that Pessoa's adherence to communism dates from around 1940.

40 See newspaper clippings in the Samuel Barnsley Pessoa Papers, Centro de Apoio à Pesquisa em História, Departamento de História, USP.

41 Rodrigues, "PCB."

42 Ridenti, "Brasilidade Vermelha." On the political trajectory of the PCB between 1943 and 1964, see Segatto, "PCB."

43 Pessoa, *Parasitologia Médica*. Editions from the mid-1970s on were coauthored with Amilcar Vianna Martins, a leading parasitologist from the state of Minas Gerais and leader of what was to become the Minas Gerais School of Parasitology. Martins, also affiliated with the PCB, was forced to retire by the military regime.

44 Pessoa was the PCB's seventeenth-most-voted candidate, with 3,003 votes in his state of São Paulo, which sent four PCB deputies to the National Assembly.

45 Feltrim, "Perseguição da Delegacia de Ordem Política e Social"; Oliveira, "Vigilância do DOPS-SP." The archives of the DEOPS, in the Public Archives of São Paulo contain, as of 2010, extensive documentation about the surveillance of individuals considered to be Communist in the 1950s, including Samuel and Jovina Pessoa and other USP professors and scientists.

46 Krementsov, *Cure*.

47 Nussenzweig and Nussenzweig, "Cura do Câncer."

48 Pessoa, *Problemas Brasileiros de Higiene Rural*.

49 Pessoa, *Problemas Brasileiros de Higiene Rural*, 537.

50 Pessoa, *Problemas Brasileiros de Higiene Rural*, 539–46.

51 Willems as cited by Pessoa, *Problemas Brasileiros de Higiene Rural*, 548.

52 Pessoa, *Problemas Brasileiros de Higiene Rural*, 548. The term *caboclo* refers to a type of mestizo peasant from the Brazilian hinterland.

53 Pessoa is probably referring to Manoel José Ferreira, who also worked for the International Health Division (renamed in 1927) in the campaign against *Anopheles gambiae* in the Brazilian Northeast (1938–1940).

54 Pessoa, "Medicina Rural e Socialização da Medicina," in *Ensaios Médico-Sociais* (1960), originally published in *Revista Paulista de Medicina* 39 (1951). This more radical article was not reprinted in the 1978 edition of *Ensaios Médico-Sociais*. The Special Public Health Service was created as a bilateral agency following the 1942 Brazil–United States Washington Accords. See Campos, *Políticas Internacionais de Saúde na Era Vargas*.

55 Pessoa, "Pauperismo, Subnutrição e Verminoses Intestinais no Nordeste Brasileiro," in *Ensaios Médico-Sociais* (1960), 201–2. This article was not included in the 1978 edition. It was originally published in 1958 in the Marxist-oriented *Brasiliense* journal. See Limongi, "Marxismo, Nacionalismo e Cultura."

56 Hochman, "From Autonomy to Partial Alignment"; Farley, *To Cast Out Disease*, especially chapters 16 and 17.

57 Pessoa, "Medicina Rural e Socialização da Medicina."

58 Pessoa, "Medicina Rural e Socialização da Medicina," 191–92.

59 Kinoshita, "Organização Comunista na América Latina."

60 Ribeiro, "Combatentes da Paz." In its September 30, 1950, issue, p. 10, the journal *A Voz Operária* announced that two million signatures had been collected.

61 See Pessoa's "Consequências Médicas das Explosões Atômicas" (lecture given in April 1955 and published in 1956), in *Ensaios Médico-Sociais* (1960), 215–40.

62 See documents now available in the state branches of the secret police (DEOPS) in the Public Archives of São Paulo and Rio de Janeiro.

63 Invitation letters dated May 8, 10, 1952, are in the Samuel Barnsley Pessoa Papers, Centro de Apoio à Pesquisa em História, Departamento de História, USP.

64 See Pessoa's "A Guerra Bacteriológica e o Congresso dos Povos pela Paz," in *Estudos Médico-Sociais* (1978), 325. The *Report of the International Scientific Commission for the Investigation of the Facts Concerning Bacterial Warfare in Korea and China* (Beijing, August 31, 1952) concluded that "the peoples of Korea and China have indeed been the target of bacteriological weapons. These have been employed by units of USA armed forces" (124).

65 On Needham's role, see Buchanan, "Courage of Galileo." On the lawsuits filed against American citizens who reported and supported the conclusions of the ISC, see Neil O'Brien, *American Editor in Early Revolutionary China*. On the HUAC hearings on the ISC, see U.S. Congress, *Hearings before the Committee on Un-American Activities*.

66 See, for example, the spat between Endicott and Hagerman, authors of *The United States and Biological Warfare*, in Leitenberg, "False Allegations of U.S. Biological Weapons Use."

67 *A Voz Operária*, September 27, 1952, 1; *Imprensa Popular*, September 15, 1952, 1 and 3.

68 *Imprensa Popular*, October 10, 1952, 1.

69 *A Voz Operária*, October 10, 1952, 4.

70 *A Voz Operária*, September 27, 1952, 4.

71 Luiz Hildebrando Pereira da Silva, "Samuel," in Pessoa, *Ensaios Médico-Sociais* (1978): 23–27.

72 *O Correio da Manhã*, September 17, 1952, 4.

73 *O Correio da Manhã*, July 24, 1953, 2.

74 *O Globo*, September 24, 1952, 1, 9.

75 *Imprensa Popular*, November 2, 1952, 1. The newspaper protested this summons.

76 "Nossa Política: As Resoluções de Viena, Instrumento de Luta pela Paz e a Independência Nacional," an editorial written on the Vienna Congress, published in the PCB journal *Problemas-Revista Mensal de Cultura Política* 44 (January–February 1953): n.p.

77 See "Falando Perante 2000 Representantes de 80 Países no Congresso de Viena," 5. Broader repercussions of the Vienna Congress were overshadowed by the death of Josef Stalin in March 1953.

78 U.S. Congress, *United States House Select Committee to Investigate Tax-Exempt Foundations*.

79 Mueller, "Rockefeller Foundation." For an early critical view of the activities of the commission in 1954, see Gideonse, "Congressional Committee's Investigation of the Foundations."

80 Mueller, "Rockefeller Foundation," 120. During this period, Rockefeller employees were obliged to check the political and ideological background of applicants for grants and funding.

81 Robert Briggs Watson to John C. Bugher, October 1955, in Pessoa's Fellowship Card, RAC/RF/RG 10.2 Fellowship Cards, box MNS, folder Brazil, Pessoa.

82 Declarations by Luiz Rey and Luiz Hildebrando Pereira da Silva, in Pessoa, *Ensaios Médico-Sociais* (1978).

83 *Diário de São Paulo*, May 10, 1944, newspaper clipping in the Samuel Barnsley Pessoa File, Centro de Apoio à Pesquisa em História, Departamento de História, USP.

84 The position had been held by renowned parasitologist Amilcar Vianna Martins, who was leaving to direct the Institute of Rural Endemic Diseases of the Ministry of Health during the Juscelino Kubitschek administration (1956–1961).

85 Robert Briggs Watson to John C. Bugher, October 1955, in RAC/RF/RG 10.2 Fellowship Cards, box MNS, folder Brazil, Pessoa, Samuel B.

86 "The President's Review," in Rockefeller Foundation, *Annual Report, 1953*, 27.

87 RAC/RF/RG 10.2 Fellowship Cards, box MNS, folder Brazil, Pessoa, Samuel B. See also Marinho, *Norte-Americanos no Brasil*.

88 *O Correio da Manhã*, December 19, 1958, 2.

89 On February 25, 1956, Soviet leader Nikita Khrushchev gave a "private" speech decrying Stalinism at the twentieth Congress of the Communist Party of the Soviet Union. The speech, "On the Cult of Personality and Its Consequences," was leaked and by June was published in the *New York Times*; its contents rapidly became widely known.

90 Fernando Silva and Santana, "Equilibrista e a Política."

91 Fernando Silva and Santana, "Equilibrista e a Política."

92 *Imprensa Popular*, March 15, 1953, 3.

93 The main collaborators to *Brasiliense* were not part of the political core of the PCB. Pessoa was one of the most frequent contributors to the journal, with twelve works in ten years, according to Limongi, "Marxismo, Nacionalismo e Cultura."

94 See document (OS) 1930 vol. 28–A. 10/10/1958, "Relatório: Informação Reservada sobre Reunião Cultural Sino-Brasileira," Acervo Arquivo do Estado de São Paulo, Projeto Violência Institucional e Autocracia de Estado.

95 Pessoa, "A Luta contra as Endemias Parasitárias na Nova China," and "A Acupuntura (Método Chinês de Tratamento de Doenças)," in Pessoa, *Ensaios Médico-Sociais* (1960): 267–84, 285–96.

96 Between 1958 and 1964, communism was legalized de facto. See Fernando Silva and Santana, "Equilibrista e a Política," 124.

97 Hochman, "Brasil Não é Só Doença."

98 In his 1963 book, *Endemias Parasitárias da Zona Rural Brasileira*, Pessoa even praised the work of Brazilian sanitarian Mário Pinotti, minister of health during the Kubitschek government (1958-1960).

99 Montenegro, "Ligas Camponesas e Sindicatos Rurais."

100 Hochman, "Vigiar e, Depois de 1964, Punir."

101 Motta, *As Universidades e o Regime Militar*.

6

Revolutionizing Cuban Psychiatry

The Freud Wars, 1955–1970

JENNIFER LYNN LAMBE

"We have to respect that Freudian anachronism somehow," psychiatrist Gregorio Rivera Núñez informed his colleagues at a July 1966 meeting at the Hospital Psiquiátrico de La Habana. "Freud," he said, "is like those stars that are already opaque—dead for a century—but we still see their light on earth."[1] Rivera offered this grudging defense of Freud in response to a discussion that had broken out at the hospital. Following his presentation on the clinical study of anxiety, several of his colleagues, dismayed at the guest appearance of Freud in Rivera's summary of the topic, had bemoaned the persistence of psychoanalytic errors in the field. Edmundo Gutiérrez Agramonte, a leading psychiatrist at the hospital, pleaded with his colleagues to jettison psychoanalytic Freudian fictions and adopt responsible Pavlovian views. Responding to his concerns, Rivera agreed that Freud was an anachronism, but one that necessarily endured. After all, he argued with a curious Marxist flourish, wasn't Freud the "dialectical base" of the "process" that his work had initiated?[2]

During the 1960s, debates about Freud were standard fodder in meetings and presentations at the Hospital Psiquiátrico. The facility was the heir to the nation's notorious mental asylum, popularly known as Mazorra. In January 1959, Dr. Eduardo Bernabé Ordaz, an anesthesiologist and comrade of Fidel Castro in the revolutionary struggles of the *sierra*, was appointed by Castro to run the hospital and undertake a monumental rebuilding effort there. Mazorra's post-1959 reconstruction was emblematic of a new age in Cuban psychiatry that exalted scientific commitment and humanitarian principles. Nevertheless, early formulations of a revolutionary psychiatry were more oriented to rebuilding hospitals and reaching beyond the bounds of the discipline than driving Freud out of the picture. Psychiatric and revolutionary discourses passed through a period of vigorous cross-pollination that, in these early years, drew few doctrinal lines around efforts to forge the revolutionary "New Man."

By 1963, however, theoretical questions had moved into the foreground of conversations among Cuban psychiatrists. At the crux of over a decade of debate was the Freud-Pavlov polemic, which buttressed efforts to establish a psychiatry that was both scientific and revolutionary. Throughout the 1960s and 1970s, these battles would reorient the mind sciences in Cuba to the work of Ivan Pavlov, the Russian physiologist famous for his experiments with conditioning in dogs. Decades earlier, Pavlov had been centered in orthodox formulations of Soviet science, and this was an example that a group of Cuban psychiatrists pushed their colleagues to follow. Relatively quickly, their campaign led to the disappearance of orthodox psychoanalytic practice from the island, as those Freudians who remained in Cuba began to assimilate other theoretical and methodological approaches.[3] It would be another decade before a renewed opening for Freud emerged as a result of dialogue with Latin American and international colleagues.

Much to the chagrin of Pavlov's Cuban partisans, however, psychological perspectives—and even a few orthodox Freudians—stubbornly hung on. Advocates of the new Sovietized psychiatry found themselves running up against the so-called eclecticism of their colleagues, who, long accustomed to adapting foreign psychiatric theory, did not afford different treatment to orthodox Pavlovianism. As I examine, some continued to utilize psychodynamic techniques and perspectives that retained the most useful elements of Freudianism while discarding those that did not fit their professional and political realities. Even as the psychiatric profession retreated from the Freudian barricades, at least in name, an unorthodox mélange of psychodynamic concepts and logic infused the project to create a revolutionary subject throughout the 1960s. Revolutionary psychiatry could officially jettison Freud, but his imprint would remain.

Cuba's Freud-Pavlov debates thus represent an illustrative node in a broader geography of Cold War intellectual exchange. Across geographical and political contexts, science and medicine assumed a heightened political status as symbols of national supremacy and even ideological apotheosis. Governments East and West, not to mention North and South, dedicated unprecedented funds and institutional support to research in the service of national defense. In this context, scientists and doctors increasingly strayed beyond their laboratories and clinics, embracing the patronage of the state and the resulting politicization of their work. That urgency was felt in a particularly acute way in the countries most directly implicated in macropolitical struggles of the period, not only the United States and the Soviet Union, but Cuba, too, where the revolutionary government magnified and hyperbolized the nationalist implications long attached to science and medicine.[4] In Cuba, as in other "Global South" countries, the Cold War knowledge race would intersect in dramatic ways with the domestic imperative for scientific and economic development.

When compared to the military-academic-industrial complex, theoretical debates over two long-dead scientists might seem arcane, to say the least. Yet the Freud-Pavlov polemic took on ideological significance well beyond its limited therapeutic consequences. These debates manifested a clear theatrical spirit, as well as a ritual function: to purge Cuban psychiatry of its alleged bourgeois trappings in preparation for an imminent socialist future. Absent direct pressure from revolutionary officials, leaders of the field hoped to parlay self-purification into vanguard status; "we Stalinized ourselves," as one practitioner told me. They did so, nonetheless, in a context of widespread self-policing and intolerance for political inconformity, a deliberately cultivated strategy of revolutionary officials.[5]

The energy devoted to theoretical difference might suggest rigid political lines. Strikingly, however, the Freud-Pavlov divide was never as absolute as psychiatric leaders wished to depict it. By foregrounding change and continuity within the Cuban psychiatric field, I hope to reorient attention to the messy, often conflicted, nature of the revolutionary project during its tumultuous first decade. This snapshot of intellectual evolution in process exposes the halting and hybrid path that it could take, even in politically explosive circumstances. Theoretical eclecticism might thus represent a de facto challenge to hardened divides between Freudian and Pavlovian, capitalist and Marxist, U.S. and Soviet. While the eventual waning of Freud highlights the force behind Pavlov, the intellectual path to that endpoint suggests a more complicated reality: the inconsistencies in the very notion of ideological incompatibility.

Yet these theoretical battles also reflect back onto the political context in which they emerged. Politicization has long been something of a dirty word in medicine, including in Cuba, where in prerevolutionary times it was associated with widespread corruption in public health administration. Generation after generation of reformers thus returned to the fundamental imperative to separate medicine and politics, even as many of them were swept up in political mobilization.[6] Elsewhere, medical and scientific practitioners attempted to shield themselves through dutiful empiricism and practiced objectivity, even as objectivity itself became a politicized Cold War object. In revolutionary Cuba, however, scientificity *and* politicization were presumed to evolve in concert.

The scientific vanguard here met the political one with mutually aggrandizing effects, as Cuban psychiatrists sought to enact their professional relevance and scientific authority in a new revolutionary moment.

Pavlov and the Soviets

The historic confrontation between psychoanalysis and Marxism-Leninism has been neither static nor uniform, and its eventual collision with the Cuban Revolution was far from inevitable.[7] The framework for arguments about Freud had been established in the Soviet Union during the decades following the Bolshevik Revolution, and Soviet interlocutors made frequent appearances in Cuban conversations on this question. In the 1960s and 1970s, many Cuban psychiatrists, guided by official pronouncements and pressure, determined that Pavlovianism was the most scientific and Marxist approach to the study of the mind. Freud, in contrast, was responsible for theoretical mystifications and political abominations. The Pavlovian approach, as had been established in the Soviet Union, was exalted for its orientation to laboratory experimentation and its political compatibility with dialectical materialism, which framed the relationship between human beings and the world around them as one of direct reflection rather than unconscious mediation.

On the most fundamental level, the Freud-Pavlov wars of the 1960s dramatized a long-standing tension within the psychiatric field between what can be characterized as *functional* and *organic* perspectives. Functional understandings highlight the psychological or emotional roots of mental pathology. Organic paradigms, on the other hand, point to underlying somatic or biological causes. These framings—often abbreviated as "psyche" versus "soma"—have carried important implications for treatment as well. While psychotherapy (and, within that, psychoanalysis) would be the classic example of a functional approach, somatic therapeutics have varied widely over the course of the last three centuries, from bloodletting and purging to the so-called "shock therapies" and psychopharmaceuticals. These different understandings of the relationship between mind and body have also provoked acrimonious debate within the field of psychiatry, particularly beginning in the late nineteenth century. The rise of neurology in this period sparked heightened enthusiasm for the organic understanding of mental illness as rooted in biological causes. The later development of radical somatic treatments for mental illness, such as insulin therapy, electroshock therapy, and psychosurgery, would endow this framework with renewed legitimacy within the psychiatric field.[8]

In the late nineteenth and early twentieth centuries, the work of Russian physiologist Ivan Pavlov had offered a novel variation on the organic view of mental functioning. Grounded in the Russian neurological tradition, Pavlov's famous experiments on laboratory dogs, in which he succeeded in inducing salivation after associating the sound of a bell with food, led him to the notion of the "conditional reflex." According to Pavlov, the conditional reflex would form in the newest parts of the brain, which had evolved throughout human history to encompass "lower" and "higher" zones. Brain reflexes, he argued, function on several levels of increasing complexity as a response to "excitation" and "inhibition" from the outside world. Essentially, however, all mental activity responds to a physiological prompt. The theoretical camp that follows Pavlovian thinking on mental functioning is known as the "reflexological" school.[9]

On the other hand, the functional view of mental illness also received a boost in the late nineteenth century with the rise of psychoanalysis. Psychodynamic approaches, in which emphasis was placed on internal psychological conflict, predated "talk therapy" by many decades, if not centuries.[10] But Freud was among the first to offer a synthetic vision of the "dynamic" interaction between conscious and unconscious forces and emotions. The consolidation of psychoanalysis would propel the establishment of multiple schools and techniques within the fields of both psychiatry and psychology, many of which departed from the tenets of orthodox psychoanalysis.[11]

The back-and-forth between these two conceptions of mental function guided the evolution of psychiatry throughout the twentieth century. In practice, however, few psychiatrists were as theoretically exclusivist as this distinction might imply. Everyday clinical practice often demanded a more expansive therapeutic approach, which reached to both psychological and biological theories of mind. Yet the importance ascribed to these battles stretched well beyond the medical domain. Both in Cuba and beyond, mental health practitioners took up the "psyche versus soma" problematic in order to make *political* interventions as well. As we will see, the very terminology associated with this divide was thus not always deployed in a scientifically consistent or obvious way.

Indeed, the intellectual split between organic and functional schools of psychiatry had acquired broader political significance in the aftermath of the 1917 Bolshevik Revolution. The early 1920s actually represented a period of growth for psychoanalysis in Russia, with the founding of the Russian Psychoanalytic Society and the Moscow Institute. As Martin Miller has argued, this receptiveness correlated with the experimental spirit of the Lenin years and the New Economic Policy. Soviet officials and psychoanalysts, however, had also discovered that they shared intellectual and social interests in the fields of child psychology and pedagogy. These tensions led to a strange paradox: Russia's psychoanalysts, belatedly admitted to the international community of Freudians, belonged to the only state-financed psychoanalytic field in the world. Though it remained subject to the whims of the state vis-à-vis its project to establish a "Marxist psychology," Soviet psychoanalysis pursued a number of routes to rapprochement between Marxism and Freudianism in the early 1920s, the most interesting of which regarded them as complementary systems of thought.[12]

By 1928, however, psychoanalysis had come under attack in the Soviet Union, as Stalin's rise brought ideological experimentation to a halt. At the 1930 Congress for Human Behavior, psychoanalysis was branded bourgeois, "cosmopolitan," and anti-Soviet.[13] If Soviet psychiatrists had previously dreamed of mobilizing their expertise to create the society conjured up by the Bolshevik Revolution, henceforth their role would be significantly curtailed.[14] The year 1936 also marked the death of Pavlov himself and the subsequent officialization of the "dialectical materialist" vision of the mind, in which mental processes were understood to be dependent not only on bodily functions but also—critically—on social context or, more precisely, class conflict.[15] After the Communist Party reined in the psychiatric field in 1936, Pavlovianism remained the official scientific doctrine in the Soviet Union, in spite of Pavlov's own opposition to communism.[16] The 1951 "Pavlov Session" represented the high point of this Pavlovian orthodoxy, as psychiatrists, like physiologists before them, exhorted themselves and their colleagues to adopt responsible Pavlovian views.

New work on the Pavlovian orthodoxy has nonetheless offered a more bounded view of its reach, stressing the possibility for varied interpretations in practice, as well as the determining role of local context in shaping its spread throughout the Soviet Union.[17] This drama, as it played out under Stalin during the most repressive years of Soviet history, prefigured the theoretical and political conflicts that would surface in the Latin American Cold War. In places like Argentina, Brazil, and Chile, psychoanalysis would be pulled in divergent political directions, sometimes appropriated by authoritarian governments of the right to naturalize conservative values, other times claimed by the activist left as a "revolutionary tool," what Mariano Ben Plotkin refers to as a "complement for politics, an instrument to make sense of it, and a way to articulate the public and the private dimensions of the self."[18] As Jane A. Russo argues, that "plasticity" inhered in psychoanalysis; diverse groups had long found it to be "reasonably adaptable and capable of harboring a good measure of political ambiguity."[19] In 1970s South America, there was notable expansion of a "psy" culture in the seemingly unpropitious context of authoritarian dictatorship, even as psychoanalysis also became an important touchstone for some members of the organized left.

In many ways Cuba represents a dramatically different case: one of the only successful revolutionary governments to prevail during the Cold War in spite of the most aggressive opposition of the United States. How would psychoanalysis, then, evolve in response to revolutionary governance? Given the ideological and political proximity of the Soviet example, one might imagine the straightforward implantation of Pavlovian models, as Soviet psychiatrists traveled to Cuba to offer Pavlovian instruction and Cubans in turn journeyed to the Eastern Bloc to witness Soviet psychiatric practice for themselves. Promoting Pavlov, however, was not a simple matter. Though many psychiatrists of an organicist bent welcomed reflexological perspectives even before 1959, others presented psychoanalytic objections to the Soviet advance. On one hand, a tradition of therapeutic and theoretical openness among Cuban mental health professionals—what Pavlovians would denounce as "eclecticism"—rendered unilateral approaches unappealing for some. A venerable strand of psychodynamic thinking in Cuban psychiatry also guaranteed that Soviet predominance would not come easily. Particularly troublesome, in fact, was the recent arrival of formal psychoanalysis to Cuban shores.

Freud in the Tropics

On the eve of revolution, the Cuban psychoanalytic field was mostly incipient. A narrow focus on orthodox psychoanalysis, however, obscures a broader climate of interest that preceded its consolidation by several decades. Though many early twentieth-century Cuban psychiatrists had at least a passing familiarity with psychoanalysis, the most sustained attention germinated at the intersection of the fields of pedagogy, psychology, and mental hygiene, and it tended to be more theoretical than practice-oriented. By the late 1920s, some Havana psychiatrists had adopted a more serious attitude toward the study of Freud, though their orientation was far from exclusivist.[20] A variety of non-Freudian psychodynamic theories and psychological tests, particularly the Rorschach, which featured ambiguous images to be analyzed by the patient, also proved influential later on.[21] Among a small but influential cohort of Cuban psychologists, interest in psychoanalysis had also become well established across the political spectrum.[22]

By the 1940s and 1950s, attention to psychoanalysis within the "psy" disciplines was matched by Freudian enthusiasm among Havana's better-heeled classes, as reflected in psychiatrists' complaints about the patients who stormed their private practices complaining of Oedipal complexes. While the cost and duration of analysis limited its appeal to a broader spectrum of Cuban society, politically inclined psychologists like Juan Guevara Valdés had already undertaken efforts to expand access before 1959.[23] Popular middle-class magazines like *Bohemia* and *Carteles*, which had long covered the basic tenets of Freudianism, also fomented popular psychoanalytic consciousness, though more extensive coverage was afforded to organicist developments. The attraction of psychoanalysis as an emblem of modernity for the upper-middle classes was, nonetheless, mitigated in some cases by their Catholic faith, as manifested by the rise of an anti-Freudian cohort of Catholic psychiatrists.

At the same moment, interest in Freudianism within psychiatry prompted initial forays into analytic training, often through the intellectual and touristic circuits linking Cuba to the United States, Europe, and other parts of Latin America. Finally, in the late 1940s, Italian psychoanalyst Spartaco Scarizza, a graduate of the University of Bologna, turned up in Cuba.[24] After arriving in Havana, Scarizza contacted the Colegio Médico Nacional to request permission to practice and teach psychoanalysis in Cuba.[25] Several of Havana's most prominent psychiatrists entered analysis with Scarizza shortly thereafter.

The expanding interest in psychoanalysis coincided with the first efforts to organize within the psychiatric profession along doctrinal lines. The Sociedad Cubana de Psicoterapia, founded in 1951 with José Angel Bustamante as its first president, brought together thirteen Havana psychiatrists interested in a psychodynamic approach, and the group met regularly to host presentations and discussions.[26] Bustamante then traveled to London to call on Ernest Jones, Freud's British ally and biographer. With his support, they solicited the help of Leo Bartemeier, an influential U.S. psychoanalyst. Bartemeier, a devout Catholic who had sought and received Pope Pius XII's blessing to assume the presidency of the International Psychoanalytical Association (IPA), subsequently presented biyearly seminars while on vacation with his family in Cuba.[27] With Bartemeier's backing, the Cuban contingent was officially recognized as a Psychoanalytic Study Group at the 1955 Congress of the IPA in Geneva.[28] Finally, another faction of seventeen psychiatrists, again presided over by Bustamante, established the Sociedad Psicoanalítica Cubana in 1955.[29] In the same year, the Sociedad Cubana de Psicoterapia kicked off a psychoanalytic seminar series with a lecture on the unconscious by Scarizza.[30] Meanwhile, a separate group of the psychoanalytically inclined had congregated those psychiatrists who had received analytic training outside Cuba, some through direct engagement with Anna Freud.[31]

In practice, however, even Cuba's most psychoanalytically inclined psychiatrists were broad reaching when assembling their therapeutic arsenals, consisting of both suggestion and analysis on one hand and shock and pharmaceutical treatments on the other.[32] Most Cuban commentators agree that in the years leading up to the revolution, the Freudian camp had the edge on its organicist counterpart, in terms of both organization and popularity.[33] Nevertheless, the field was far from uniform, and well before 1959, critiques of psychoanalytic theory and practice had already emerged from a variety of quarters.

The strongest challenge to the embryonic field came from the Pavlovian camp. Since the 1920s, psychiatrists in Cuba had expressed interest in Pavlovian reflexology. The first significant proponent was Rodolfo Guiral, who began his medical career planning to focus on ophthalmology. His interest in the somatic side of medicine remained strong even after he decided to specialize in psychiatry.[34] In the 1920s, Guiral won a professorship in the Cátedra de Enfermedades Nerviosas y Mentales (Department of Nervous and Mental Illnesses) at the University of Havana, where he became an influential mentor for a generation of organicists, including those who would realign the emphasis of the field in the early years of the revolution. Guiral's famous lectures, which emphasized medical approaches to psychiatry, nonetheless gave due attention to psychological considerations. Many patients would enter a psychiatrist's office suffering from a functional rather than organic illness, Guiral reminded his students. Freudian consciousness, moreover, was all around them, and they ignored its content at their own peril.[35] From the beginning of his career, Guiral had thus been an amphibious practitioner of both psychotherapeutic and somatic techniques.

At the height of his professional maturity, Guiral refused to accept any paradigm in an exclusivist fashion. Celebrating recent therapeutic advances, including electroshock, insulin therapy, and neurosurgery, he told Dr. Diego González Martín in a *Bohemia* feature that he regarded the Pavlovian School as the logical realization of Freud's efforts: "Pavlov's School gives a physiological foundation to Freud's School. . . . Freud oriented himself to the psychological aspect; Pavlov saw the anatomical-physiological foundation."[36] It was thus necessary to consider both the "spirit" (*alma*, function) and the nervous system (structure) with an eye to social and historical context. Universalist concepts, Guiral told González Martín while perusing a book of Rorschach tests, had to be weighed against Cuba's "national reality."[37]

Guiral's rejection of orthodox Freudianism was bold and uncompromising. He stood fast even at the cost of losing patients who, he bemoaned, sought to have their Oedipal complexes examined. Freudian concepts, he suggested, were more historical artifact than scientific fact: "Before Pasteur the fear of microbes did not exist, and today we do not see Charcot's case of hysteria, nor do we find people who believe they have been turned into wolves."[38] Critiquing his own early years as an orthodox Freudian, Guiral proposed that it was time for psychiatrists to do away with "preconceived ideas" and immerse themselves in their own cultural context.

There was no more vocal or public opponent of Freudian psychoanalysis in the 1950s than Dr. Diego González Martín himself, who publicly condemned Freudianism as a "reactionary fraud." Unlike other Cuban psychiatrists of a Pavlovian bent, González Martín's opposition to psychoanalysis stemmed from political commitment. For this reason, he would become a leading figure in the post-1959 psychiatric field, celebrated for being the first in Cuba to bring a "Marxist focus" to the "sciences of the psyche."[39] The roots of González Martín's political consciousness developed early in life. Growing up, he bore witness to the treatment his father suffered as a working-class Canary Island immigrant in Cuba. Biographers trace his early political involvement to his childhood experiences and his revolutionary self-education. González Martín was a founding member of the Ala Izquierda Estudiantil (Student Left Wing), a radicalized and anti-imperialist breakaway group from the student organization that had formed at the University of Havana to combat dictator Gerardo Machado (1926–1933). He also worked with the Confederación Nacional Obrera de Cuba (National Worker's Federation of Cuba) and was a member of the Cuban Communist Party beginning in 1932.[40]

González Martín's involvement with the Communist Party deeply influenced his early adoption of Pavlovianism. In 1953 he undertook a "clandestine" trip to the Soviet Bloc, including occupied Austria and Romania, where he first explored reflexology. His Marxist orientation to psychiatry had crystallized even earlier in his doctoral thesis on "Economic and Social Factors in Mental and Nervous Illnesses," where he emphasized the "hegemony of the economic-social factor in the production of neuro-psychical disturbances."[41] His trip to Romania, however, inspired a subsequently combative approach to Cuban psychoanalysis. He related that upon his return, he spoke about Pavlovianism for "nearly four hours, well into the early morning" at the Cuban Society of Neurology and Psychiatry, leaving his "opponent," José Gurri, only ten minutes to "congratulate" him at the end.[42]

As the leading polemicist for Pavlov in Cuba, González Martín frequently engaged in professional debates. His most avid antagonist and close friend was Dr. Roberto Sorhegui, a confirmed Freudian and leftist, who sustained strong ties with the revolutionary leadership up to his death in 1959. By the time of the revolution, Sorhegui had begun to move toward a critical reassessment of Freud in light of Pavlov's contributions, a synthesis that he believed Freud himself had anticipated.[43] Following González Martín's 1956 presentation on "Rational Psychotherapy," Sorhegui opined that he did not consider his exposition to be either "rational or reflexological."[44] José Angel Bustamante, another Freudian-leaning psychiatrist, challenged González Martín to render the "union of the physiological with the social" more clearly, a riposte from the theoretical "left," as it were.[45] While Edmundo Gutiérrez Agramonte, a Guiral student, spoke sympathetically on his behalf, the other replies to the presentation were notable, not for their dogmatic insistence on Freudianism, but rather for their exploratory take on the matter. Several suggested that the very distinctions being raised between different approaches to psychotherapy were new to them and encouraged more study of the topic. Dr. Enrique Collado, on the other hand, seemed to despair of the profusion of theoretical schools, arguing that "all roads lead to Rome when it comes to Psychotherapy."[46]

González Martín's commitment to Pavlov inspired conferences, published work, and even courses on reflexology in the 1950s. He offered one such class at the University of Havana's Escuela de Verano (Summer School), where his students were primarily workers from the Centro Benéfico-Jurídico de Trabajadores de Omnibus, a clinic for workers in the transportation sector that was directed by the Cuban Communist Party.[47] His Pavlovian campaign culminated in the publication of *Experimentos e Ideología* (Experiments and Ideology) in 1960. Dr. Ernesto González Puig, a professor of psychology at the University of Havana after 1959, characterized the work as "a completely Marxist book before the Revolution."[48] González Martín wrote the first part of the text in the final years of the Batista dictatorship and finished it while teaching in Venezuela after the revolution. The work strikes an uncompromising theoretical position from its opening words: "It is frequently asserted that great coincidence exists between the distinct psychological schools of the present. The opinion of the author is completely opposed to that view. It is said, for example, that the Pavlovian and Freudian schools converge in many fundamental questions. And that is incorrect. The simple fact that one is the product of experimental investigation and the other the speculative result of observation, already establishes an abyss between them."[49]

González Martín insisted that "eclecticism," "contemporizing," and "confusionism of hybrid postures" stood firmly opposed to the advance of "Science." As depicted by González Martín, "Science"—read: Pavlovian reflexology—stood at the apex of the field's upward march away from the "Tower of Babel" haphazardly erected by the "byzantine" agglomeration of psychological schools.[50]

Pavlovianism was the correct materialist path, González Martín held, because it provided, through laboratory experimentation, an "absolutely objective" understanding of brain function through conditioned reflexes in dialogue with social context.[51] Moreover, it promised to unveil the essential nature of the psyche as the "dialectical union between social superstructure and the supergranular tissue of the human cerebral cortex."[52] By discarding notions of the unconscious and its autonomy, a society could even achieve meaningful change in social consciousness. No "stereotypes" remained beyond the grasp of a "rational psychotherapy" buttressed by a new social order, González Martín averred, not even the "conditioned reflexes" of racial discrimination, per Fidel Castro's own phrasing of the problem.[53]

González Martín's hopeful gesture toward the revolutionary climate in Cuba in 1959 anticipated a professional and ideological shift in his discipline. In many respects, he served at its vanguard, and Pavlovian perspectives finally received their due in professional and official circles. The transition from a psychoanalytical to a reflexological emphasis, however, was neither immediate nor absolute. In some cases, it followed the politicized trajectory modeled by González Martín, who carried out experiments at the newly founded Instituto de Investigaciones Fundamentales del Cerebro (Institute of Fundamental Investigations of the Brain) and was widely celebrated for being a revolutionary Pavlovian avant la lettre. In others, however, the revolution merely provided a propitious historical climate for the triumph of long-held, mostly apolitical, organicist views. And, finally, even as orthodox Freudian analysis officially disappeared, psychoanalytic ideas survived not only among the psychodynamically minded professionals who remained in Cuba, but even in psychiatric and official visions of revolutionary subject formation. These dynamics, however, cannot be understood outside of a broader Cold War climate. Freudianism, particularly associated with the imperialist behemoth to the north, had to be abandoned, at least in name.

The Cold War

Given the then-recent expansion of Freudianism in Havana, the Cuban psychiatrists who welcomed their Soviet colleagues to Havana after 1959 were primed to have a meaningful debate on psychoanalysis. Though their knowledge of and interest in Pavlov were less profound, the establishment of a new revolutionary psychiatry did not amount to the straightforward implantation of Soviet models. Throughout the 1960s, anti-Freudianism was virulent, but not quite compulsory, rigid, or even univocal. Meanwhile, the attack on psychoanalysis was pervasive, but strangely unofficial and even haphazard.

By 1962, however, a more formal line of critique had surfaced within the psychiatric field, especially at Havana's Hospital Psiquiátrico. This critical momentum also inspired some psychiatrists to turn to intellectual dialogue with Soviet mental health professionals. In many cases, reflexology, already a standard part of their theoretical vision, led them to Soviet interlocutors. Edmundo Gutiérrez Agramonte was the key representative of this group and, beginning in 1962, led a course on reflexological psychotherapy at the Hospital Psiquiátrico. In his seminar, Pavlovian, though not necessarily Soviet, models predominated. Nonetheless, until 1962, strictly reflexological perspectives had a more muted presence in the official publication of the Hospital Psiquiátrico, and a motley crew of organicist and psychodynamic viewpoints continued to prevail. It is telling that, in late 1962, a seminar on psychoanalytic theory was offered alongside Gutiérrez Agramonte's course, sandwiched between a seminar on insulinotherapy and a series of conferences on the history of hysteria and psychological tests.

By 1963, the penetration of Soviet Pavlovianism into Cuban circles accelerated considerably, capping the maturation (and occasional disruption) of political ties between Cuba and the Soviet Union. This process dated back to a proposal made to the Ministry of Public Health two years earlier by hospital director Eduardo Bernabé Ordaz. With the goal of "improving the scientific level" of the facility, Ordaz had requested that two professors of Soviet psychiatry be invited to come to Cuba and teach a course on psychiatry.[54] While insisting that the conferences would be only for those employees who "spontaneously and voluntarily" decided to attend, Ordaz highlighted the scientific superiority of Pavlovian reflexology over the "idealist" bias of the hospital's psychiatrists. In September 1963, I. T. Victorov, professor at the Leningrad Institute of Medicine, and D. N. Isaev, professor of child psychiatry at the Institute of Pediatrics in Leningrad, began offering seminars at Cuba's Colegio Médico and the Hospital Psiquiátrico. The famed Communist psychiatrist Florencio Villa Landa of Spain, who had left his country for the Soviet Union following the Spanish Civil War, served as interpreter in linguistic and, likely, theoretical matters.[55] Victorov and Isaev remained in Cuba for roughly a year and a half and were regular participants in the life of the discipline during that time. The intellectual imperative of the visiting Soviet psychiatrists was to offer a dialectical materialist assessment of Freud and introduce Pavlov to their Cuban colleagues.

Victorov and Isaeiv belonged to a reenergized generation of Soviet Pavlovians who were once again discussing and debating Freud. After three decades of Pavlovian orthodoxy, Stalin's death in 1953 created an opening, not for the reclaiming of Freud, but rather for the renewed and more informed denunciation of psychoanalysis. As the Cold War escalated, greater political significance was attached to critiquing Freudianism, now linked to the exploding U.S. psychoanalytic community rather than the European Jewish psychoanalysts of yore. F. V. Bassin, one of the emblematic figures of this turn, had, like his mentor Dimitri Uznadze, returned to the notion of the unconscious in order to take back areas of the mind claimed by and thus thrown out along with Freud.[56] The work of Bassin and other members of a rejuvenated anti-Freudian cohort would later be republished in revolutionary Cuba; in some cases these Cuban editions represented the first Spanish-language translations of the Soviet authors.[57]

Even González Martín, Cuba's organic Pavlovian intellectual, joined in the process of rectification. Though he had refused to even consider Freud in his previous writings, in 1965 he penned a sustained critique of psychoanalysis in the pages of *Cuba Socialista*. There, he continued to decry the "metaphysical determinism," ahistoricism, and political conservatism of psychoanalysis. Nevertheless, the article also recognized Freud's contributions to psychiatry, particularly his foregrounding of the unconscious and his valorization of a dynamic, rather than mechanistic, understanding of mental functioning.[58] Like his Soviet counterparts, González Martín believed that the vital question of the unconscious had to be taken on through a critical engagement with both Freudian and Pavlovian antecedents. He maintained that this discussion, however, could transpire only in light of the historical motion away from Freud that had already occurred in Cuba, as the Oedipal complex, once a fashionable touchstone among wealthy patients in Havana, had finally been cast among the smoldering embers of a prerevolutionary past. Taking on Freud was, nevertheless, no fait accompli but rather an explicit challenge to the "scarce" but persistent group of "revolutionary Freudians" who continued to cling to the Viennese master.[59]

As Victorov and Isaeiv discovered in 1963, psychodynamic holdouts persisted across the theoretical spectrum of Cuban psychiatry. Freudians and non-Freudians alike were more than prepared to acknowledge Freud's flaws but reluctant to adopt one-dimensional solutions to the problem.[60] Freudians in the group were already versed in the reflexological critique of psychoanalysis in the work of Guiral and González Martín, among others. The construction of anti-Freudianism in Victorov's and Isaeiv's presentations, however, was explicitly yoked to the tenets of dialectical materialism.

Over the course of the conference cycle, Soviet and Cuban adherents to Pavlovianism maintained that only Pavlov had correctly portrayed consciousness as a physiological process of reflection, in which the objective content of the outside world was processed in the brain through sensation, perception, and thought. Laboratory and clinical investigation would elucidate these physiological processes and provide a grounded, scientific understanding of the brain. In contrast, Freudianism and other psychodynamic approaches were "idealist" and unscientific, a lucrative swindle perpetrated by analysts in capitalist countries. Moreover, they argued, the "sociologization" of psychoanalysis, particularly in the United States, bolstered a reactionary political system, in which the essential character of the class struggle was obscured through psychologization.[61] On this score, there was no room for compromise: Freudians, neo-Freudians, Jungians, psychodynamicists, and psychobiologists were equally culpable of denying the fundamentally physiological character of cognition and consciousness.

Nevertheless, one element of this critique was specific to its Cuban setting: namely, the critical role played by the United States in elevating and disseminating Freudianism. Victorov lampooned the popularity of Freudianism in the United States, where, he asserted, people greeted each other by asking after the other's "unconscious." The "contaminating" effect of U.S. psychoanalysis had proven particularly damaging for Cuba, Victorov argued; Freudianism, in both its theorization and its costly practice, properly belonged in reactionary, bourgeois countries. Wandering through Cuban bookstores, he was thus dismayed to find that, "of ten books, nine were dedicated to intersexual [presumably, he means "homosexual"] relationships," framed by a sort of popular Freudianism.[62] U.S. influence in prerevolutionary Cuba, he lamented, had imprinted psychoanalysis everywhere.

Nevertheless, Victorov and Isaeiv also acknowledged the marginal utility of the psychological perspective. Their Cuban interlocutors constantly pushed them to public recognition of this fact, forcing them to consider the possibility of plurality. José Angel Bustamante, a leading, though not uncritical, proponent of psychoanalysis before 1959, urged Victorov to accept Freud's place in a therapeutic genealogy leading up to the present. Diagnosing himself as a non-"sectarian" psychotherapist with twenty-four years of experience, Bustamante admitted Freud's errors but refused to deny him his due: "We have to take some things from Freud and revise them, and even reverse them. But we have to take them."[63] Voicing his own sympathies for the physiological point of view, he pushed inclusiveness in another discussion with Victorov, in which he finally responded that, "through a very lively discussion," the Soviets had indeed reached the agreement that research into personality had to be carried out through both "physiological and psychological" methods."[64]

Victorov's admission was an oblique reference to the unofficial "return" of psychological tests to the Soviet Bloc, where they had been banned by the Central Committee of the Communist Party in 1936 along with mental hygiene.[65] Soviet authorities had condemned projective psychological testing as unscientific and reactionary, perpetuating class inequality by normalizing it. In the post-Stalin era, however, psychological tests had quietly resurfaced, prompting doubts as to whether they had ever really disappeared. At least one Cuban psychologist, Gustavo Torroella, had witnessed this firsthand in his travels throughout the Soviet camp in the mid-1960s.[66]

But lingering trauma around psychological "tests," rendered as such in Spanish, also provoked debates among Cuban psychiatrists and psychologists employed at the Hospital Psiquiátrico. The first had erupted following a presentation by Elsa Pradere about her use of the Machover ("draw a person") test together with the Rorschach. In response, Ernesto González Puig, a psychologist from the University of Havana, admitted that the topic "made his hair stand on end."[67] In his comments, he tried to reconcile a continued reliance on psychological tests with the ideological implications of that use:

> The School of Psychology has an orientation that we try to keep as closely in line with the philosophy of our Revolution and our State as possible. So it's something like that, without having ever been set out concretely, that the Rorschach and in general all of the projective instruments to investigate the personality, run up against the Marxist-Leninist focus and dialectical materialism. These are the things that one hears, that people put out there, and we sincerely don't think they're true, for a very simple reason: the phenomenon of projection is a fact and, as a result, any kind of instrument based in that phenomenon, well it's an instrument that can legitimately be used.[68]

Advocating an open approach in both practice and instruction, Puig added that students in the Department of Psychology would learn Rorschach and Machover, but that the emphasis overall would be on Pavlov.

Psychological tests, however, remained a controversial subject. While psychologists advocated for their guarded use, the Pavlovian challenge led to more infrequent testing in practice.[69] By 1967–1968, however, the conversation had come full circle. A measure approved at a meeting of the hospital direction "reminded" the three hospital psychologists to use *more* tests, noting that only twenty-five tests had been performed in the preceding trimester.[70] Later in 1968, psychologist Gustavo Torroella reported that the use of psychometric testing had "resumed . . . with official backing."[71] Unlike their "traumatized" Soviet counterparts, Cuban psychologists even dared to call the tests by name.

In other cases, however, disagreements between the Soviet psychiatrists in Havana and their Cuban counterparts touched on more fundamental differences. Victorov's most vociferous critic was Juan Portuondo, director of the hospital's Department of Psychology, who would eventually leave Cuba for Spain. Yet the first debates had broken out between Portuondo and Gutiérrez Agramonte, who clashed following a 1963 Gutiérrez Agramonte presentation on reflexological psychotherapy. Presumably in response to these disagreements, Gutiérrez Agramonte extended a special invitation to Portuondo to attend a forthcoming installment of the Soviet conference cycle, an offer that Portuondo accepted.[72] From that point on, Portuondo became the most unyielding psychodynamic holdout in these meetings, leading Victorov to characterize the state of their relationship after the first conference attended by Portuondo as something of a "cold war."[73]

Victorov came prepared to the first conference attended by Portuondo: he had studied Portuondo's work on the topic of autism in order to issue an informed critique. His presentation dismissed the "mystical" and sexualized Freudian treatment of autism. In response, Portuondo aimed more broadly. In a thorough rejoinder to Victorov, he ranged widely over the arguments presented throughout the conference cycle. Disavowing philosophical stances in science as a distraction from the scientific method, he also took issue with the Soviet characterization of Freud as an "idealist." He contrasted this view with the one he had encountered while he was a student at a Catholic university, where Freud's materialism was denounced. Priests, he prodded, "know quite a lot about philosophy."[74] In any case, Portuondo insisted that the relevant question was not one's philosophical stance but the explanatory power of a theoretical paradigm.

Victorov, in turn, disputed Portuondo's claims of ideological disavowal; Portuondo, he warned, had merely rendered his own ideology invisible to himself. Furthermore, if an ideological perspective on scientific questions was inevitable, Victorov preferred to be on the side of dialectical materialism, "not only because it is the ideology of the working class, but also because dialectical materialism correctly reflects the general laws of natural and societal development."[75] While he stumbled over a more specious claim that the pope was using Freudianism to declare war on materialism by labeling it as such, Victorov's reply was as energetic as Portuondo's challenge.

And the battle continued. Following another Victorov presentation in 1965, Portuondo offered the following critique: "The reality continues to be one: man and his shadow, it's all physiological, it's all psychical, it's a circle. If you look at it from one side, you see the psychical, if you look at it from the other the physical. Until man achieves unity (*unidad*) we'll keep fighting for the sake of it."[76] Indeed, Portuondo was arguing less for an orthodox psychoanalytical approach than one that retained psychology as part of the picture. In this admission, he found little room for compromise with his interlocutor, who, following Harry K. Wells, condemned Freudianism as "one of the greatest errors" of humankind.[77]

A Picture of Freud

These skirmishes ended inconclusively, and both Victorov and Portuondo soon departed Cuba. Nevertheless, the conversation continued between Cuban Pavlovians and holdout members of the psychodynamic camp. By the early 1970s, as a result of the campaign against Freud within the profession, the emphasis in the field shifted away from psychodynamic viewpoints, but Freud remained an active object of contention in discussions at the Hospital Psiquiátrico. While many of these arguments drifted ever more decisively toward a Pavlovian, or at least organicist, consensus, the debate about Freud—and even the recognition of his contributions—never entirely vanished, though these conversations came to have a rehearsed quality by the mid-1970s.[78]

In fact, capping a decade of theoretical exploration and development within the psychiatric field, in the early 1970s the Cuban Instituto del Libro had introduced Sigmund Freud to the ranks of authors published in revolutionary Cuba.[79] The publication of Freud's collected works in several volumes was a result of the initiative of Cuban psychologist Juan Guevara, who felt that the field of Cuban psychology had suffered from the absence of psychoanalytic literature.[80] But his victory was short-lived. Some of Freud's later "sociological" works were deemed problematic enough to justify pulling the book from circulation. As Carolina de la Torre recalled, this represented a "jump, from 1965 to 1971, from reading everything, publishing everything and debating everything, to recalling from circulation the recently published works of Freud or any book that grazed the image of the Soviet Union with a rose petal, or tried to insinuate a stain or polemic about the USSR or socialism."[81]

Nevertheless, a sufficient number of volumes survived to inform a revived tradition of Freudian interrogation in the 1980s.[82]

Meanwhile, there was an element of truth to psychiatrist Manuel Domínguez's contention that some former partisans of Freud had found value in Pavlov, "reassuring in some concerns that psychoanalysis had not settled."[83] More often, the Pavlovian campaign provided the intellectual framework for the broader implementation of organicist treatment methods, as psychopharmaceuticals, electroshock therapy, and other biological interventions became increasingly prevalent in revolutionary Cuba. The departure of the most committed psychoanalysts through the 1960s also contributed to this shift in therapeutic emphasis.

In other cases, psychoanalysts who did not leave Cuba in the 1960s, such as Carlos Acosta Nodal, who developed a novel model of "therapeutic film debate," remained active partisans of Freud in Cuba "until the last breath."[84] Many, however, fell somewhere between the two extremes. The most prominent representative of that orientation was José Angel Bustamante, whose explorations in transcultural psychiatry and social psychiatry pulled him away from both orthodox Freudianism and Pavlovianism. Others maintained a stronger intellectual and emotional attachment to Freudian ideas. Cuban psychiatrist José Pérez Villar, who was in Chicago training with students of Freud when the revolution broke out, had returned to Cuba to participate in the revolutionary process. More than a decade later, when Argentine psychoanalyst Juan Carlos Volnovich met Pérez Villar working at the William Soler Pediatric Hospital in Cuba, he found a photo of Freud hanging in Pérez Villar's office.[85] Though no Cuban analysts continued to practice orthodox psychoanalysis in Cuba in these years, few completely relinquished their psychodynamic leanings.

It was this brand of tenacious flexibility that troubled strict dialectical materialist observers, such as Spanish psychiatrist Fermín Galán Rubí. Galán, who was born in Moscow to parents in exile from Franco's Spain, had joined the revolutionary effort in Cuba along with his parents and undertaken psychiatric training. At the Primera Jornada Nacional de Psiquiatría, held in 1975, he critiqued his Cuban colleagues for continuing to proffer insufficiently materialist approaches. Galán blamed the influx of published materials and foreign psychiatrists and psychologists for its "corrosive" impact in Cuba, where "Marxist ideological positions are not firm."[86] In the battle against Freudianism, Cuban psychiatrists had to be vigilant against the efforts of some of their colleagues to synthesize psychoanalysis with Marxism. "It should be very clear," Galán warned, "that there is no room for intermediate positions in the ideological sphere."[87] It was less certain, however, that either government officials or mental health professionals would be willing to enforce this theoretical line.

In fact, by the late 1970s, Silvia Werthein and Volnovich, both fleeing political persecution in the Argentine dirty wars, had even initiated psychoanalytic practice in Havana. The irony of Cuban support for politically dissident Argentine psychoanalysts was not lost on the pair. Volnovich even recalls trying to question the officials processing his admission as to why they were allowing him in. Ultimately, Volnovich did not remain long in Cuba, practicing analysis precisely *because* there was no longer a psychoanalytic field, and his patients tended to be temporary residents of Cuba, especially Argentine, Chilean, and Uruguayan children orphaned by the dirty wars.[88] He has suggested, however, that explicit anti-psychoanalytic sentiment in Cuba was fairly limited.[89]

Evidently, even at its apex, anti-Freudianism was not entirely exclusivist, and the significant contingent that moved away from psychoanalysis did not necessarily become orthodox Pavlovians. Meanwhile, outside of hospital meetings, the Freud-Pavlov polemic constituted the intellectual groundwork for cooperation between the revolutionary government and mental health professionals. Though government officials inconsistently summoned psychiatrists and psychologists to the practical work of revolutionary subject formation, some medical professionals eagerly mobilized throughout the 1960s to direct the mental transformation associated with "revolutionary mystique." Having passed through a series of ideological purges in the early 1960s, the new Department of Psychology at the University of Havana embarked on a series of collaborations with the revolutionary government in the areas of labor, industry, reeducation, and revolutionary defense. Paradoxically, the overall emphasis of this work was on applied, rather than theoretical, psychology. The presumed ideological orthodoxy of revolutionary psychologists had opened a space for them to participate in revolutionary mental engineering, a project that, it turned out, had little to do with Pavlov.[90]

In this respect, some medical professionals presented themselves as mere deputies of the "enormous psychotherapy that is Revolution," as Dr. Julio Ayllón Morgan had argued before the X Congreso Médico Nacional in February 1963.[91] While acknowledging that the fall of a "rotten system" had provoked more than one personality crisis among Cuba's youth, Ayllón lauded its capacity to bring a society collectively on the verge of neurosis, particularly in the psychically depleted zones of the countryside, to mental health. Psychiatrists ought to look to the revolution, he insisted, to understand their own role.

In this spirit, Ayllón and his colleagues had gathered together the sixteen hundred students of the school where he was completing his rural medical tour of duty and carried out what can be described only as a mass session of revolutionary psychotherapy: "We explained to them the reasons behind the symptoms they were feeling, with the relationship between one's state of mind and bodily ailments, as well as nervous crises. Likewise, we exalted the courage and the sacrifice they would have to expend in order to reach the proposed goals. We valorized . . . the effort they were making and what the Revolution and the people expected of them."[92] In a mere hour, he contended, they had "cut off with a single stroke an epidemic of hysterical attacks in the girls and the tensions of the boys."[93] He expressed his faith that, in the future, they would be able to overcome their weaknesses in order to keep fighting for the revolution. This was the labor, Ayllón effused, that Fidel Castro himself was carrying out as the leader of the revolution's great psychotherapeutic exercise. In calling upon his colleagues to "imitate [Fidel] in every possible way," he too ran afoul of the campaign to bring Cuban psychiatry in line with firm scientific and, specifically, Pavlovian principles.[94]

This was the contradiction, however, that would persist at the heart of the project to revolutionize Cuban psychiatry, defying just-so stories about Cold War politics and intellectual exchange. If orthodox Pavlovianism seemed to confine them to narrow exercises of reflexological theorizing, throughout the 1960s Cuban psychiatrists proposed to extend their expertise outside the bounds of the discipline, to link the field to the revolution that, as Ayllón argued, they should try to emulate. A significant number of the Cuban psychiatrists who remained after the early years of revolution were prepared to let Freud join other artifacts of the past in the ideological cemetery of repression. Burying the tropical Freud, however, did not a Pavlovian make. While some psychiatrists joined neurology labs and subscribed wholeheartedly to the scientific, dialectical materialist position encouraged by their Soviet mentors, others continued to push out into the world the revolution had made, analyzing and fortifying its extension into individual minds.

Nevertheless, partnerships like those initiated between government officials and revolutionary psychologists were inherently unstable, and psychiatrists, whose reputation as bourgeois Freudians persisted into the revolutionary years, were inconsistently invited to participate. By the early 1970s, as the revolution entered a period of institutionalization and Sovietization, the spirit of experimentation—psychological and otherwise—began to fade from the scene. For the most part, mental health professionals retreated from the front lines of revolutionary mental engineering, and their theoretical battles seemed

Jennifer Lynn Lambe

increasingly insular. By the late 1980s, a rejuvenated generation of the psycho-dynamically minded would finally invite Freud back to the table. Yet they did so too late for their initiative to matter.

Elsewhere in Latin America, the Cold War ushered in a paradoxical psychoanalytic pluralism: forces on the right and the left claimed its vocabulary as an apt vehicle for self-definition, expanding its reach and sociopolitical relevance.[95] They thereby created a broad space for apolitical consumption and implementation, in some cases contributing to the formation of full-fledged "psy cultures." In the 1960s, Cuban psychiatrists transacted parallel battles highlighting that same "plasticity" of psychoanalysis. Freudianism, however, did not retain its predominance among psychiatric professionals, nor did it expand its reach in psychiatric practice. Even as the state, not unlike others in the region, appropriated its vocabulary to make claims about revolutionary subject formation, psychoanalysis itself receded in importance. Yet the Pavlovian orthodoxy was similarly fragile, its imprint barely visible in the realm of practice.

What, then, do we make of these battles, which seem to have affected everyday psychiatry in only limited ways? The "Freud Wars," I argue, are best viewed as a compelling stage of the scientific Cold War, a microcosm of contemporary struggles over revolutionary belonging and psychiatric prerogative. Their outcome was in some ways less important than their inherent drama, namely, the performative assertion of professional relevance. This is not to imply, however, that Cuban battles over Freud and Pavlov were merely another variation on the timeworn soma-and-psyche theme. Rather, the very intensity of this struggle—its seeming centrality to the mission of a revolutionary profession—highlights not only psychoanalytic plasticity, but also psychiatric *politicization*. Against the ostensible intentions of both Freud and Pavlov, their theories have persistently buttressed nonscientific paradigms and programs, providing the tools with which Cuban psychiatrists, like many of their professional predecessors, could wage politics.[96]

Notes

I am grateful for the thoughtful feedback and contributions of Michael Bustamante, Lillian Guerra, David Minto, Robin Wolfe Scheffler, Marco Ramos, Belinda Zhou, Adrián López Denis, Raúl Necochea López, Anne-Emanuelle Birn, John Warner, Mariola Espinosa, Ethan Pollock, and participants in the New York Cuban Studies

Workshop. I would especially like to thank Cuban colleagues and psychiatrists who shared their memories of these debates as well as the archivists and librarians at the Archivo Nacional de Cuba, Museo Histórico de las Ciencias Carlos J. Finlay, Biblioteca Nacional de Cuba José Martí, New York Academy of Medicine, and National Library of Medicine. This is a condensed and adapted version of an article published in the *Bulletin of the History of Medicine* 91, 1 (2017): 62–93.

1   Rivera Núñez, "Estudio Clínico de la Angustia."

2   Rivera Núñez, "Estudio Clínico de la Angustia."

3   Unlike some of their Latin American colleagues, first-generation Cuban analysts tended to be fairly committed Freudians; Melanie Klein and others were less influential there. For another account of these battles, see Marqués de Armas, *Ciencia y Poder.*

4   On this connection, see Funes Monzote, *Despertar del Asociacionismo Científico en Cuba*; Hirschfeld, *Health, Politics, and Revolution in Cuba*; Espinosa, *Epidemic Invasions*; Rodríguez, *Right to Live in Health.*

5   See Guerra, *Visions of Power.* On the complex overlap between biomedical debates and the Cold War, see also Hochman and Paiva's chapter in this volume.

6   See Gacetilla, "Diciembre 21"; Herminio Portell Vilá, "Politiquería y Medicina"; Rodríguez, "To Fight These Powerful Trusts."

7   For an account of similar debates in Argentina with a different outcome, see Plotkin, *Freud in the Pampas*, 166–90. A more recent effort to bring together Marx and Freud in the Latin American context can be found in Bosteels, *Marx and Freud in Latin America.* The literature on psychoanalysis in Latin America is broad and growing. For a representative sample, see Vezzetti, *Aventuras de Freud en el País de los Argentinos*; Taiana, "Transatlantic Migration of the Disciplines of the Mind"; Plotkin, "Psychoanalysis, Race Relations, and National Identity"; Ruperthuz Honorato, "Retorno de lo Reprimido."

8   This section draws primarily on Valenstein, *Great and Desperate Cures.*

9   See Zajicek, "Scientific Psychiatry in Stalin's Soviet Union"; Todes, *Pavlov's Physiology Factory.*

10   On the long history of the unconscious, see Ellenberger, *Discovery of the Unconscious.*

11   See Makari, *Revolution in Mind*, esp. 239–446.

12   Martin Miller, *Freud and the Bolsheviks*, 53–69.

13   Martin Miller, *Freud and the Bolsheviks*, 94–104.

14   See Zajicek, "Scientific Psychiatry in Stalin's Soviet Union"; Zajicek, "Insulin Coma Therapy."

15   See Zajicek, "Scientific Psychiatry in Stalin's Soviet Union."

16   Zajicek, "Scientific Psychiatry in Stalin's Soviet Union." See also Rose, Levold, and Hiltzik, "Ivan Pavlov on Communist Dogmatism."

17   Zajicek, "Scientific Psychiatry in Stalin's Soviet Union"; Zajicek, "Insulin Coma Therapy"; Marks and Savelli, "Communist Europe and Transnational Psychiatry"; Doboş, "Psychiatry and Ideology."

18 Plotkin, "Diffusion of Psychoanalysis under Conditions of Political Authoritarianism," 203–4. See also Ramos, "Psychiatry, Authoritarianism, and Revolution."

19 Russo, "Social Diffusion of Psychoanalysis," 165.

20 For example, Juan Portell Vilá, "Psicoanálisis y Su Aplicación al Estudio del Niño." José Angel Bustamante, *Psiquiatría en Cuba en los Ultimos Cincuenta Años*, cites "Dr Lavette [*sic*]" as the first practitioner of psychoanalysis in Cuba.

21 See Potts, "Apuntes para Una Historia de la Psicoterapia de Grupo"; Potts, "Factores Emocionales en los Grupos Humanos"; Potts, "Patrones de Conducta en los Grupos Terapéuticos."

22 For example, Alfonso Bernal del Riesgo was a cofounder of the Cuban Communist Party who, while in exile in Vienna, became a student of dissident psychoanalyst Alfred Adler. See Bernal, "Dr. Alfonso Bernal del Riesgo: Cronología."

23 See Juan Guevara, "Mesa Redonda."

24 Scarizza made the pilgrimage to Cuba after apparently falling in love with a Cuban actress aboard a cruise ship on which he was employed as a physician, or, according to another account, for the purpose of giving psychoanalytic instruction. Humberto Nagera, interview by the author, Tampa, July 3, 2011. Nagera related the cruise ship story to me, while Ángel Arturo Otero Ojeda highlights the "expressly . . . pedagogical" function of the visit. See Otero Ojeda, "Carlos Acosta Nodal."

25 "Actas de la Sociedad Cubana de Neurología y Psiquiatría."

26 Sociedad Cubana de Psicoterapia, Archivo Nacional de Cuba, Registro de Asociaciones, series 56, folder 191, file 4189.

27 "In Memoriam: Leo H. Bartemeier." Nagera told me that this story was known among his colleagues.

28 José Angel Bustamante, *Psiquiatría en Cuba*, 58; Nagera interview.

29 Sociedad Psicoanalítica Cubana, Archivo Nacional de Cuba, Registro de Asociaciones, series 56, folder 167, file 3183. In order to become a member, one needed to have met the following qualifications: ten years of medical practice, five years of psychotherapy practice, and completion of analysis with a psychiatrist belonging to an IPA-recognized group. Humberto "Nájera" now uses the "Nagera" spelling of his last name.

30 "Seminario Psicoanalítico," *Diario de la Marina*, February 22, 1955, 3-A.

31 Nagera interview.

32 See Sagredo Acebal, "Tratamiento Somatopsíquico de una Neurosis Obsesiva." This is hardly surprising given the orthodox medical training of all psychiatric residents at the University of Havana. Nagera recalls a division of labor whereby once those leaning toward psychotherapeutic approaches established private practices, they sent patients with more severe illnesses or psychoses to other clinics for somatic treatment.

33 See Triana Noa, "Diego González Martín." Several psychiatrists who began their careers in the 1950s echoed this characterization in interviews.

34 Guiral had also trained in the United States in the late 1920s under Robert Foster Kennedy, an Irish American neurologist based at Cornell University.

35 Rodolfo J. Guiral, "Conferencia VIII," Tomo I (class lecture, "Psychiatry," Cátedra de Enfermedades Nerviosas y Mentales, University of Havana, 1944). This mimeographed copy of the lectures was made by Dr. Rafael Larragoiti and is held at the Biblioteca of the Museo Histórico de las Ciencias Médicas Carlos J. Finlay.

36 González Martín, "Grandes de la Medicina Cubana."

37 González Martín, "Grandes de la Medicina Cubana."

38 Guiral, "Medicina Psicosomática."

39 González Serra, "González Martín," 74.

40 González Serra, "González Martín." He served as a political commentator for the Communist Party newspaper *Noticias de Hoy* and later *Bohemia*.

41 González Martín, "Desarrollo," 669. This citation and some of the details are also provided in González Serra, "González Martín."

42 González Martín, "Desarrollo," 669.

43 See Sorhegui, "Algunas Correlaciones Psicoanalítico-Físicas en la Estructuración de la Personalidad."

44 "Sesión Ordinaria el 2 de Agosto de 1956," 53.

45 "Sesión Ordinaria el 2 de Agosto de 1956."

46 "Sesión Ordinaria el 2 de Agosto de 1956."

47 González Martín, "Desarrollo," 669.

48 Triana Noa, "Diego González Martín," 216. Triana Noa and González Serra celebrate González Martín for having reached the same conclusions as the classic Soviet bibliography on the topic without having read it.

49 González Martín, *Experimentos e Ideología*, 17.

50 González Martín, *Experimentos e Ideología*, 50.

51 González Martín, *Experimentos e Ideología*, 61.

52 González Martín, *Experimentos e Ideología*, 190.

53 González Martín, *Experimentos e Ideología*, 189–90.

54 Ordaz, "Editorial."

55 Villa Landa (1912–1992), a member of the Spanish Communist Party, moved to the Soviet Union at the invitation of the Red Cross after serving as a medic for the Republican forces in the Spanish Civil War. In the Soviet Union, he studied neuropsychiatry and Pavlovianism. In 1957, he emigrated to Mexico, where he was responsible for translating a number of important Soviet psychiatric texts into Spanish. From Mexico, he was invited in 1961 to serve as a professor of psychiatry at the University of Havana, an invitation that he eagerly accepted. He left Cuba for the Soviet Union in 1973 and finally returned to Madrid in 1978. See "Florencio Villa Landa"; Igual, "Florencio Villa Landa."

56 See Martin Miller, *Freud and the Bolsheviks*, 132–36. See also Angelini, "History of the Unconscious in Soviet Russia." The career of Jewish psychologist Sergei Rubinstein, ostracized under Stalin but later rehabilitated, exemplifies this turn. See Martin Miller, *Freud and the Bolsheviks*, 110–12.

57 Bassin, *Problema del Inconsciente* (1980). While Bassin's work was published only later on, other Soviet authors appeared much earlier. See Rubinstein, *Ser y la Conciencia*; *Psicología Soviética*; Leontiev, *Problemas del Desarrollo del Psiquismo*. Transla-

tion and publication efforts did not focus solely on Soviet authors in these years. Jean Piaget's 1945 *La Formation du Symbole chez l'Enfant: Imitation, Jeu et Rêve, Image et Representation* was published by the Cuban Instituto del Libro in 1967, and Gordon Allport was also later republished and eventually withdrawn from circulation due to a reference to Soviet brainwashing. In the early 1960s, translated works by Soviet authors most commonly appeared in article form in the *Revista del Hospital Psiquiátrico de la Habana*, alongside the translated conference cycle.

58 González Martín, "Algunas Consideraciones Críticas sobre la Teoría Freudiana."

59 González Martín, "Desarrollo," 671. Many members of the Psychoanalytical Society ultimately left the island, even as some of the most prominent members, particularly Bustamante, Acosta Nodal, Pérez Villar, and Córdova, remained. See Marqués de Armas, *Ciencia y Poder*, 180, 317. The society was officially canceled on July 22, 1960, along with most prerevolutionary organizations.

60 See discussion following Fernández Martí, "Comentarios sobre los Problemas Transferenciales en los Esquizofrénicos."

61 Victorov, "Carácter Idealista y Reaccionario."

62 Victorov, "Análisis de las Bases Teóricas del Freudismo," 485.

63 Victorov, "Análisis de las Bases Teóricas del Freudismo," 488.

64 Victorov, "Exposición de las Relaciones Mutuas entre la Teoría de la Actividad Nerviosa Superior."

65 See Zajicek, "Scientific Psychiatry in Stalin's Soviet Union."

66 See Torroella, "Situación Actual de las Pruebas o Exámenes Psicológicos en los Países Socialistas."

67 Pradere, "Machóver como Técnica Complementaria del Diagnóstico de Rorschach."

68 Pradere, "Machóver como Técnica Complementaria."

69 See Portuondo, "Diagnóstico a Través del Test de Rorschach."

70 "Acta No. 78, Sesiones del Consejo de Dirección."

71 Torroella, "Estado de la Psicometría en la URSS."

72 "Acta No. 26, Sesiones del Consejo de Dirección."

73 Victorov, "Pensamiento Autista, Autismo y Delirio Autista," 584–87.

74 Victorov, "Pensamiento Autista, Autismo y Delirio Autista," 584.

75 Victorov, "Pensamiento Autista, Autismo y Delirio Autista," 585.

76 Victorov, "Patofisiología de la Esquizofrenia y su Patogénesis según Autores Soviéticos."

77 Victorov, "Trastorno del Pensamiento y de la Inteligencia." Victorov frequently referred to Wells's *Sigmund Freud*, presumably believing that an American critique of Freud would be more familiar to his Cuban counterparts.

78 Some of the most aggressive Pavlovian partisans continued to express limited approbation for certain concepts or schools of Freudianism; see, for example, Nogueira Rivero, "Psicoterapia y Principales Escuelas Psicológicas."

79 The publication utilized the first Spanish translation of Freud's works by Luis López Ballesteros, which had been released in seventeen volumes by the Biblioteca Nueva de Madrid between 1922 and 1934. The 1971 publication is extremely

rare, and I was not able to locate the final volume, which includes the most controversial sociological writings, at the Biblioteca Nacional José Martí in Havana.

80 Due to his long-standing involvement with leftist politics, Guevara was far from an uncritical reader of Freud. See "Mesa Redonda."

81 Nevertheless, de la Torre, who has been one of the key proponents of a retrospective critique of anti-Freudianism in the 1960s and 1970s, insists that psychology was one of the only fields that was not pulled into the cultural "gray years" of 1971–1976, though the Department of Psychology at the University of Havana had experienced a process of ideological purification in the early 1970s due to the concerns of some faculty members that they had strayed too far from strict Marxist perspectives. See "Palabras de Carolina de la Torre en el Homenaje a los Graduados"; de la Torre Molina, "Historia de la Psicología en Cuba."

82 The return of psychoanalysis to revolutionary Cuba is usually dated to the Encuentros Latinoamericanos de Psicología Marxista y Psicoanálisis, which began in 1988. There, Cuban psychologists debated their Marxist—but Freudian and Lacanian—Latin American colleagues. See Dueñas Becerra, "Ciencia Psicológica Cubana." The presence of leftist and Marxist psychoanalysts and health professionals like Monika Krause and Marie Langer in Cuba also helped to create a renewed opening for discussions of psychoanalysis.

83 Manuel Domínguez, "Conceptos Actuales de la Psiquiatría."

84 See Dueñas Becerra, "Profesor Carlos Acosta Nodal"; Otero Ojeda, "Carlos Acosta Nodal"; Rodríguez Mesa, "Recorrido Histórico de los Modelos de Psicoterapia Utilizadas [sic] en Cuba." The retrospective valorization of holdouts against Pavlovianism can obscure some of the complexity of the historical moment.

85 See Emilia Cueto, "Entrevista a Juan Carlos Volnovich."

86 Galán Rubí, "Ideología y Salud Mental," 80.

87 Galán Rubí, "Ideología y Salud Mental," 84. In 1973 the Marxist Spanish psychiatrist J. Solé Sagarra noted the predominance of the Soviet school but with the continued influence of U.S., East German, Czech, French, English, and Spanish psychiatry. See Sagarra, "Psiquiatría en Cuba y Otros Países Socialistas."

88 Hollander, Uprooted Minds, 57.

89 See Emilia Cueto, "Entrevista a Juan Carlos Volnovich." See also Werthein, "Palabras en la Mesa de Apertura." For more on psychoanalysis under authoritarianism in Argentina, see Plotkin, Freud in the Pampas; Ramos, "Psychiatry, Authoritarianism, and Revolution." On Volnovich and Werthein, see Hollander, Uprooted Minds, 33–61.

90 For more on these collaborations, see Lambe, Madhouse, 140–98.

91 Ayllón Morgan, "Algunos Casos de Neurosis," 25.

92 Ayllón Morgan, "Algunos Casos de Neurosis," 24. Ayllón considered this exercise to be Pavlovian in nature despite its evidently sui generis character.

93 Ayllón Morgan, "Algunos Casos de Neurosis," 24.

94 Ayllón Morgan, "Algunos Casos de Neurosis," 25.

95 See, for example, Ramos's chapter in this volume.

96 On the diverse uses of Freud, see Zaretsky, Political Freud. Other recent work in this vein includes, for example, Antic, "Therapeutic Fascism."

Part III

Health Politics and Publics, with and without the Cold War

7

From Cold War Pressures to State Policy to People's Health

Social Medicine and Socialized Medical Care in Chile

JADWIGA E. PIEPER MOONEY

It is not possible to provide health and knowledge to a malnourished people, dressed in rags and working under merciless exploitation. . . . It is necessary that the well-off contribute without haggling, for their own security. It is necessary that each and every one of our citizens support the gigantic task of lifting our country economically, health-wise and culturally, and thus bring the most dignified and effective benefit for the republic.

—Chilean health minister Salvador
  Allende, 1939

I have the deep conviction that we are not yet fully grasping the severe importance of these initiatives . . . and that only time will tell the impact that they will have on the defense of our race, on the protection of human capital, and in terms of overcoming the tremendous injustices that derive from the existence of social divisions in the country.

—Senator Salvador Allende, on the
  proposed creation of the Servicio
  Nacional de Salud, 1950

Chile's National Health Service, the Servicio Nacional de Salud (SNS), was established in 1952—thanks in large part to medical doctors such as then-Senator Salvador Allende and epidemiologist Benjamín Viel—only to be torn down over two decades later, after Augusto Pinochet's bloody coup d'état deposed Allende three years after his democratic election to the presidency. Yet the story of the SNS, from its lead-up in 1952 to its demise in 1979, is not only one of domestic Chilean politics. Medical authorities who advocated for both social medicine and the SNS negotiated crucial questions in their day-to-day work: which health system could best protect the health of Chile's people, and how should the design and implementation of social medicine take into account the contemporary debates around political ideology?

Drawing from the ideas and practices of public health doctors across distinct time periods in twentieth-century Chile, this study traces the fears and concerns brought about by the politically and ideologically fraught relationship between social medicine and socialized medicine. In these contexts, *social medicine*—an understanding of illness as inherently linked to the social origins of disease, thereby requiring an integrated medicosocial approach to treatment—was contested and conflated with *socialized medicine,* defined as a state-organized and regulated health system with equal and universal access for all of a country's citizens.[1]

This chapter begins by analyzing the origin of these debates prior to the Cold War, when Chilean physicians began to forge a systematic response to the country's growing health crises. In the late 1930s, Salvador Allende, as a newly minted minister of health, and many of his colleagues both supported the practice of social medicine and proposed an expanded role for the state in public health. These experts crafted and sent to Congress legislation modeled after Allende's blueprint developed in his 1939 book *La Realidad Médico-Social Chilena (Chilean Medical-Social Reality).*[2] The proposed law sought to strengthen the medical and health infrastructure, extend the benefits of social security to workers' entire families, and unify all health institutions under one agency. While many doctors were prepared to support these changes, others feared that the status of *funcionario* (full-time state employee) would significantly limit their professional freedoms and their income. Given the tense sociopolitical climate and the ambiguity of medical professionals' positions, the proposal for a unified, state-led health system for all citizens initially failed to garner sufficient congressional support.[3]

The second part of the chapter traces subsequent developments in which doctors used existing national and community-based initiatives to make a case for social medicine and socialized medicine and to protect their professional interests in a changed political environment—now with the support of the newly founded College of Physicians of Chile (1948).[4] In 1952, Salvador Allende, now from his position as senator, helped push through a bill modeled after a plan by epidemiologist Benjamín Viel and economist Francisco Pinto, once again promoting a unified health system for all Chileans. In this second round of health policy debates, we can trace the footprints of a Cold War discourse that no longer differentiated between social and socialized medicine and linked both to the dangers of communism, compulsory state control, and the absence of individual freedoms. In the United States, for example, physicians and politicians cast debates over health care reform in terms of a political and ideological conflict between the public duty to provide medical goods and services, and freedom (for doctors and the public) from the alleged threat of state "control."[5] But in Chile, the anticommunist discourse of the U.S.-led Western Bloc did not inevitably determine national policies. In Benjamín Viel's activities, for example, we find evidence of a social medicine praxis that expediently managed both to avoid some global political paradigms (such as ideological competition between capitalism and communism) and to engage with others (such as the Neo-Malthusian discourse of overpopulation) in promoting a public health approach to serve the needs of the Chilean nation.

Popular Front Politics and Chile's Medical-Social Reality

In the 1930s, Chilean doctors and policymakers from distinct political-ideological quarters pushed for an increased role of the state in medical care, following 1920s social security legislation that covered only urban industrial workers. Most prominently, health ministers Dr. Eduardo Cruz Coke (1937–1938), a conservative, but one influenced by Christian social thought, and Dr. Salvador Allende (1939–1942), a Socialist, proposed the reorganization of public health and prioritized concerns about the loss of "human capital"—productive workers—through disease.[6] Cruz Coke's initiatives spurred new social welfare regulations and health programs that strengthened the role of the state in the provision of health services, as, for example, through the Chilean Preventive Medicine Act.[7] Cruz Coke, whose interpretation of social medicine differed from Allende's in that it favored health interventions to improve labor productivity—as opposed to seeing public, universal health care as a matter of social justice—first sent his bill to Congress in September 1937. It passed in January 1938 with the support of fellow physicians who endorsed the design of a health care system with increased "direction from above," including compulsory medical exams and regulation of doctors' prescriptions. In Cruz Coke's words, "planned medicine" was expected to lower mortality and morbidity rates by combining regular checkups, preventive rest, and curative action. He promoted his campaign for preventive medicine in the name of workers' health and Chile's economic progress, as reflected in increased productivity of the industrial working class.[8] Many doctors approved of increased state responsibility for public health, although the specific characteristics of government direction from above—as well as the role doctors should play in shaping the politics of health—remained the subject of much debate.[9] Reformers such as Cruz Coke focused on the industrial working class, sidestepping issues of poverty, inequality, and uneven access to health services that Allende, in the opening section of *La Realidad Médico-Social Chilena*, referred to as "tremendous injustices that derive from the existence of social divisions in the country."[10]

Prior to his role as health minister, Allende had been a medical student activist and leader of the Chilean Medical Association, the Asociación Médica de Chile (AMECH), founded in 1931.[11] Association members addressed the role of social medicine and the responsibilities medical doctors could—and should—assume in the politics of public health. These duties extended well beyond clinical care to include the promotion of social and socialized medicine. At the association's national convention in 1935, participants endorsed the national reorganization of medical care.[12] Their recommendations included placing public health under one ministry, integrating health prevention and social security policies, and transforming medical education to emphasize the social aspects of health and disease, especially regarding the widespread problems of alcoholism, syphilis, and tuberculosis.[13] These ideas informed the plans that Allende advocated a few years later as minister of health.

In 1939, while rising German aggression in Europe commanded increasing international attention, Chile was in the midst of a decidedly domestic political experiment. The newly elected Popular Front president, Pedro Aguirre Cerda, together with his young health minister Salvador Allende, offered a revolutionary plan for public health involving a central role for the state. Aguirre Cerda's government conveyed an innovative spirit through the slogan, "To govern is to educate and to give health."[14] Allende's books and articles as well as his proposals explicitly linking poverty with disease and unequal wealth distribution with the nation's poor health were radical contributions to public health policymaking in the Chilean context.

Allende, one of the leading contributors to Chile's "golden age" of social medicine, was himself influenced by nineteenth-century German pathologist Rudolf Virchow's ideas concerning the fundamental political underpinnings of health and the state's responsibility for ensuring the public's health.[15] Allende had studied under German physician and Virchow disciple Max Westenhöfer, who taught social medicine at the University of Chile. Like Virchow, Westenhöfer insisted that the effective practice of medicine was inseparable from the study of the social origins of disease.[16] Virchow first advanced this position in 1848, when the Prussian government sent him to investigate a typhus epidemic in the poverty-stricken province of Silesia. During this mission Virchow connected the patients' poverty, lack of education, and political disenfranchisement to their vulnerability to disease, concluding that socioeconomic conditions explained the prevalence of deadly epidemics among the poor.[17] He insisted that many outbreaks of disease were, in reality, "artificial epidemics," manifestations of the gap between rich and poor, and the result of misguided political leadership, which he believed should be remedied through civil society actions and responsive government initiatives, including closing the gap between rich and poor.[18]

Reflecting Virchow's insights, Allende promoted the need for political change on a larger scale when he introduced the key elements of social medicine to his compatriots. In his now-famous book, *Chilean Medical-Social Reality*, he discussed the links between disease and poverty, arguing that doctors' efforts to heal the medical ills of the nation had to include the economic and social contexts of disease. Allende emphasized high poverty rates and class divisions as primary obstacles to the health and well-being of all members of Chilean society, and he proposed substantial political remedies. From his perspective, only a new political strategy, one that closed the wide gap between rich and poor, would bring about a healthy and prosperous nation. He envisioned income redistribution, economic reforms, and broadscale social and political transformations to abolish class-based differences in access to health care services. Allende began with a proposal to reform what he considered an outdated social security system, then outlined a public health system to centralize health services for all Chileans under a single agency.[19]

At the time, Allende and other doctors in Chile were seeking to address multiple health crises that had intensified through decades of increased industrialization and urbanization. The growing industrial sector in the capital, Santiago, attracted thousands of migrants each year, leading its population to nearly double during the first decades of the twentieth century, reaching 712,533 residents by 1930.[20] Many urban migrants endured overcrowded and unsanitary living conditions, while officials documented rising rates of crime, prostitution, and domestic violence. Doctors were concerned about typhus, tuberculosis, alcoholism, and venereal disease but were most of all alarmed at soaring infant mortality rates, which reached 212 per 1,000 live births in 1930.[21]

In response to these crises, Allende argued that only a centralized national health care agency could competently set political priorities and guarantee access to health services to those citizens who most needed them. He pushed for a system that would help alleviate the nation's social ills by "mak[ing] it possible to provide preventive and curative care to the three million Chileans who, as a matter of law, are going to receive medical care." This arrangement, in turn, would foster the realization of a national plan "with a central vision" for addressing "the problems of our social pathology." Allende supported state-led medical intervention because, in his opinion, it would both strengthen labor productivity and help accomplish the humanitarian goal of improving the health of all citizens.[22]

In 1940, despite the support of left-leaning Chilean physicians, Chile's Congress rejected Allende's blueprint for a national health service. Scholars have cited both economic and political reasons to explain this outcome. Legislators were concerned about the financial burden the proposed system would pose, and some doctors feared possible professional restrictions due to government control. Additionally, the government's evolving stance on communism, which culminated in the outlawing of the Partido Comunista de Chile (PCCh, Communist Party of Chile) in 1948, may have contributed to the rejection of centralized, state-led initiatives.[23]

Indeed, anticommunism played a growing role in health policy debates through the 1940s, mounting with the rise of Cold War tensions on a global scale. Although the impact of anticommunism varied—with only sporadic denunciations, and accusations against those holding communist convictions initially left untouched socialists and militants of the Partido Socialista de Chile (PS, Socialist Party of Chile)—an anticommunist climate nonetheless shaped political negotiations around social medicine and socialized medical care.

These factors—as well as the ideological distance between the Chilean PS and Moscow—help explain why Allende, a Socialist by political affiliation, avoided public persecution during the anticommunist backlash, while others, even some who had not been party militants, were harassed for their alleged political beliefs. The PS had been founded only in 1933, "impos[ing] a unified party structure on a bewildering kaleidoscope of microparties, factions, and splinter groups," representing various socialist orientations.[24] The new group identity of the PS originated partly as a result of its members' unanimous rejection of affiliation with the USSR, in contrast to the PCCh's close ties to Moscow, likely contributing to the greater persecution of the latter than the former in 1940s Chile. Whether the distinction was imagined or real, Chilean political and economic elites helped construct Communists as the main enemies: landowners depicted labor organizers and rural agitators as PCCh militants who represented a threat to the nation. Subsequent denunciations of "unpatriotic" forces singled out Communists rather than Socialists or other militants of smaller left-wing political parties.[25]

By the late 1940s, denunciations of communists drew not only from the anticommunist rhetoric that gathered steam at the beginning of the Cold War but also from a new "Law for the Defense of Democracy." In September 1948, President Gabriel González Videla, who had come to power in 1946 with the support of the PCCh, outlawed the party. This move improved his relationship with the United States—which went on to bankroll much of the country's economic development through loans and investments in this period—and allowed González Videla to target a wide range of political agitators who threatened to delegitimize his government.[26]

At times, denunciations of alleged communists resulted in the discrimination or firing of doctors employed as civil servants. In March 1948, for example, primary-school teacher Jorge Cancino denounced two physicians to the Puente Alto Police Department in Santiago, accusing Raúl Cantuarias Bernal and Manuel Zorrilla Moreira of unlawful communist activity. Both doctors worked with community health projects and held key administrative positions in the local government—Cantuarias Bernal as the director of the Puente Alto Health Center and Zorrilla Moreira as its head of pediatrics. Cancino claimed that both had regularly attended meetings with PCCh members and communist sympathizers. In his accusation, he also listed the names of other alleged communists involved in such gatherings.[27] Anticommunism, now legally sanctioned by the 1948 law, inspired Cancino and others to report purported communist activities at local police stations.[28]

Cancino's accusations were consistent with the larger picture of newly sanctioned denunciations. Accusations ranged from current or prior membership in the PCCh to spreading communist propaganda. Without clear evidence, some were accused simply for failing to demonstrate political distance from communism. Certain allegations deliberately sought to control or block the actions of organized labor, resulting, for example, in the forcible removal of those suspected of communist activities to locations where political organizing was impossible. Others seem to have been based on personal antipathies, with accusers using the new law for personal gain to retaliate against rivals or resolve long-standing conflicts.[29] Many alleged communist agitators were doctors and/or health officials employed in government offices, hospitals, or public health centers.

Cancino's action offers merely a glimpse into the complex and charged political climate in which individuals' putative politics could threaten their careers. Although some Chileans made ample use of the practice of denunciations, others refused to join the anticommunist witch hunt and defended the accused, risking their own credibility and livelihoods. Indeed, renowned physicians like surgeon Dr. Sótero del Río and epidemiologist Dr. Enrique Laval defended the reputation of Cantuarias Bernal and Zorrilla Moreira, insisting that their colleagues were not communists but reputable and dedicated professionals. Even priests joined the long list of those who defended the two doctors and vouched for their impeccable "moral" character.[30] This episode illustrates the connections drawn between communism and socialized medicine, which had already begun to shape similar debates elsewhere.[31] Jeopardizing the lives and careers of some doctors even before the passage of Chile's anticommunist legislation, it drew attention to social/socialized medicine in ways that would become extremely dangerous for some of its advocates and practitioners.

The 1948 Chilean law that outlawed communist activity, and the capitalist rhetoric that warned about the spread of communism during the Cold War, fed existing anxieties about the possible loss of autonomy in a state-led health system. Industrial workers, for example, feared that proposed reforms would increase state control or co-opt their existing social insurance benefits; organized labor routinely rejected any outside regulation of their pension and health funds that might potentially undermine control of the funds by mutualist organizations.[32] White-collar workers refused to embrace socialized medicine reforms, concerned that the extension of social rights might result in being equated with the "lower" industrial working class.[33] Chilean elites' entrenched belief in "natural inequality" and concern that a universal health system would lead to greater social equality also heightened fears of comprehensive health reform.[34]

Many doctors remained uneasy about the possible consequences socialized medicine could have on their professional role.[35] Physicians fretted that status as employees in a state system would limit their autonomy and lower their incomes. They had grown accustomed to working for several employers, in addition to running their own private practices. They were uneasy about the implications of joining a single large organization (the state) without first negotiating their position under a new organizational structure. These tensions lessened in 1948, when the medical professional guilds helped create a new institution, the College of Physicians of Chile, as the principal body representing doctors' interests. Because the college lobbied on behalf of members, doctors were reassured that their interests would not be threatened under a unified health service. This development helped pave the way for passage of the SNS.[36]

Throughout these larger contextual shifts, both in terms of Cold War anticommunism and political and economic conditions in Chile, individual doctors committed to social medicine managed to create certain spaces for progressive medical praxis, community projects, and policy changes. Benjamín Viel's approach and activities offer a case in point.

Negotiating Social Medicine and Community Health Projects in the Cold War

Unlike Allende, Benjamín Viel, an epidemiologist with a keen interest in the organization of public health, was not affiliated with any political party, deliberately operating outside the realm of partisan politics. Viel's vision of social medicine was shaped by his experiences both in Chile and abroad, and he used his international relationships as a powerful asset in advancing his career and policy interests. In 1939 Viel was awarded the first of several fellowships by the Rockefeller Foundation's International Health Division; over the years he cooperated closely with the foundation as it broadened its activities in Chile.[37]

Viel earned a master's degree in public health from Harvard University in 1940 and a doctorate from Johns Hopkins in 1944. Upon his return to Chile, and still supported by the Rockefeller Foundation, he began to explore ways of incorporating social medicine into an expansion of community health units in urban areas. Viel used his expertise and international connections to find new approaches to reducing infant and maternal mortality among the urban poor. Quinta Normal, a working-class district of Santiago, became a testing ground for physicians, nurses, and midwives to cooperate and work closely with the local population.[38] Viel emphasized that the Rockefeller-funded public health units could inspire collaboration between people from the community and health personnel, under the latter's close supervision. The project Viel's team set up in Quinta Normal became an early, unofficial prototype for the primary health care model that would attract international attention in the 1970s.[39] The project promoted an effective health delivery system based on lessening the social and physical distance between doctors in hospitals and their patients' living environments. It also prioritized the use of only those medical technologies that were beneficial and accessible to the poor.[40]

Health posts were built close to the populations in need of service, to substitute for services formerly available only at distant hospitals. Local lay health personnel were involved in public health campaigns. Physicians, nurses, social workers, and midwives worked closely with the local population across all activities. Community leaders helped coordinate and organize services and facilitated interaction between doctors and patients.[41] Viel's team in Quinta Normal documented remarkable success, especially in treating alcoholism and preventing infant deaths by linking interventions to the social and physical environment of patients and communities. Public health statistics and testimonials confirmed the success of this social medicine praxis.[42] A Rockefeller field officer noted that "improvement is evident, mothers are more interested, more request service, [and] babies are better cared for."[43]

The Quinta Normal experience not only enhanced Viel's administrative expertise but also amplified his national and international reputation as a health official eager to help resolve the financial and organizational challenges of the practice of social medicine, potentially via socialized medicine. In 1950, the British Council of Cultural Relations invited Viel to visit England and Scotland to observe how the British National Health Service (NHS) functioned. Viel himself saw the NHS as a "classic" system of socialized medicine in which all medical and hospital services were administered by the state.[44] He had been impressed by the achievements of the NHS and the work of British economist and social reformer William Beveridge, whose 1942 report *Social Insurance and Allied Services* served as a model for a "comprehensive policy of social progress," including a set of health care services available to all citizens, funded through taxes.[45] Beveridge's sweeping proposal for a welfare state promised to end the Depression era and wartime austerity for all Britons and fulfill high working-class expectations for the postwar period. In 1945, the Labour Party, supportive of Beveridge's plans, won its first majority government in a landslide electoral victory. The party's campaign manifesto stated, provocatively, that "the Labour Party is a Socialist Party, and proud of it." With the Labour Party's commanding place in British politics, socialized medicine could weather the implications of being associated with socialism, which would have proven impossible in the United States.[46]

Back in Chile, meanwhile, Benjamín Viel's intentional detachment from the politics of "left and right" facilitated the success of some of his health projects. Viel and economist Francisco Pinto published a study on social security reform that included Viel's blueprint for a centralized health care system. Viel's plan, adapting aspects of the British approach, resembled Allende's model but was less provocative to political conservatives. Both men linked health reforms to the need to protect "human capital," but unlike Allende, Viel considered the redistribution of wealth and the end of class differences to be a secondary concern. Instead, he allayed the fears of those who held that socialized medicine would engender socialism by framing health as a contributor to economic productivity and national development. Viel and Pinto advanced a market capitalist logic similar to Cruz Coke's in 1938, with health integral to the ability to work. Workers, according to Viel and Pinto, were collectively powerful yet individually unable to pay for the benefits of medical science. Extending health care to all workers would not only prevent human suffering and misery but also increase the strength and productivity of the labor force. Viel and Pinto's proposal made clear that workers "should receive care not only because they are human beings, but also because the survival of the community depends on their existence, their physical and mental state."[47] While they recommended a state-led system of socialized medicine to create equal access to health care for all people, Viel and Pinto left class differences intact.[48]

Law 10.383 was passed in August 1952, creating Chile's Servicio Nacional de Salud (SNS), a conscious echo of Britain's NHS nomenclature. Through it, the state assumed responsibility for public health. However, Congress had approved the SNS only after making a number of significant modifications to the Viel-Pinto plan. Rural laborers, domestic and self-employed workers, and employees in private and public white-collar jobs remained excluded from what Pinto and Viel had originally envisioned as a universal system.[49] As a result, industrial workers in urban areas stood to benefit the most from the new policy. It was an improvement, to be sure, yet one that did not fully address the inequalities that health reformers had been pointing out for decades.

Socialized Medicine in the United States and the USSR: Cold War "Models"

Even after the creation of the SNS, the Cold War backdrop to Chile's debate on social and socialized medicine persisted. By then, renowned public health advocate Benjamín Viel had spent ample time in the United States and had moved up from his role as a Rockefeller-funded medical student to become an international expert. In the United States, he witnessed a public, symbolic, and charged critique of socialized medicine—the outcome of historical processes linked to early communist-capitalist rivalries. President Franklin D. Roosevelt, for example, had been adamant about adding public health legislation to the Social Security Act in the 1930s. However, amid pervasive propaganda depicting socialized medicine as a communist plot, Roosevelt and his advisers were apprehensive about the reaction of the conservative American Medical Association and of private insurance companies. This resulted in the delay and eventual removal of comprehensive health coverage from Roosevelt's New Deal agenda.[50] By the mid-1940s, as historian Beatrix Hoffman explains, "health reformers' insider status made them vulnerable to opponents who saw a Soviet-inspired conspiracy for 'socialized medicine' at the very heart of the federal government."[51]

Indeed, when President Harry Truman announced his advocacy for a national health care system in 1947, he insisted that he did not, by any means, promote "socialized medicine."[52] In 1950, economist and educator Melchior Palyi, a U.S. citizen of Hungarian descent and an internationally recognized educator, published a book on "compulsory medical care," a text that reflected the tone of critiques of socialized medicine in the Cold War United States. In his attack on both the welfare state and socialized medicine, Palyi argued that "all modern dictators—communist, fascist, or disguised—have at least one thing in common. They all believe in Social Security, especially in coercing people into governmentalized medicine." He warned of "Marxian Totalitarianism" and "Bismarckian Social Security," allegedly the true creeds of medical socialism.[53] Though it remains unclear how many people actually read Palyi's book—or other studies that emphasized the dangers of "medical socialism" loosely defined—the fear of state "controlled" and allegedly dangerous "compulsive" health services deeply affected a range of social policies in the Western Bloc.

In 1960, Viel was invited to the Soviet Union to observe the country's approaches to health care organization—and used the occasion to do fieldwork for a comparative study of socialized medicine in Great Britain, the Soviet Union, and Chile. His Soviet hosts, according to Viel, were eager to showcase what they considered to be socialized medicine successes, while Viel himself put forth a mix of concerns and praise. In his comparative volume published the following year, Viel emphasized the theme of patient-doctor relations over that of political management of physicians.[54] As a firm believer in the right of patients to choose their own physicians, he condemned what he perceived to be Soviet statist doctrine denying patients that right.[55] Observing medical education and the bureaucratic organizational structure of public health, he also criticized the Soviet system of "overspecialization" and its subdivision of public health into smaller units. He believed this arrangement prevented a holistic social medicine praxis, such as the one established at the Universidad de Chile's School of Public Health.[56]

Nonetheless, Viel praised other components of the Soviet health system. He was particularly impressed with the importance the Soviets assigned to fertility regulation. Viel approved of the attention that socialist countries gave to birth control and acknowledged that the doctrine of Marxism-Leninism recognized almost dogmatically that every woman has the right to decide and determine the number of children she wants to have.[57] Viel praised maternity clinics in the Soviet Union and the birth control information and materials made readily available to women there. He was well-disposed to—at one and the same time—learn from socialist models and apply for funding from sources espousing capitalist values to implement those models. Viel's promotion of family planning in Chile exemplified this attitude.

New Directions: From Social Medicine Praxis to Family Planning Programs

The family planning domain, starting in the 1960s, saw considerable reverberation of Cold War rivalries in Chilean health politics. While the Soviets had legalized abortion and advocated for women's own decision-making regarding their fertility, these discussions were more fraught in the United States, with legalization and public funding trailing philanthropic and popular interest. In 1965, however, the administration of Lyndon Johnson made a robust new commitment to support family planning programs anywhere in the world, provided such assistance was requested by national governments. Through the U.S. Agency for International Development, the State Department relentlessly promoted the use of birth control technologies and the crafting of population limitation policies in developing nations through the 1980s.[58] This strategy was predicated on the belief that rapid population growth in these nations exacerbated poverty, which, in turn, might increase popular sympathy for communism at a time when the Cuban Revolution made securing the allegiance of Latin American regimes a central geopolitical goal of the United States.[59]

Viel's population initiatives did not equate rapid population growth with an alleged communist threat, yet he drew from the Neo-Malthusian positions espoused by joint U.S.-Chile funded family planning programs. In the mid-1960s, Viel published a book, later translated into English, on what he called the "demographic explosion" in Latin America.[60] He alerted readers to the rapid population growth in the region overall and in Chile, where the population had more than doubled over the course of five decades, going from 3,731,593 people in 1920 to 8,884,768 in 1970.[61] Most dramatically, Santiago's population had increased fivefold in the same period due to declining mortality rates and growing immigration.[62]

Moved by such arguments about Chile's rapid population growth, Viel and other physicians and social scientists produced new research using census data, mortality statistics, and the personal histories of women from specific poor neighborhoods. They identified two main crises: high maternal mortality rates due to self-induced abortions and a threat of economic deceleration caused by rapid population growth in urban areas.[63] To justify new family planning programs, researchers and policymakers adopted a strategy designed to save the lives of women who relied on self-induced abortions as the only method of birth control available to them.

Crucially, the research leading to this strategy did not single out medical interventions as the sole solution to a complex social problem. Following in Virchow's social medicine footsteps, Viel and his colleagues began to tentatively portray rising maternal mortality at the intersection of poverty, sexual abuse, women's anxieties about the moral condemnation of childbearing out of wedlock, and the absence of birth control technologies. Physicians emphasized the last of these as they addressed what compelled many women to seek backstreet abortions, often without medical assistance.[64] A solution, therefore, could not lie exclusively in the biomedical realm. In fact, according to medical researchers, avoiding dangerous abortions would best be accomplished by "the prevention of unwanted pregnancies via adequate education campaigns that inform women about the use of contraceptive technologies adapted to their cultural and economic realities."[65]

Thus, the fieldwork studies of the 1960s, combined with women's testimonies, supplied evidence to correlate access to family planning education and services, the prevention of unwanted pregnancies, and a decrease in self-induced abortions and their gruesome consequences. Such studies validated earlier lessons about delivering education and resources suited to the needs and interests of the population served. Furthermore, because medical researchers linked their efforts to prevent abortions and maternal mortality to broader Cold War debates about the dangers of overpopulation in the developing world, they were able to secure the financial support of international agencies from capitalist nations, predominantly in the United States.

In 1965, these studies, combined with political activism, led to the creation of the Asociación Chilena de Protección de la Familia (APROFA, Chilean Association for the Protection of the Family). Viel's international contacts, as well as his advocacy of family planning as an economic development strategy, helped secure the backing and collaboration of the International Planned Parenthood Federation/ Western Hemisphere Region (IPPF/WHR) in New York, which provided financial and technical support of APROFA campaigns, including educational materials and contraceptives. The association's educational initiatives sought to reach the public, men as well as women, to support family planning programs and their goals—preventing abortions and maternal mortality, controlling population size, and protecting domestic economies from child-rearing expenses.[66] Under Viel's guidance, APROFA became the first private entity to establish family planning services in the country. Navigating complex waters, APROFA both strengthened its international ties and cooperated with the SNS. Yet the association's private status ensured that its family planning programs would be run by health officials and family planning educators not beholden to the government.[67] Keeping APROFA's leadership at arm's length from the government bureaucracy was important because, despite the persuasive campaign in favor of birth control that Viel and his colleagues spearheaded, the issue continued to be controversial in Chile, particularly among politically influential sectors such as the military and the Catholic Church.[68] As such, government agencies were best served by keeping a certain distance from family planning organizations.

The program's achievements were notable. Public health officials and practitioners encouraged women to use both APROFA services and those of Chile's

SNS. The collaboration was fruitful. By 1966, there were 102 APROFA family planning centers addressing women's needs nationwide, and more than 58,000 women had received contraceptives free of charge.[69] In September 1966, APROFA attained a significant distinction when it became a full member of the IPPF/WHR and, at the same time, received juridical personhood status from the Chilean government. The latter legalized the institutional and economic independence of APROFA clinics, paving the way to make the association into a self-financing organization.[70] Viel continued to work for APROFA for decades to come. With only a short moratorium on its activities imposed by the military dictatorship in the 1970s, APROFA endures to this day as the single most active institution promoting family planning and making birth control available to Chilean women and couples.

Viel's merit lay in his pioneering style of harnessing the new U.S. interest in population limitation during the tense Cold War and adapting it to address a dramatic health problem in Chile. Still, even though the prevention of self-induced abortions through family planning positively affected maternal health, the lessons of social medicine could have been even more radical. Most importantly, Viel and his colleagues might have used family planning initiatives to tackle other complex social problems women faced, such as the socially tolerated sexual violence that often led to unwanted pregnancies in the first place. Similarly, they failed to address the stigma attached to out-of-wedlock pregnancies, not to mention poverty itself. The popularization of birth control methods and education, in this context, was an important but only partial step to improve women's health. This is a key reminder of the constraints that local gender systems and political and economic structures—as well as global political and ideological factors—impose on health activities.

Conclusion

Cold War competition and anticommunist propaganda in the capitalist world represented an important backdrop, at times moving to center stage, for debates about social and socialized medicine. These factors determined the political variables that physicians and legislators had to consider in their deliberations on social and socialized medicine in Chile. From the 1930s on, these deliberations were marked by debates about the extent to which health should be considered as human capital, and thus indispensable for economic development.

For doctors such as Salvador Allende and Benjamín Viel, the subjects of social and socialized medicine remained on the forefront of their political and medical engagement—albeit in starkly different ways. Allende maintained a Marxist perspective that prioritized social and economic equality and transformative social change, evident in his understanding of the inseparability of poverty and ill-health, cited in this chapter's epigraphs. His vision of social medicine (and universal health care legislation) foregrounded the struggle against class differences as the underpinning of health. Viel's approach, meanwhile, offered ameliorative health programs for the popular classes based on social medicine practice (integrating medical care with attention to social conditions), community health projects, and family planning services. Allende, who asked "that the well-off contribute without haggling, for their own security," critiqued strategies that merely concealed the contradictions of modern capitalism.[71] His socialist inclination—defeated in his initial health reform proposal in the 1940s—would once again be tested in the 1970s, when socialized and social medicine was politically framed within a socialist system for the first time in Chilean history.

The Chilean experience confirms that the political variables of the Cold War—particularly the anticommunist campaign promoted in the capitalist world—limited the scope of health reforms and the implementation of socialized medicine, equating (the defense of) social and socialized medicine with an allegedly dangerous political ideology. But doctors could also negotiate these variables and mediate the consequences of Cold War constraints in the name of advancing what they defined as the nation's public health needs. The establishment of APROFA and the organization's success in obtaining SNS and foreign funds remain important evidence of the latter, at least in regard to social medicine. Still, Chile's own political structures constrained just how far some of these health programs and family planning initiatives could go.

Anne-Emanuelle Birn asserts that "the modern history of public health is perforce an international phenomenon"; indeed, the trajectory of social and socialized medicine in Chile demonstrates that we have to go beyond the geographical and political boundaries of nation-states to understand the changing politics of health.[72] Viel's international ties—in the United States, the United Kingdom, and the Soviet Union, as well as his determined nonpartisanship in his native Chile—allowed him to practice and promote (a version of) social medicine precisely because he did not equate health reform with the overturning of capitalism or with a robust challenge to class inequalities. In 1952, the newly founded state-run health care system enabled him to expand the social medicine model that he had implemented in his community health projects in the Quinta Normal neighborhood. Later, when population planners in the United States began to associate "overpopulation" with Cold War fears of communism, Viel succeeded in mobilizing both international and domestic support for family planning programs.[73] Predicting the supposed dangerous consequences of a "demographic explosion" that threatened economic development, he linked population policies both to social medicine practice and to the need for coordination between the community level and the national level through the health care system.[74]

Epilogue

In 1970, former health minister Salvador Allende became the nation's first elected socialist president. His leadership of the Unidad Popular (UP) coalition government, aiming for a peaceful road to socialism, would be short-lived. It was terminated by a September 11, 1973, U.S.-backed military coup that installed an anticommunist military dictatorship, led by Augusto Pinochet, that dominated Chilean life for seventeen years. Allende died in the government palace, La Moneda, on the day of the coup. Although Allende's defense of socialized medicine did not directly lead to his death, it is clear that his "radical" views on public health contributed to his depiction as a "subversive" political leader during the Cold War. Relative to the denunciations of communists in the 1940s, which led to discrimination and firing from public service, the dictatorship's 1970s anticommunism not only affected wider swaths of the population but also inflicted unprecedented violence upon its victims.

Like the 1940s witch hunt, the Pinochet dictatorship's persecution of the political left in Chile also affected health care workers. While Benjamín Viel had accepted a leadership position at the IPPF/WHR in New York City in 1970 and continued to live abroad in the 1980s, many of his collaborators were arrested, incarcerated, "disappeared," or sought political exile. In the eyes of the military, community health workers and social medicine practitioners were enemies of the state, regardless of their actual ideological and party affiliations. Consistent with this position, almost immediately after the coup, the military leadership purged the University of Chile's School of Public Health of its "leftist" faculty and officially terminated the Quinta Normal community health project. Dr. Gilda Gnecco, who had worked with Viel for many years and remained deeply immersed in Quinta Normal, remembered the sense of helplessness and defeat she felt upon finding the post shut and abandoned by military orders issued after the coup.[75] Many doctors, like Gilda Gnecco, lost their positions and struggled to survive the dictatorship.[76] As a consequence of the radical restructuring of the health system by the military regime, the School of Public Health lost not only much of its staff but also its historical connection to the community in Quinta Normal and its position of leadership in national public health policymaking.[77]

Cold War divisions and the politics of eliminating people and projects with social medicine ideas and alleged leftist ties continued to have repercussions on Chilean national realities and physicians' lives for decades to come. Although social medicine was not considered as great a threat as socialized medicine in the early Cold War, in later years, authoritarian and anticommunist forces regarded both as suspect and dangerous. Indeed, in Chile and across much of the world, social medicine has remained conflated with the purported dangers of socialized medicine, a reality that places boundaries on the reach of social policy changes and the implementation of adequate health systems in the twenty-first century.

Notes

Epigraphs: Allende, "Chile's Medical-Social Reality," 153, 155; cited in Illanes, "*En el Nombre del Pueblo, del Estado y de la Ciencia,*" 385.

1   This classic definition of "social medicine" can be traced as far back as 1848 in the writings of Rudolf Virchow. The basic features of "socialized medicine" as a state-controlled system of health insurance and care emerged between the 1880s and the 1910s, first in Germany and later in Scandinavian countries, France, and Switzerland. See Virchow, "Excerpts from 'Report on the Typhus Epidemic'"; Starr, *Social Transformation of American Medicine.*

2   In general, medical doctors were supportive of the bills, which involved the extension of social security benefits to the entire family of the worker and the unification of all health institutions under one agency, thereby strengthening medical and health infrastructures. See Rosselot, "Reseña Histórica de las Instituciones de Salud en Chile"; Allende, *Realidad Médico-Social Chilena.*

3   The interests of medical doctors were represented by the Medical Union (Sindicato Médico), founded in 1924, and the Chilean Medical Association (Asociación Médica de Chile, AMECH), founded in 1931; AMECH was the immediate predecessor of the College of Physicians of Chile (1948). See Molina, "Orígenes de la Asociación Médica de Chile." All of these organizations sought to defend the political and economic interests of medical doctors and to regulate medical practice, and their different degrees of involvement as well as specific demands and involvement in political campaigns were closely linked to the changing political landscape in Chile. For example, AMECH raised concerns about the diminished salaries that would be paid by public agencies and about the loss of the doctor-patient relationship as a result of institutionalized care. Its propositions were at

times contradictory. While AMECH made policy recommendations that sup-ported social and socialized medicine, it also backed policies that prioritized the privileges of medical doctors. Scholars have argued that the political positions—and related actions—of medical associations showed the ongoing ambiguous relationship between those proposals that favored social medicine and others that defended the professional (corporate) interests of physicians. See Lagos Escobar, *Cien Años de Luces y Sombras*.

4 AMECH emphasized that the College of Physicians of Chile and the Statutes of the Physician as Civil Servant (Colegio Médico de Chile y Estatuto del Médico Funcionario) were critical preconditions to any other organizational changes that could take effect. The former was needed to create the legal basis for ensuring the fair economic and professional treatment of the Medical Corps.

5 Marmor, "Right to Health Care."

6 The term "human capital" has a complex history. Here, I follow its definition adopted by economic development experts in the early twentieth century as intrinsically linked to the health of workers. In his 1939 book, *La Realidad Médico-Social Chilena*, Salvador Allende called human capital "the fundamental base of economic prosperity of a country" and asserted that "any governmental plan requires a dense and healthy population, capable of working towards a thriving industrial and economic development. This is the mission of human capital." See Allende Gossens, *Salvador Allende Reader*, 40. See also Goldsmith, Gutiérrez, and Sanhueza, *Country Profiles*, 1–2; Cifuentes, "Etapas del Proceso Sanitario Chileno," 25.

7 Cruz Coke's model of Christian social thought was expressed, for example, in the encyclical *Rerum Novarum*, that sought to mediate the "Rights and Duties of Capi-tal and Labor." This entailed the peaceful integration of the working class into the political and economic system and the acknowledgment of the voice of trade unions and other labor representation in the welfare state in Chile. Some scholars have argued that Eduardo Cruz Coke's political contributions to the develop-ment of public health and welfare and his specific (and changing) expressions of Christian social positions not only contributed to the shaping of the Chilean welfare state but also helped legitimize Christian social thought in the nation. In 1946, Cruz Coke was nominated by the Conservative Party as a candidate in the presidential election, and his campaign—based on Christian social thought—became an important step in the development of Chile's Christian Democratic Party. See Huneeus and Paz Lanas, "Ciencia Política e Historia"; see also Cruz Coke, *Discursos*.

8 Cruz Coke, "Chilean Preventive Medicine Act," 185, 188. See also de Viado, "Aims and Achievements of the Chilean Preventive Medicine Act."

9 Romero, "Hitos Fundamentales de la Medicina Social en Chile"; Molina, "An-tecedentes del Servicio Nacional de Salud"; Molina, *Institucionalidad Sanitaria Chilena*. See also Illanes, *"En el Nombre del Pueblo, del Estado y de la Ciencia"*; Salinas, "Salud, Ideología y Desarrollo Social en Chile." Benjamín Viel addresses the sub-ject in *Medicina Socializada y Su Aplicación en Gran Bretaña, Unión Soviética y Chile*.

10 Cited in Illanes, *"En el Nombre del Pueblo, del Estado y de la Ciencia,"* 385.

11 On the history of AMECH, see Illanes, *"En el Nombre del Pueblo, del Estado y de la Ciencia"*; Valdivia Ortiz de Zárate, *La Milicia Republicana*; Molina, "Orígenes de la Asociación Médica de Chile."

12 For the history of AMECH and its role as a pioneering organization whose members addressed questions of social and socialized medicine, see Molina, "Orígenes de la Asociación Médica de Chile."

13 For a list of propositions at the conference, see Díaz P., *Escuela de Salubridad de la Universidad de Chile*, 2. See also Chile, *Proyectos de Leyes*; Filerman, "Exploratory Field Study of the National Health Service," 41.

14 See Allende, "Chile's Medical-Social Reality," 151.

15 Waitzkin, "Social Medicine Then and Now"; Waitzkin, "Commentary."

16 See Manríquez, "Professor Max Westenhöfer." On Allende's student activism, see Tedeschi, Brown, and Fee, "Salvador Allende."

17 On this point, Virchow was also influenced by Friedrich Engels's devastating critique of the effects of capitalist exploitation on the health of the working class. See Engels, *Condition of the Working Class in England*, also discussed in Birn and Brown, "Making of Health Internationalists," 16–20.

18 Goschler, "Wahrheit zwischen Seziersaal und Parlament." See also Ackerknecht, *Rudolf Virchow*.

19 See Pieper Mooney, *Politics of Motherhood*, 28–29. On Allende's proposals and responses to such ideas, see "Dr. Allende nos Expone la Acción Desarrollada."

20 De Ramón, *Santiago de Chile*, 185.

21 Collier and Sater, *History of Chile*, 177. On infant mortality and its link to the fundamental disjuncture of patriarchy without patriarchal households, see Milanich, *Children of Fate*, 18.

22 In Bol. Congreso, Dip. Extraord., 25 de Diciembre de 1950, 1445–1522, cited in Illanes, *"En el Nombre del Pueblo, del Estado y de la Ciencia,"* 385.

23 Mardones Restat and de Azevedo, "Essential Health Reform in Chile"; Labra, "Medicina Social en Chile"; Labra, "Poder Médico y Políticas de Salud en Chile."

24 Corkill, "Chilean Socialist Party and the Popular Front," 261.

25 For patterns of denunciation of "unpatriotic" forces, see Pavilack, *Mining for the Nation*.

26 Kofas, "Politics of Foreign Debt." Indeed, the "law in defense of democracy" prevented all "agitators" from voting. For evidence that the new illegality of the Communist Party of Chile was not only about communism, see G. J. B., "Politics and Economies in Chile"; Venegas Valdebenito, "La 'Ley Maldita.'" Brian Loveman argues that anticommunism was reinforced after 1946 with the Chilean armed forces' participation in the Rio Pact (1947) and received the benefits of arms transfers and military educational opportunities in the United States. Loveman, *For La Patria*, 127.

27 Inspectoría de Puente Alto, *Informe providencia estrictamente reservada, sobre actividades comunistas de los médicos que se indica*, no. 15, Puente Alto, 12 de Marzo de 1948.

28 Some scholars see this as the second wave of anticommunism in Chile, linked
    to increased fear of communist agitation with the election of the first Popular
    Front government. See Bohoslavsky, "Anticomunismo en Chile." See also Venegas
    Valdebenito, "Anticomunismo y Control Social en Chile."
29 Huneeus, *Guerra Fría Chilena*.
30 See Huneeus, *Guerra Fría Chilena*, 267–68.
31 See Brickman, "Medical McCarthyism and the Punishment of Internationalist
    Physicians."
32 Illanes, *Historia del Movimiento Social y de la Salud Pública en Chile*; Illanes, *"En el
    Nombre del Pueblo, del Estado y de la Ciencia"*; DeShazo, *Urban Workers and Labor
    Unions in Chile*; Pavilack, *Mining for the Nation*. See also Góngora, *Ensayo Histórico
    sobre la Noción de Estado en Chile*.
33 On white-collar workers' unwillingness to be associated with the "lower" indus-
    trial working class, see Viel, "Medicina y Calidad de Vida."
34 In fact, Chile's old ruling elite had made efforts to combat communism long
    before the Cold War through charity, repression, and social legislation. See Rosem-
    blatt, "Charity, Rights, and Entitlement." See also Morris, *Elites, Intellectuals, and
    Consensus*.
35 Viel, *Medicina Socializada*, 149–50.
36 See also Villarroel and Venturini, "Contribución del Colegio Médico"; Molina,
    "Orígenes de la Asociación Médica de Chile."
37 For evidence of Rockefeller strategies and the clash of cultural values that at
    times troubled the interactions between Rockefeller missionaries of science and
    their Latin American counterparts, see Marcos Cueto, *Missionaries of Science*. For a
    critique of the Rockefeller campaigns, see also Birn, *Marriage of Convenience*.
38 Pinto, Francisco, and Viel, *Seguridad Social Chilena*, 10–11. Viel's Quinta Normal
    community health project was not unique in Chile. Dr. Alejandro del Rio, for
    example, led a similar project in Puente Alto. But Quinta Normal was special as
    it attracted the most foreign funding and institutional attention. See Filerman,
    Exploratory Field Study of the National Health Service, 43. For a discussion of the
    origin and application of similar interventions in other Latin American regions,
    see Birn, "Unidades Sanitarias."
39 World Health Organization, *Declaration of Alma-Ata*.
40 On related pilot health projects in the community, see also Ramos's chapter in
    this volume.
41 The Quinta Normal project also relied on funding from the Josiah Macy Founda-
    tion from the United States and the Patronato Nacional de la Infancia in Chile.
    See Viel, "Medicina y Calidad de Vida." On the functioning of one of these
    centers, the Centro de Atención Materno Infantil Integral Ismael Valdés, see also
    Vargas Catalá, *Historia de la Pediatría Chilena*.
42 Cabello González, "Influencia de la Unidad Sanitaria de Quinta Normal en la
    Reducción de la Mortalidad Infantil de la Comuna"; Salomón Rex, "Organización
    y Funcionamiento de Una Unidad Sanitaria."

43   J. H. Janney, Annual Report 1947, 84, International Health Division, Chile, February 25, 1948, Folder 1339, Rockefeller Archive Center, Sleepy Hollow, NY, record group 5, series 3, box 104.

44   Viel, *Medicina Socializada*, 11.

45   Beveridge, *Social Insurance and Allied Services*.

46   Dale, *Labour Party General Election Manifestos*, 55.

47   Pinto, Francisco, and Viel, *Seguridad Social Chilena*, 90.

48   Labra, "Medicina Social en Chile," 218.

49   Labra, "Medicina Social en Chile," 218. On the functions of the National Health Service, see *Vida Médica* 2, 13 (1952): 20–33.

50   Hoffman, "Health Care Reform and Social Movements in the United States"; Knoblauch, "Campaign Won as a Public Issue Will Stay Won."

51   Hoffman, "Health Care Reform and Social Movements in the United States," 77. See also Derickson, "House of Falk."

52   See Starr, *Social Transformation of American Medicine*; Geselbracht, *Civil Rights Legacy of Harry S. Truman*, 131; Truman, *Strictly Personal and Confidential*, 96.

53   Palyi, *Compulsory Medical Care and the Welfare State*, 18, 135.

54   Viel, *Medicina Socializada*. In his written assessment, Viel directly addressed the dangers of the propagandistic tone that most international publications on the subject had adopted in light of the rising superpower rivalry. He used Henry Sigerist's study of *Health Work in the Soviet Union* as a key source to help him evaluate Soviet practices, along with the works of Fraser Brockington and T. F. Fox, which highlighted the perspectives of social and preventive medicine practitioners. Viel cites his readings in *Medicina Socializada,* 107. See also Brockington, "Public Health in Russia"; T. F. Fox, "Russia Revisited."

55   Viel's position on this subject was reminiscent of the changed outlook of Chilean medical doctors in the 1960s: some physicians began to reject the statist tendency typified by Allende and others prior to the Cold War. Instead of seeing state-run medicine as the solution to health problems or to problems afflicting the profession, selected doctors campaigned for the principle of *libre elección*, the freedom for the patient to choose their doctor and pay a fee for their treatment directly to the physician. See Larrañaga Jiménez, "Estado Bienestar en Chile." This approach threatened previously dominant notions about the role of the state in health organization and appeared to prioritize a private and individualist form of care that contradicted Viel's general emphasis on collective and public health treatment in the community. It is likely that Viel's evaluations were informed by the 1959 restructuring of the Chilean SNS, when its base of operations was shifted away from local health clinics and moved to the hospital complex. This reorganization created new spaces for private and individualist form of care and for independent doctor-patient relationships that catered to middle sectors who could pay for specialized treatments. For references to the earlier history of medical doctors' complicated relationship with private practice, see Vargas Cariola, "Médicos."

56   Viel, *Medicina Socializada*, 133.

57 While Viel acknowledged that women's right to regulate their fertility was invoked with the onset of the Russian Revolution, he also documented the "practical" approach to fertility regulation by the Soviet leadership. In the context of the enormous death rates in the Second World War, for example, the use of contraceptives was declared "an expression of bourgeois selfishness." According to Viel, the tolerant attitude toward contraception and abortion was reinstated in 1955. See Viel, *Explosión Demográfica*, 115–16; Viel, *Demographic Explosion*, 113. See also Viel, *Medicina Socializada*, 144–45.

58 On the role of Puerto Rico as a laboratory for family-planning research, see also Necochea López's chapter in this volume.

59 For evidence of the impact of this strategy in different national contexts, see Necochea López, *History of Family Planning in Twentieth-Century Peru*; Hartmann, *Reproductive Rights and Wrongs*; Pieper Mooney, *Politics of Motherhood*.

60 Viel, *Explosión Demográfica*; Viel, *Demographic Explosion*.

61 Martínez, *Situación y Tendencias*.

62 Viel, "Family Planning in Chile"; Viel, "Population Explosion in Latin America."

63 On the political context of the institutionalization of family planning, see Pieper Mooney, *Politics of Motherhood*; Zárate and González Moya, "Planificación Familiar en la Guerra Fría Chilena"; Rojas Mira, "Global y lo Local en los Inicios de la Planificación Familiar en Chile." For a general introduction to the history of fertility regulation in Chile, see also Jiles Moreno and Rojas Mira, *De la Miel a los Implantes*; Zárate, *Dar a Luz en Chile, Siglo XIX*.

64 Romero, Medina, and Vildósola, "Aportes al Conocimiento de la Procreación." For women's explanations of their own abortions, see Armijo and Monreal, "Epidemiology of Provoked Abortion in Santiago"; Armijo and Monreal, "Factores Asociados a las Complicaciones del Aborto Provocado."

65 *Revista Ercilla* 1453 (1963): 17.

66 Armijo et al., "Problem of Induced Abortion in Chile"; Hall, "Hombres y la Educación."

67 See Rosselot, "Regulación de la Natalidad en el Servicio Nacional de Salud de Chile."

68 For details on military restrictions to family planning, see Pieper Mooney, *Politics of Motherhood*, chapter 5. Religious influences have changed dramatically with the increased involvement of Opus Dei in Chilean politics. See Monckeberg, *Imperio del Opus Dei en Chile*.

69 Hankinson and International Planned Parenthood Federation, *Proceedings of the Eighth International Conference of the International Planned Parenthood Federation, Santiago, Chile*, 181.

70 The government granted APROFA *persona juridica* status Decree 2194, September 5, 1966. See Avendaño, *Desarrollo Histórico*, 13–14.

71 Allende, *Realidad Médico-Social Chilena*, 155.

72 Birn, "Nexo Nacional-Internacional na Saúde Pública," 676.

73 Viel suggested that socialized medicine could effectively tackle the problem of "overpopulation," arguing that top-down control of population policies would

further Chilean development. See, for example, Viel, *Medicina Socializada,* especially 44–45. Viel also took advantage of a shift within the Rockefeller Foundation away from public health campaigns toward population growth concerns. See Larraín, *Sociedad Médica de Santiago.*

74 Pinto, Francisco, and Viel, *Seguridad Social Chilena*; Viel, *Medicina Socializada*; Viel, *Explosión Demográfica*; Viel, *Demographic Explosion.*

75 Gilda Gnecco, interview with the author, Santiago, Chile, January 2013.

76 Gilda Gnecco continued to work in multiple "underground" health projects as well as with the Vicariate of Solidarity.

77 Pino and Solimano, "School of Public Health at the University of Chile."

8

"Psychotherapy of the Oppressed"

Anti-Imperialism and Psychoanalysis in Cold War Buenos Aires

MARCO RAMOS

In 1972, a group of British and Argentine psychiatrists came together to conduct a rather bizarre experiment in the Belgrano neighborhood of Buenos Aires. An outsider would have hardly recognized it as an experiment at all. It did not involve medical facilities, psychological testing, or psychiatric treatments. Instead, the experiment consisted of filling a large house—called simply "La Casona"—with twenty-five young people, several of whom had been diagnosed as psychotic. These "research subjects" lived together with the organizer of the experiment, British psychiatrist David Cooper, and several prominent Argentine psychiatrists, including Eduardo Pavlovsky. Argentine mental health professionals had invited Cooper to Buenos Aires to share his new vision of "antipsychiatry," a growing movement that attacked the legitimacy of traditional psychiatric practice.[1] Through the development of antipsychiatric communes in Argentina, like La Casona, Cooper believed he could prove that schizophrenia was not a condition that should be stigmatized, pathologized, or treated in mental institutions. In fact, the schizophrenic, Cooper argued, was not ill or sick at all, but had a lot to teach psychiatrists and Western society. These antipsychiatric communes, Cooper and his followers argued, would reform social and political relations in Argentina and even launch a "Third World revolution."

Despite the initial promise of antipsychiatry in Argentina, Cooper's "politico-therapeutic" experiment in La Casona ultimately failed. Leftist psychiatrists in Buenos Aires objected to the neocolonial underpinnings of antipsychiatry and Cooper's countercultural, hippie lifestyle. "What for the

Europeans is counterculture," wrote prominent psychiatrist Hernán Kesselman in an article on antipsychiatry, "for Argentines and Latin Americans in general should be counter-colonization."[2] Despite Cooper's insistence that his "antipsychiatric experimentation" was an "attack on imperialism," Argentines accused the project of cultural colonialism.

I take this outlandish failed experiment as a starting point for examining conflicting global visions of anti-imperialism and the "Third World" in Buenos Aires during the late Cold War. Much of the literature on Argentine psychiatry, particularly psychoanalysis, has emphasized the strong, transnational connections forged between European and *porteño* (Buenos Aires) practitioners in the second half of the twentieth century. Scholars have traced the diffusion of the work of British psychoanalyst Melanie Klein, French psychoanalyst Jacques Lacan, French philosopher Louis Althusser, and more recently Soviet psychologists such as Lev Vygotsky.[3] As psychoanalyst Luis Hornstein recently pointed out, Argentine psychoanalysis is often situated "between Vienna, London, and Paris," reflecting and reinforcing the commonplace view that Buenos Aires is an outpost of European culture, a "Villa Freud," in a Southern continent.[4]

However, psychiatry in Buenos Aires was far more than a receptacle for the diffusion of Euro-American and Soviet thought in the 1970s. In this chapter, I argue that psychiatry in Buenos Aires provides an invaluable window into the imagined political and medical futures of the Third World during the middle-late Cold War. With the emergence of Peronist nationalism on the political left in the 1970s, psychiatrists in Buenos Aires used their profession to expose the neocolonial violence of the Cold War superpowers and to imagine an independent Argentine nation, liberated from the clutches of U.S. and Soviet imperialism. Psychiatrists in the openly Marxist Federación Argentina de Psiquiatras (FAP)—the largest psychiatric organization in Argentina in the 1970s—read not only Europeans like Klein and Althusser, but also anticolonial, Third World thinkers, such as Frantz Fanon, Paulo Freire, Ernesto "Che" Guevara, and Mao Zedong.[5] They situated Buenos Aires not as a European capital below the equator, but as a site of anticolonial, Third World struggle in solidarity with Havana, Algiers, and Beijing.

Rather than tracing global *connections* between Argentine and European practitioners, this chapter follows a series of transnational *desencuentros* (failed encounters), as leftist psychiatrists in Buenos Aires critiqued U.S. and Soviet psychiatry on anticolonial grounds. In the first two sections, I discuss anti-imperial attitudes in Buenos Aires toward First World psychiatry (in the guise of Cooper) and toward U.S. capitalism (in the form of psychodynamic critiques of dependency linked to the penetration of U.S. factories in Argentina and of ambivalence around reliance on U.S. philanthropic funding). The third section moves to the Second World and explores another desencuentro, this time between leftist Argentine psychoanalysts in the FAP and F. V. Bassin, a Soviet psychiatrist in Moscow. Though the meeting was somewhat productive, FAP psychoanalysts and Bassin ultimately diverged in their belief in the revolutionary potential of psychoanalysis. Bassin maintained that psychoanalysis reduced socioeconomic realities to intrapsychic conflict, while Argentine analysts concluded that Bassin privileged laboratory-based, Soviet theories of the mind over the psychodynamic study of the unconscious.[6] The final section discusses nationalist, Third World visions of psychiatry in Buenos Aires, as psychiatrists inspired by leftist Peronism grounded their profession in the history and culture of the Argentine nation. Throughout this story, we see leftist mental health professionals in Buenos Aires walking a fine anti-imperial line as they attempted to secure resources, both material and ideological, from the superpowers while also imagining a sovereign, nationalist future without them.

Beyond the historiography on Argentine psychoanalysis, this chapter also contributes to the emerging literature on science and medicine in the global Cold War. A large and growing body of work has demonstrated that science, medicine, and health are fertile ground for the exploration of Cold War imaginaries in the U.S. and Soviet superpowers.[7] The Space Race, atomic power, the "defeat" of infectious disease with antibiotics, "wonder drugs," CIA and KGB brainwashing techniques—the list goes on—all reflected and reinforced Cold War dreams of terrestrial (and extraterrestrial) domination.

Less attention, however, has been paid to how Cold War medicine can provide insight—not into superpower dominance, but into Third World revolution and anti-imperialism.[8] After all, the revolutionary Guevara, who makes an appearance in this story, was an Argentine physician, and Frantz Fanon, also present here, was a Martinique-born psychiatrist who had worked under French colonial medical service in Algeria. As I discuss, leftist psychiatrists in Buenos Aires traveled to Havana to visit Guevara and Fidel Castro in the 1970s and elaborate politico-medical visions of a revolutionary Latin America. Another group of leftist psychiatrists in Buenos Aires created the "Fanon Group" to connect struggles against European colonialism in Africa with revolutionary nationalism in Argentina as a "dependent economy" of the United States.

However, for all the passionate talk of anti-imperial revolution in the field of Argentine mental health, I conclude that "anti-imperialism" was at best a vague, shifting concept in the 1970s, more likely to result in misunderstandings, desencuentros, and contradictions than synthesis and action. Without a doubt, anti-imperial discourse inspired activism, psychiatric research, and transnational travel, but it never coalesced intellectually as a unified theory, politically as a leftist revolution, or professionally in a dedicated psychiatric organization. Rather than provide answers, the discourse of anti-imperialism was the language with which leftist Argentine psychiatrists raised questions about the meaning of "Argentina" as a nation and its position relative to broader political and scientific developments in the global Cold War. Should psychiatrists in Argentina turn to radical thinkers, like Cooper, who were from the First World but claimed to be "anti-imperial" supporters of the Third? Was Soviet psychiatry, which had already gone through its own revolution, a better match for Argentine mental health? Or should Argentine psychiatrists eschew the imperialist thinking of the First and Second Worlds altogether to ground psychiatry in their own nation's deep history and culture? Anti-imperialism was not the answer to these questions—rather, it was the discourse in which they were articulated. This chapter focuses on Marxist psychoanalysts, "hippie" gurus, and European *tiersmondistes* to show how Cold War health in Latin America was drawn not only along East–West lines but also around diverse, often conflicting North–South visions of the Third World as a promising escape from U.S. and Soviet neocolonialism.

Revolutionary Psychoanalysis in Argentina

In the early 1970s, Argentine psychoanalysis was in the midst of a leftist radicalization. The official psychoanalytic organization in Argentina, the Asociación Psicoanalítica Argentina (APA), had recently witnessed the defection of two vocal groups, Plataforma and Documento, from its ranks. The reasons cited for the fracture were nothing less than a political awakening. The manifesto of Plataforma read, "As scientists and professionals, we propose to put our knowledge at the service of the ideologies that question, without compromise, the system in our country that . . . exploits the oppressed classes."[9] Both Documento and the more radical Plataforma objected to the "neutrality" that had characterized the psychoanalytic profession throughout the 1950s and 1960s, and both groups pledged to break from tradition and put psychoanalysis at the service of the people.[10] In triumphant language, they claimed that they were the "first in the history of the world to break from a psychoanalytic society for politico-ideological reasons."[11] The member list of Plataforma and Documento contained some of the most prestigious and influential psychoanalysts in Argentina, including an original founder of the APA, Marie Langer.

This leftist awakening in the psychiatric field was inspired by political mobilization in Argentina at large.[12] In 1969, students and workers in the city of Córdoba, Argentina, launched a civil uprising against the dictatorship of General Juan Carlos Onganía. Onganía's military government (1966–1969) was the first in a series of U.S.-backed dictatorships in Argentina, culminating in the 1976 dictatorship of Jorge Rafael Videla, which used terror against its citizens to stem the tide of "communist subversion." The 1969 "Cordobazo" revolt, as it affectionately came to be called, demonstrated the presence of popular support for violence against the military regime, strengthened revolutionary guerrilla movements, and became a rallying cry for leftist intellectuals, including psychoanalysts. "The Cordobazo woke us up as an institution," noted Marie Langer.[13] In 1971, Langer published an influential essay, "Psychoanalysis and/or Social Revolution," in which she argued that analysts should not separate political commitment from their psychoanalytic practice.[14] Led by Langer, practitioners in Plataforma argued that psychoanalysis would no longer serve as a tool of social control that adapted citizens to the norms of those in power; instead, it would facilitate a revolution. Throughout the early 1970s, efforts to unite Freud with Marx became the central theoretical and clinical project for a generation of Argentine psychoanalysts.[15]

British psychiatrist David Cooper arrived in Argentina in 1970 amid this radicalization of the psychoanalytic field. The director of the Asociación Argentina de Psiquiatría Social (Argentine Association of Social Psychiatry), Mauricio Goldenberg—who was arguably the most prominent psychiatrist in Argentina at the time—had arranged for Cooper's visit to Buenos Aires. Goldenberg's interest in Cooper, at least from a clinical perspective, concerned the British psychiatrist's world-famous therapeutic community, called "Villa 21," at the Shenley Hospital in Hertfordshire, England. Therapeutic communities were a new psychiatric approach in the 1960s that emphasized patient participation in mental health care by promoting a democratic, inclusive institutional culture. Largely inspired by Cooper's service at Villa 21, therapeutic communities were popping up across the globe in the 1960s and 1970s, in the United States, Italy, and France, as well as Argentina. Argentine psychiatrists Raúl Camino and Wilbur Grimson, for example, founded prominent therapeutic communities in and outside of Buenos Aires that were based on the work of Cooper and fellow British psychiatrists Maxwell Jones and Thomas Main.[16]

Progressive psychiatrists flocked to hear Cooper speak about Villa 21 at the famous Psychopathological Service at Lanús in Buenos Aires. Cooper told Argentine mental health professionals that he had flattened the clinical hierarchy at Villa 21, generating a "progressive blurring of the role between nurses, doctors, occupational therapists, and patients."[17] Cooper now questioned the need for and function of roles like "the sick patient who needs treatment," "the healthy doctor who has a cure," and even the category of "mental illness" itself. He wondered, "Can patients treat each other? Can staff acknowledge their own 'illness' and need for 'treatment'? If they did, what would happen next? Were not these categories of 'illness' and 'treatment' themselves ultimately suspect?"[18] These experiences at Villa 21 led Cooper to center his latest book around the concept of "antipsychiatry" or the rejection of the fundamental categories and practices that grounded traditional psychiatric care.

Cooper was a sensation in Buenos Aires, as much for his provocative thinking as for his eccentric personality. Covering one of his talks, the Argentine popular magazine *Panorama* stated that Cooper had "seduced" young mental health professionals in Buenos Aires. "They swooned at [his] black sweater and the frayed pants, the curly red hair and the interminable beard."[19] Scandalizing Argentine sensibilities, which he described as "too formal," Cooper sat on the floor with his shoes off to give his talk at Lanús.[20] Argentine psychiatrist Wilbur Grimson, who ran one of the major therapeutic communities in Buenos Aires, remembers Cooper less as a health professional, and more as a charismatic "guru."[21] "Before the diffusion of concepts or theories," Grimson recalled, "Cooper appeared to consider the models of life concordant with his ideas. . . . Those who surrounded themselves with the persona of Cooper noted . . . the force generated by his detachment from all social comforts, which opened new ways of living and being."[22] Grimson argued that antipsychiatry for Cooper was more than an academic idea or clinical orientation. The British psychiatrist also *performed* antipsychiatry in his everyday life through his countercultural sensibility and style of being.[23]

Beyond an interest in his clinical work, leftist psychiatrists in Argentina—especially those involved in the Plataforma and Documento movements—were drawn to Cooper's radical politics, particularly his attempts to unite socialist revolution with psychiatric practice. From the start, psychoanalysts in Plataforma considered their relationship to European thinkers, like Cooper, and their position within global knowledge networks. In fact, the Plataforma movement actually began in Europe in the climate of May 1968, when a group of European and Argentine psychoanalysts broke off from the 1969 International Psychoanalytical Association Conference in Rome for politico-ideological reasons. "Platform" movements emerged not only in Buenos Aires but also in Austria, Italy, and Switzerland in the aftermath of the congress.[24] In an early Plataforma piece, "Psychoanalysis and Anti-imperialism," Hernán Kesselman noted with a mixture of irony and pride that Europeans were recognizing Latin America not for its delicious "beef nor for its *fútbol,* but because of its profound anti-imperialist and anticapitalist vocation that characterizes the struggle of our peoples in the Third World."[25] Kesselman may as well have been describing Cooper. The British psychiatrist was part of a growing movement of New Left intellectuals in New York, Paris, and London who romanticized the Third World during the Cold War as a promising alternative to an unsatisfying First and Second World dichotomy. Many of these tiersmondistes thinkers objected to the colonialism of their European homes and traveled south in the 1970s to interact firsthand with anticolonial revolutionary movements in Africa, Asia, and Latin America. For example, Cooper's closest English colleague, R. D. Laing, who was a major force in the international antipsychiatry movement, traveled to India several times throughout the 1970s. French philosopher Jean-Paul Sartre visited Castro in 1966, and the Italian radical psychiatrist Franco Basaglia followed in Cooper's footsteps and traveled to Argentina later in the decade.

Cooper claimed an especially intimate relationship with the Third World and a personal stake in anticolonial struggle. In an interview with the Argentine newspaper *La Opinión,* Cooper pointed out that he had been born in South Africa in 1931 and moved to England only after medical school, to complete his psychiatric training. "From a very personal point of view, I am in Buenos Aires because I passed the first quarter of a century of my life in the Third World," he proudly stated.[26] Because of "obvious reasons," presumably the apartheid regime, Cooper felt he could not return to South Africa, but he saw his "return to Argentina [as] something like a 'home-coming.'"[27] Cooper framed his trip to Buenos Aires as a struggle against "cultural neo-imperialism," and in an interview with the newspaper *Panorama,* he stated, "It was time for the First World to look to the Third World!"[28] In Buenos Aires, Cooper planned to establish an "International Center for the Third World," as he called it, where First World psychiatrists would come to "Third World Argentina" not to teach, but to learn. He criticized the "political inertia of the British system" he had left behind—the fact that England was firmly planted in First World democracy and capitalism. He argued that advances in (anti)psychiatry would emerge not in the "politically inert" spaces of Euro-America, but amid the revolutionary volatility of Third World spaces such as Argentina.[29]

While Europeans were romanticizing the Third World in New York, Paris, and London in the 1970s, leftist intellectuals in Latin America were negotiating their relationship to anticolonialism and the Third World. Latin American states were not "postcolonial" in the same sense as African and Asian ones that were forging new nations for the first times in their histories, but concepts such as "cultural and economic imperialism" and "structural dependency" helped connect revolutionary struggle in Latin America to the decolonizing projects of their southern neighbors.[30] For example, the Uruguayan leftist thinker Eduardo Galeano, who published the influential *Las Venas Abiertas de América Latina* in 1971, helped draw analogies between the Cold War exploitation of Latin America and the formal colonialism of the past, as well as Caribbean, African, and Asian decolonization in the present.[31] The insights of the Economic Commission for Latin America and the Caribbean provided a political-economic framework for the Non-Aligned Movement, which sought to unite countries in Africa, Asia, and Latin America against the neo-imperialism of the Cold War superpowers in the second half of the twentieth century.[32]

Leftist psychoanalysts connected their revolutionary struggles in Buenos Aires to anticolonial movements across the Third World. In the FAP, one group organized itself around a fellow psychiatrist fighting for social liberation in Africa, Frantz Fanon. Written in 1969, the manifesto of the "Fanon Group," as it called itself, cited at length Fanon's 1956 letter of resignation from the French colonial psychiatric service and his call to arms against the violence of colonization in Algeria. The group wrote, "[Fanon] marks the destiny . . . of [Argentina] . . . by exposing the exotic 'other context' of faraway peoples in wars of social and national liberation. [These other contexts] actually reflect our own daily pulse . . . and reality."[33] The Fanon Group linked the distant struggles of psychiatrists navigating decolonization in North Africa to the everyday realities of Argentina as a "dependent economy." As Fanon had shown, psychiatry could provide a critical framework for justifying a revolution that was already happening in Africa, and that many psychiatrists believed was just on the horizon in Argentina.

Putting psychoanalysis at the service of the people and anti-imperial interests required scientific labor and institution building. After the split from the APA, which had served as the major psychoanalytic training center in Argentina, members of Plataforma and Documento needed alternative sites of instruction. Founded in 1972, the Marxist Centro de Docencia e Investigación (CDI) was designed to fill this gap and was created in line with the goals of the Plataforma and Documento groups.[34] In the early 1970s, a generation of young, generally leftist psychologists, psychiatrists, social scientists, and activists trained and taught at the CDI, which was divided into three areas. Area 1 was devoted to historical and dialectical materialism. Courses were taught primarily by Marxist university professors in sociology, history, and anthropology. Area 2 focused more squarely on psychoanalysis.

Specifically, there were courses on psychoanalytic theory, nosography, and psychoanalytic psychopathology. Finally, Area 3 attempted to translate the theory from Areas 1 and 2 into action within the local political world in Buenos Aires. In this more "applied" area of the CDI, concrete experiences with "workers" in diverse institutions were encouraged as part of the learning experience.[35]

A paradigmatic example of the anti-imperial dimensions of the CDI's work was a research study conducted by leftist psychoanalysts Hugo Vezzetti and Guillermo Pecheny on the psychodynamic effects of economic dependency in the U.S. Standard Electric Plant in San Isidro in the province of Buenos Aires.[36] Published in the popular leftist cultural journal *Los Libros* in 1973, the study approached the plant as a site of colonial penetration. Through interviews and meetings with Standard Electric workers, the authors gathered evidence about the psychodynamic effects of U.S. economic imperialism on Argentine workers and citizens. "The function of the repressive order [in the plant]," they argued, "points to a totalizing mode of control that encompasses the [workers'] means of communication . . . , their values, and attitudes, that is to say, a true ideological and psychological conditioning [of the worker]."[37] Vezzetti and Pecheny argued that "totalizing" control on the plant floor—including the regulation of bathroom visits, mandated silence, unequal promotion of workers to sow dissent, deliberate circulation of rumor, demanding work hours, monotonous labor, and so forth—could not be explained through economic analysis alone. Outside of the simple maximization of profit, there existed a dimension of power essential to production that *psychologically* conditioned and disciplined the factory worker to the behaviors and thinking appropriate to the proletariat. Vezzetti and Pecheny claimed the goal of their study was not simply to trace the psychodynamic effects of the labor environment in one industrial plant, but rather, at a more general level, to understand the emergence of compliant proletariat subjectivity in exploited and dependent economies. For Vezzetti and Pecheny, the psychological effects of the imperialist penetration of Standard Electric in Argentina went beyond the lives of the workers within the plant. The "deforming impact of imperialist penetration," they argued, affected large sectors of society and caused a breakdown in the psychophysical development of Argentina as a nation.[38]

The published version of Vezzetti and Pecheny's Standard Electric study was framed by a quotation from a participating worker. I quote it in full here as it offers a particularly clear vision of how both psychologists and factory workers envisioned the work of revolutionary research at the CDI in the early 1970s:

What is new in this [research] is the chance for the Standard Electric workers . . . to see a new type of science that is different from the . . . science that serves our bosses. [It is] a science that can help the working class to see more clearly the condition and situation in which they live. . . . Around that reality, [we can] construct together a new science that fundamentally aids the revolutionary process, helps deepen the level of consciousness of factory workers, and connects scientists themselves with concrete reality.[39]

By connecting psychology with the lived experiences of workers, mental health professionals at the CDI hoped to construct a new brand of science that worked not as a tool of imperialism and capitalism, but in the interests of national revolution.

The tiersmondiste Cooper and leftist psychiatrists in Buenos Aires, then, shared not only an interest in progressive psychiatric techniques, but also an anticolonial orientation, valorization of the Third World, and a leftist belief in psychiatric revolution. This shared understanding provided the foundation for the rather bizarre experiment described at the beginning of this chapter. During his time in Buenos Aires, Cooper was introduced to the leading Plataforma psychiatrists Hernán Kesselman and Eduardo Pavlovsky, who lived together in a large house called La Casona in the Belgrano neighborhood of Buenos Aires. The three psychiatrists agreed to conduct an "antipsychiatric" or "politico-therapeutic" experiment at La Casona, envisioned primarily by Cooper, sometime in 1972. The experiment involved twenty-five people living in the house, including Cooper and Pavlovsky. Most of the people living there had passed through "some type" of psychiatric institution, including individuals "currently classified as 'psychotic.'" Cooper stated that communalism and free love—sharing everything from personal property to "the sexual"—should reign in the commune. Everyone would also share in the betterment of their own and everyone else's mental health without any semblance of a "doctor-patient" relationship. Finally, he proposed an "exterior guide," between the ages of twenty-five and thirty-five, who did not live in the house, to supervise the whole process.[40]

These communes were at the center of Cooper's ambitious *foquismo* (focal point) theory of psychiatric revolution. In his second major book, *The Grammar of Living*, which was written while in Argentina in the early 1970s, Cooper argued that these communes could serve as Guevarist-style *focos* that would spark a revolution, not through armed conflict, but through the transformation of microsocial relations.[41] His communes would allow Argentine citizens to develop "new ways of living in a pre-revolutionary society," through the interaction with madness outside of a medical context. These interactions would let Argentines extend the notion of politics beyond "the macrosocial, [beyond] politics at the scale of political parties, national states, and geopolitics." Citizens would learn to explore the "micropolitical . . . in groups where one encounters the other face to face."[42] The overturning of micropolitical relations in the daily life of his *foquista* communes, Cooper argued, would eventually ignite "revolutionary activism," spilling into the macropolitical realm and overturning the structure of Argentine society.

The La Casona Experiment and First World Imperialism

Progressive psychiatrists in Argentina saw Cooper's proposed experiment at La Casona as a potentially significant step in the evolution of therapeutic communities as a psychiatric technique in Argentina and abroad. Cooper's attention to the politics of microsocial relations in psychiatric institutions and his antipsychiatric efforts to blur the boundaries between doctor, staff, and patient were clearly rooted in his own experiences working in therapeutic communities, particularly Villa 21, in England.[43] His radical proposal to create not a therapeutic community but a *politico*-therapeutic commune at La Casona piqued the interest of Argentine psychiatrists who—whether politicized or not—had been involved in efforts to democratize psychiatric care since the 1960s and who wanted to gain insight into the latest developments in progressive community psychiatry from England.[44]

However, despite its initial promise and the interest it garnered among Argentine psychiatrists, the experiment at La Casona ended in failure. Much of the criticism leveled at the experiment—from Pavlovsky, Kesselman, and Grimson, among others—was directed at Cooper's *hippismo*. Antipsychiatry for Cooper was more than just a politico-therapeutic orientation—it was a way of being in the world that infused his everyday life and personal interaction with others. In fact, in *The Grammar of Living*, Cooper formalized this aspect of antipsychiatry as a "μ-shift" (mu-shift), which designated the "bi-directional movement" between the radical reform of microsocial relations among individuals and macropolitical revolution in Argentine society at large.[45] Within La Casona, this microsocial reform manifested itself as "*hippie* counterculture," according to Pavlovsky. "In [La Casona, Cooper] was in love with a very young girl. She made [him] crazy there," Pavlovsky recalled. Strangers passed in and out of the house daily, and Cooper slept on a mattress on the floor to "declass" himself and lower his social status. Pavlovsky remembered, "It was madness [*una locura*] in the house: I lived with David Cooper and the ideological move-ment of '60, the *hippismo*. . . . The other [Argentine psychoanalysts]—Emilio Rodrigué, Armando Bauleo, and Hernán Kesselman—came to La Casona but did not live there, which was dangerous because I was left alone to deal both with an irrational love relationship and with Cooper's friends." While Pavlov-sky and Kesselman, among others, entertained Cooper's experiment for a few months, eventually they grew tired of the project, and it ended abruptly some-time in late 1972.[46]

Despite all the potential points of convergence—from an emphasis on progressive therapeutic communities to anticolonial movements in the Third World—leftist Argentine psychoanalysts were, in the end, critical of Cooper and his antipsychiatry. After his experience in La Casona, Kesselman, for ex-ample, doubted the revolutionary potential of hippismo in the Third World. He wrote, "The counterculture that we recognize as one of the most accessible means of combat for the youth of the 'developed' countries, extrapolated me-chanically as a banner of struggle to our environment and our reality, would be another form of Europeanizing and colonizing penetration."[47] It is hard to imagine that Cooper—the most obvious referent for First World hippismo in Buenos Aires in 1972—was not on Kesselman's mind as the representative of this "colonizing penetration." Others directly challenged Cooper's contention that a countercultural reform of microsocial relations in Argentine society could ever develop into a more general revolution. The psychiatrists Antonio and Nicolás Caparrós, who advocated for political militancy in the field of mental health during the 1970s, directly targeted antipsychiatry in their work. Later, the Caparrós cousins would publish the influential book *Psicología de la Liberación* (Psychology of Liberation), a key reference for the liberation psy-chology movement that developed in Latin America in the 1980s and 1990s.[48] Concerning antipsychiatry, they remarked dismissively in 1973, "The formal proposals of Antipsychiatry in relation to problems . . . of the Third World, would lead to the elimination of the growing participation . . . of the popular strata and consequently to sterile marginalization."[49] Antipsychiatry's "indu-bitable hue of individualism," which was "typical of the metropole," prevented the collective action that was necessary for revolution in Argentine society.[50] Cooper's communes were not revolutionary focos, according to Caparrós, but the colonial outposts of a First World "guru."

Though Cooper insisted that First World scholars should learn, not teach, in the Third World, Argentine mental health practitioners pointed out that he had difficulty following that rule himself. Cooper clearly came to Argen-tina to teach, lead, experiment, and prescribe. This is evident from his stance on the legalization of marijuana. Consistent with his ties to counterculture, he advocated for the legalization of marijuana in the First World, but in the Third World he encouraged its prohibition. In a newspaper, Cooper wrote that marjiuana's "illegality engenders vigilance, and its generalized use halts the revolutionary process."[51] Argentine psychologists/historians Enrique Carpintero and Alejandro Vainer criticized the double standard and paternalism of Cooper's position: "[Cooper implied] that the revolution was for the countries of the Third World, while the developed countries should go on being capitalist."[52] Cooper may have advocated First World learning from the Third World, but his readiness to prescribe the right actions for Argentines overshadowed his "anti-imperialist" intent.

The rejection of Cooper was also related to divergent views of the revolutionary politics of sexuality. In Western Europe and the United States, the New Left aligned itself with sexual revolution and the "politics of Eros" during the Cold War. As German Freudo-Marxist philosopher Herbert Marcuse argued, a "polymorphous sexuality" was necessary for revolution against authoritarianism. "The fight for Eros," Marcuse famously wrote, "is the *political* fight."[53] However, many on the revolutionary left in Argentina rejected Marcuse's call from Europe to embrace eroticism, pleasure, and sexuality. As the leader of the revolutionary Unión Nacional de Estudiantes put it succinctly: "Marcuse can go to hell."[54] Without a doubt, as historian Eric Zolov has compellingly argued regarding Mexico, young people on the "New Left" in Argentina heeded countercultural calls for a hippismo, drug use, rock music, and a "liberated" sexuality.[55] But for the most part, leftist psychoanalysts were not among them. As a whole, psychoanalysts tended to belong to an older generation of upper-middle-class professionals whose traditional, family-based values often clashed with those of the younger *náufragos* and *roqueros* who participated in the liberatory sexual movements of the New Left. Far more conservative in their sexual politics, many leftist psychoanalysts argued that the sexual revolution was a "false" revolution that diverted important energy away from "true political revolution," namely mobilization of the working class against the established capitalist order. In a leftist journal in 1971, one Argentine psychoanalyst argued that eroticism was merely a tactic that consumer capitalism used to distract "true revolutionaries," so that their liberatory work would be confined to the "safe realm of sexuality."[56]

Local psychiatrists' relationship to Cooper's antipsychiatry, then, was ambivalent, layered, and complex. On one hand, Cooper—as well as other European (anti)psychiatrists who visited Argentina, such as Basaglia—represented potential intellectual resources and allies. These New Left Europeans shared with their *porteño* counterparts an orientation toward progressive psychiatric reform, socialist revolution, and anticolonial movements in the Third World. From this perspective, the encounter with Cooper reflects the pervasiveness of anticolonial discourse among psychiatrists during the Cold War not only in Buenos Aires, Havana, and Algiers but also in Paris, New York, London, and Moscow.

But on the other hand, Cooper—in his actions and lifestyle—represented exactly the "cultural imperialism" that he promised to subvert. The almost circular logic at play—where Cooper's "rebellion" against First World imperialism was rebuffed precisely because he was a First World imperialist—reflects the complexity of anti-imperial discourse in these transnational desencuentros. Could techniques, knowledge, and resources from the First (or Second) World actually be used to combat cultural and economic imperialism, as Cooper claimed? If so, how? Or was First and Second World knowledge, like antipsychiatry even when it masqueraded as "anticolonial," a sort of Trojan horse, as Kesselman argued—just one more example of the cultural imperialism it promised to challenge? As we will see in the remainder of the chapter, there was no single answer to these questions within the leftist world of mental health in Buenos Aires. Goldenberg and Langer, for example, maintained a closer relationship with potentially useful First and Second World allies, while others, such as the more radical Caparrós, argued that the independent future of the Argentine nation depended on divorcing itself from the imperialist superpowers.

The ambivalent attitude toward the First World manifested itself not only intellectually but also materially, at the level of funding, particularly from the United States. Though leftist intellectuals in Buenos Aires in the 1970s used psychoanalysis to combat imperialism—from its countercultural hippies to its transnational factories—the rejection of the First World in the field of mental health was by no means complete or wholesale. Times were tough and resources scarce for Argentine psychiatrists. As the state steadily decreased funding for health services through the 1970s, directors of psychiatric services increasingly turned to privatization, funding from pharmaceutical companies, and grants from the First World to keep their services running. In this period, some psychiatrists at the University of Buenos Aires School of Medicine received financial support from the Rockefeller and Ford Foundations, as well as the U.S. military, especially to fund laboratory research.[57]

Cooper's visit itself reflected the tension between economic realities and anti-imperial imaginaries. Although Cooper fashioned himself as an anticolonial ally, his trip to Argentina was funded, rather ironically, through a grant from the U.S.-based Ford Foundation. Mauricio Goldenberg, an internationally recognized leader in community psychiatry in the 1970s, used this Ford Foundation grant not only to invite First World psychiatrists, like Cooper, to Argentina, but also to run his influential, reformist psychiatric service at Hospital Lanús in Buenos Aires. Psychiatrists on Goldenberg's service, particularly Hernán Kesselman, objected to the imperialist penetration of Goldenberg's service through U.S. financing. While Kesselman, among others, supported the reformist psychiatric orientation of Goldenberg—centering around his therapeutic community approach—they could not support his ties to the First World. Kesselman and others vocally resigned from Goldenberg's psychiatric service in the early 1970s. The United States represented an oppressive colonial power, and Kesselman stated that he could not be merely an "intellectual of dissent."[58]

A Second World Desencuentro

In the early 1970s, critique of neocolonialism was by no means confined to First World capitalism or hippismo in Argentine psychiatry. While much of the anti-imperialist discourse originated in Bolshevik texts—Vladimir Lenin's *Imperialism: The Highest Stage of Capitalism,* for example—many leftist Argentine mental health professionals similarly found dimensions of orthodox communism from the Second World problematic, and even "imperial."[59] Although Soviet and Argentine psychiatrists all spoke the language of anticolonialism, as in the case of Cooper, they seemed to speak past each other.

In 1972, Marie Langer wrote that there was a *guerra fría* (cold war) between psychoanalysis and Soviet science.[60] For one, the Soviet Union had formally banned psychoanalysis for decades because Soviet psychiatry was Pavlovian reflexology. In Argentina, psychiatrists who belonged to the official Partido Comunista Argentino (PCA) generally stuck to the party line and rejected the leftist brand of psychoanalysis emerging in the Argentine *mundo-psi* (psy-world) in the late 1960s. But because there was not a strong reflexology movement in Argentina—and psychoanalysis in *consultorios* (private offices) was out of the question—Communist psychiatrists instead participated in traditional asylum-based care and paradoxically aligned themselves not with the emerging generation of leftist psychoanalysts, but with conservative asylum psychiatrists on the political right. Emiliano Galende, the secretary general of the FAP in the 1970s, remembers that the Communists were one of the exceptions to the general rule that "people on the political left were involved in psychiatric reform, while people on the right were involved in traditional psychiatry."[61]

As attempts to unite Freud and Marx came to dominate the field of Argentine mental health in the late 1960s, many psychoanalysts felt that communism's Pavlovian vision of psychiatry, and its ties to retrograde asylum practice, were out of touch with the political changes sweeping the nation.

The rejection of Soviet Communism, however, was incomplete and uneven in Argentine mental health. The Second World superpower did not offer as much as the First World in the way of funding in Argentina, but ideologically, the USSR was a more useful resource. Having undergone a socialist revolution, the Soviet Union was operating (at least what appeared to be) a successful national mental health service. Several Argentine mental health practitioners received professional degrees in Moscow in the 1970s, funded in part by the Instituto de Relaciones Culturales Argentina-USSR (Institute of Argentine-Soviet Cultural Relations).[62] A group of thirty FAP psychiatrists, led by psychoanalyst Marie Langer, traveled to the Soviet Union in 1972 to examine the functioning of a psychiatric system under socialism. The most important and substantive interaction on the trip was a series of meetings with Soviet psychiatrist F. V. Bassin.[63] The USSR had recently relaxed its ban on psychoanalysis, and Bassin represented a new generation of Soviet psychiatrists who did not dismiss psychoanalysis categorically. Initially, the visit with Bassin seemed promising. Langer, among others, believed Argentina was at the turn of its own revolution, and Bassin offered valuable insight on the alignment of psychiatric services with Marxist ideology.

However, rather quickly it was clear that Bassin and the Argentines disagreed fundamentally about Freud.[64] While Bassin did not reject psychoanalysis out of hand, he argued that all of the significant portions of Freud's theory of the unconscious could be reduced to Soviet theories, such as set theory or the experimental psychology of Georgian psychologist Dimitri Uznadze. Both the Argentines and Bassin agreed that the unconscious could serve as an object of scientific investigation, but they differed on *how* to go about investigating it. For Langer and her colleagues, the answer was psychoanalysis, but for Bassin, the only way forward was Soviet-style laboratory psychology. Although the visit to the Soviet Union was cordial and mildly productive—it led to the Spanish translation of Bassin's book on the unconscious in Argentina—the differences between the two sides ultimately prevented further collaboration.[65] On one side, Bassin believed psychoanalysis was fundamentally reactionary, because it reduced socioeconomic realities to intrapsychic conflict. On the other, Argentine analysts concluded that Soviet psychiatry, even at its most charitable, diluted the study of the unconscious by privileging alternative, Soviet theories of the mind.[66]

Soviet Communism in Argentina also suffered for reasons outside of, though related to, psychoanalysis in the early 1970s. Many leftist intellectuals in Argentina had long been suspicious of Soviet anti-Semitism. In the General Assembly of the United Nations (UN) in 1965, the Soviet Union formally proposed that Israel be linked to colonialism and racism and rejected a proposal from the United States and Brazil to include anti-Semitism in the UN's campaign against racial discrimination. The USSR's support for Syria and Egypt against Israel in the Six-Day War in 1967 only seemed to confirm Soviet prejudice, and the sweeping Israeli victory in the war also contributed to feelings that the USSR was ineffective in international politics. In Argentina, the Central Committee of the PCA followed Moscow's lead, describing Israel as *nazi-fascista* and adding the nation to the list of "imperial" countries.[67]

The anti-Israel rhetoric of the PCA had a profound effect on the Argentine world of mental health, particularly after the Six-Day War, alienating many Jewish psychoanalysts and institutions that were otherwise sympathetic to communism. For example, in the late 1960s, José Itzigsohn, a Jewish reflexologist who had been a crucial motor for the diffusion of Soviet neurophysiology in Argentina, broke from the PCA because its leaders asked him to sign a proclamation denouncing Israel. He joined the famous Jewish psychoanalyst José Bleger, who had also been expelled from the PCA, and together they helped to make anti-Semitism a major topic and area of study in the Argentine mundo-psi.[68] Bleger was a member of the APA committee that organized the 1963 annual conference entitled "Psychoanalysis and Anti-Judaism," which investigated the psychodynamic roots of anti-Jewish sentiment.[69] For instance, several papers from the conference explored circumcision and argued that "Jewish phobia" was actually fear of the circumcised Jew, because the practice of circumcision triggered the latent fear of castration in society.[70]

Five years after the conference, Bleger and Itzigsohn worked together to publish an influential edited volume entitled *Israel: Un Tema para la Izquierda*. Therein they denounced the Soviet characterization of Israel as an imperialist nation and criticized the USSR's political orientation toward the Middle East.[71] The collaboration between Itzigsohn and Bleger was remarkable because, as noted above, at the time the worlds of reflexology and psychoanalysis generally did not mix in Argentina. However, for these two leftist psychiatrists, questions of anti-Semitism and Jewish identity in socialist politics were significant enough to transcend their professional differences and galvanize their resistance against the diffusion of Soviet politics and psychology in Argentina. Their Jewish identities and ideological solidarity with Israel also became entangled with psychiatric practice. For his part, Bleger attempted to launch an ambitious mental health project in Israel in 1967 designed to provide psychological assistance to soldiers and civilians involved in the Six-Day War. Though it seems never to have been fully realized, the "Project for the Creation of an Israeli Institute for Research and Teaching of Psychological and Psychotherapeutic Sciences" planned to prevent mental illness generated by the conflict, as well as aid in the cultural adaptation of Jews to the native population of the Israeli territory.[72]

The international politics of the Soviet Union was problematic not only for its rhetoric against Israel, but also for its tenuous relationship with revolutionary movements in Cuba and China. An illustrative example is the case of Antonio Caparrós, mentioned above for his anticolonial critique of Cooper in 1972. Throughout the 1950s, Caparrós was a politically militant, card-carrying member of the official PCA. In the early 1960s, he joined the editorial staff of *La Rosa Blindada,* an influential literary magazine that published pieces on revolutionary movements in Cuba, Vietnam, and China. The magazine was the first to publish some of Guevara's essays in Argentina, including "El Socialismo y el Hombre en Cuba," and featured Spanish translations of selected works of Mao Zedong.[73] Caparrós sent one of his own articles published in *La Rosa Blindada* to Guevara in Cuba, as the Argentine physicians had known each other since medical school. Guevara secured an invitation for Caparrós to travel to Cuba in 1965, and there Caparrós spoke at length with Fidel Castro. Together, the three discussed how Caparrós might generate support in Argentina for Guevarist guerrilla activities throughout the region. With a renewed commitment to revolutionary movements across Latin America, Caparrós returned to Argentina and joined the short-lived, but ultimately influential, Vanguardia Revolucionaria, which supported Guevara's militant foquista group in Salta, Argentina.[74]

On orders from Moscow, the PCA explicitly targeted and condemned the transnational connections being forged by leftist intellectuals, like Caparrós, across Latin America. In the 1960s, the relationship between the Soviet Union and Cuba was strained at best, culminating in Guevara's harsh critique of the Soviet Union in his speech in Algiers in 1967.[75] Largely for its support of Castro's Cuba and Maoist China, the PCA expelled the Vanguardia Revolucionaria and the editors of *Rosa Blindada.*[76] Sensing that Soviet Communism was out of touch with revolutionary movements beyond its borders, Caparrós himself broke ties with the PCA shortly after. While Soviet Communism had been an influential and powerful minority position in both politics and psychiatry in Buenos Aires through the 1950s, the international politics of the Soviet Union at the turn of the 1970s—from its anti-Israel rhetoric to its position toward Cuba and China—alienated many of its strongest supporters in the Argentine capital. As we will see in the next section, many practitioners on the left, including Caparrós, would reorient their psychiatric militancy away from the Soviet Union and toward a leftist Argentine nationalism as the decade unfolded.

A Nationalist Psychiatry for the Third World

Estranged from the PCA, Caparrós—like many leftist intellectuals in Argentina— abandoned Soviet Communism to join the emerging movement of leftist Peronism in the early 1970s. The movement of Peronism in Argentina had emerged two decades earlier, under the presidency of Juan Domingo Perón (1944–1955). During his two terms as president, Perón developed a brand of nationalist populism that relied on a strong, centralized state operating in the interests of unions and workers. His administration instituted an array of public works projects, labor reforms, and welfare programs that promised social justice for the working class, and his economic policy emphasized independence from foreign interests by raising import tariffs and nationalizing foreign-owned companies. As historian Eduardo Elena has suggested, Perón was part of a cohort of strong(man) nationalist leaders who emerged throughout the Global South at mid-century that included, among others, Getúlio Vargas in Brazil, Victor Raúl Haya de la Torre in Peru, and Jorge Eliécer Gaitán in Colombia, as well as Jawaharlal Nehru in India and Gamal Abdel Nasser in Egypt.[77] While these nationalist leaders in Latin America, Africa, and Asia were different in telling ways, they shared a central preoccupation with political sovereignty and independence from Northern imperialism that called for more equitable distribution of national resources and an expanded role of the state in society.

The relationship between this early Peronist nationalism and the field of mental health, particularly psychoanalysis, was strained during Perón's presidency. The APA was founded in 1942, just as Perón was rising to power. The widespread perception of psychoanalysis as an "elitist" profession that catered to wealthy patients in the middle and upper classes clashed with emerging Peronist suspicions of intellectualism and antagonism toward universities, within a context of heightened support for working-class interests. A number of psychoanalysts claimed that Peronist groups, such as the fascist Alianza Libertadora Nacionalista, forced them out of prominent clinical and academic positions in the 1950s.[78] Though evidence of outright repression is limited, psychoanalysis would spread more easily in Argentine society in the years to come, after Perón was ousted as president and driven into a period of exile that lasted almost two decades.[79]

The relationship between Peronism and intellectual and academic culture shifted dramatically in the late 1960s, while Perón was still in exile. For one, the Cordobazo in 1969 sparked a new style of radical, left-wing Peronism that opposed the "union bureaucracy" of older trade union federations, such as the Confederación General del Trabajo de la República, that supported Perón's original rise to power in the 1940s. Unwilling to negotiate for social change, this new generation of radical young militants opted for armed struggle as a means of liberating the nation. Left-wing Peronist guerrilla groups in the early 1970s—fueled by state-sponsored violence on the political right—organized bank robberies, took over towns, kidnapped businessmen for ransom, and killed military officials and bureaucratic unionists.[80] In sharp contrast to earlier Peronist movements based on union activists, the membership of these left-wing Peronist organizations was largely students from middle- and upper-class backgrounds, including the young psychoanalysts who launched the Plataforma and Documento movements and, later, the overtly Marxist CDI training center in Buenos Aires. Inspired by thinkers such as Guevara and Fanon, these left-wing Peronists were far more sympathetic to academic culture—including the field of mental health and psychoanalysis—than their predecessors in the 1940s and 1950s.[81]

Returning to Caparrós, this emerging left-wing Peronism of the early 1970s was particularly attractive to intellectuals who had rejected Soviet Communism on grounds that it was out of touch with revolutionary movements in Latin America. Radical Peronism offered Argentine intellectuals like Caparrós the promise of socialist revolution, but with a solid, nationalist grounding in the legacy of Perón and without all the "imperialist" baggage that came with the Soviet Union. Not only in Latin America, but also in Europe and the United States, many leftist intellectuals became convinced that the Soviet Union had taken on the imperial mantle that it so vehemently claimed to subvert. The Soviet invasion of Czechoslovakia in 1968 was met with explicit accusations of imperialism in Argentina, as leftist intellectuals argued that the Soviets were no better than the United States in their colonial ambitions. In the early 1970s, Perón, who eagerly solicited support from leftist intellectuals in Argentina, made a personal appeal to Caparrós to join his cause, and afterward, Caparrós concluded, "Marxism was not in contradiction to the Peronist movement and actually complemented it."[82] Committed to Cuba and armed conflict, Caparrós divorced all his ties to Soviet Communism and decided to follow Perón. Members of both of Caparrós's organizations, the Vanguardia

Revolucionaria and *Rosa Blindada*, were intimately involved with the founding of several leftist Peronist guerrilla groups at the turn of the 1970s, including the violent Montoneros.[83]

In the illustrations of anticolonialism presented in the prior sections, leftist mental health professionals in Buenos Aires focused on leveling negative critiques at the cultural and economic imperialism of the United States and the Soviet Union. However, inspired by left-wing Peronist nationalism of the 1970s, Caparrós began to direct his critical gaze not outward against the imperial Cold War superpowers, but inward to "Argentina," as a Third World nation, culture, and people. He substituted an exclusive, negative focus on *anti*colonialism for a more positive, psychological exploration of Argentine nationalism. This vision of a "nationalist" psychiatry developed within the openly Marxist Coordinadora de Trabajadores de Salud Mental (CTSM), which was founded in 1972 in the aftermath of the Plataforma split from the official APA. The organization sought to unite all physicians, psychologists, and social workers under the banner of "mental health workers" who would serve the interests of the Argentine people. The leftist intellectual climate in the CTSM was extremely diverse, ranging from more orthodox communism to the many variations of leftist Peronism abounding at the turn of the 1970s.

Caparrós argued that the CTSM should serve as the institutional platform for a national, populist psychology specifically tailored for Argentina as a Third World nation. This psychology, Caparrós argued, would not have as its subject the universal or disembodied "Mind" or "Man," but instead would ground itself in the "specific, historical conditions" of Argentina.[84] For Caparrós, psychiatry could aid revolutionary struggle only once the very epistemology and ontology of the profession were rooted in the culture, thinking, and politics of Third World nations. In what might be called a sort of "ethno-psychiatry," Caparrós argued that psychologists needed to turn to "the preponderant models and values, the conception of life, desire, attitudes" that infused everyday life in Argentina.[85] Caparrós's anticolonialism, here, was not simply the rejection of the imperializing dimension of foreign psychiatry, but the nationalist grounding of psychiatry in the concrete realities of the Argentine nation.

Caparrós's nationalist vision of Argentine psychiatry privileged the cultural factors that affected the psyche. As historian Luciano García has pointed out, Caparrós's work was related to prevailing historico-genetic theories of the mind that sought to explain psychology in terms of early childhood development.[86] But rather than turning to the psychodynamics of the child-mother-father complex of Freud or the naturalistic reflexology of Pavlov, Caparrós argued that psychiatrists and psychologists should consider the cultural and national factors that influenced personality development. In so doing, psychologists would discover alternative, distinctly Argentine ways of thinking about behavior and the mind. However, this emphasis on nationalism did not mean that Caparrós abandoned the Soviet psychologists crucial to his own development as a Communist psychiatrist in the 1950s and 1960s. For example, he used the developmental theories of Soviet psychologist Lev Vygotsky to explore local ways of raising children in Argentina. Rather, the question for Caparrós was how elements of Soviet psychology could be adapted or "nationalized" to serve the interests of leftist Peronism in the concrete realities of Argentina as a Third World nation.[87]

A fellow psychiatrist and leftist, Peronist Alfredo Moffatt, took up Caparrós's injunction to ground psychology in the national culture of Argentina. In the 1960s, Moffatt led the development of a therapeutic community at the Hospital Borda in Buenos Aires. He also traveled to Brazil several times during the 1970s to study and work with the Brazilian educator and anticolonial thinker Paulo Freire. Inspired by his experiences with Freire, Moffatt published *Psicoterapia del Oprimido* (Psychotherapy of the Oppressed) in 1974, in which he attacked the servile relationship between Euro-American knowledge and the Argentine "psychoanalytic ghetto."[88]

Like Caparrós, Moffatt felt that only a "turn to the [country's] interior" would liberate Argentine thought from *yanqui* imperialism: "We must rethink sociology, psychology and psychiatry. . . . Instead of seeing [ourselves] as dependent servants to Europe and *yanqui* imperialism we should look to the interior of our land and, with our people, begin inverting our perspective. Frantz Fanon demonstrated that this is possible, and on October 17th, 1945, the [Argentine] people, through the Peronist movement, began this work."[89]

For Moffatt, a turn to the "interior" implied a thorough historico-psychological analysis of Argentine culture, from Spanish colonization, the genocide of Indigenous groups, and *gaucho* drama in the nineteenth century to the emergence of *tango* culture in the twentieth. Moffatt romanticized the *cultura criolla* (which adapted colonial-era Spanish elements to rural life in Argentina) in the country's Interior—outside of Buenos Aires—which, he claimed, was too European.[90] Argentines in the Interior had long possessed local ways of treating mental illness, such as religious rituals—he called such "therapy" *psicoterapia criolla*—that should inform more "scientific" efforts to treat mental illness from Europe. By "indigenizing and nationalizing" psychiatry, Moffatt argued that psychiatrists could finally produce a truly "popular psychiatry" fit for Argentina as a nation. This nationalist psychiatry would transcend the "timid, servile, and colonized" attitude that, he claimed, had defined Argentina's relationship with the First World since national independence.[91]

Moffatt's vision of a nationalist, popular psychiatry was based on his clinical experiences in the "Peña Carlos Gardel" service, which he founded at the Hospital Borda in Buenos Aires in 1971.[92] While the work at Peña Carlos Gardel was inspired, at least in part, by Cooper's experiment at La Casona, Moffat promoted "national, popular forms of culture" over the elitist, hippie counterculture that motivated Cooper. Specifically, Moffatt attempted to "resocialize" patients on his service through the model of "parties" (*fiestas*) where patients, staff, physicians, and often friends and family from outside the hospital engaged in activities linked to popular culture, including dancing, singing, *asado* (barbecue), games, and sports. According to Moffatt, Peña Carlos Gardel embraced "popular [cultural] forms, respect for self-determination, and avoided imposing 'cultured' forms of recreation associated with the more urban and intellectualized culture of doctors and hospital authorities."[93] The parties of Peña Carlos Gardel, which included hundreds of attendees, inspired patients to develop a number of organizations within the hospital, including a "university" that provided patients with support for finding jobs, as well as a theater group.

However, in 1974, the politically conservative director of the Hospital Borda, psychiatrist Carlos Sisto, closed Peña Carlos Gardel, along with the patient groups it had inspired. According to Sisto, the service needed to be shut down because of a confrontation between patients and police. Sisto believed that the "liberatory" practices of Moffatt's services threatened the authority of psychiatrists in the hospital as a whole. As Sisto proclaimed in an exasperated tone during his declaration closing Moffatt's service, "[Peña Carlos Gardel] questioned medical treatment. They questioned therapeutics. . . . The sick after [the experience of Peña Carlos Gardel] no longer want to take their medication."[94] Moffatt disputed this and claimed that the deeper reason for the closure of his service was that Sisto felt threatened by the progressive techniques employed at the Peña Carlos Gardel.[95]

The story of Peña Carlos Gardel reflected the fate of many of the progressive practices inspired by the revolutionary, anti-imperial fervor of the early 1970s. As the decade unfolded, a wave of violent military dictatorships systematically cut funding for mental health care in Argentina. Progressive psychopathological services, such as Peña Carlos Gardel and Grimson's therapeutic community, suffered. Many were shut down, often for professional or ideological reasons, turning hospitals into overcrowded *cronicarios*, long-term asylums where the condition of patients stagnated chronically without hope of recovery.

Some military officials directly targeted members of revolutionary psychiatric organizations like the CDI and FAP with paramilitary raids of offices, and over a hundred leftist mental health professionals were "disappeared" for their real or presumed ties to leftist politics. As one official stated in the popular conservative magazine *Somos*, Freud and Marx were "ideological criminals," and the psychoanalyst's couch was a "hotbed" for the production of subversive guerrilla fighters.[96] In this repressive context, many mental health professionals in Argentina retreated from their former political militancy and entered private clinical practice, believing that a turn to "psychoanalytic neutrality" would insulate them from the dictatorship's reach. Others, including prominent practitioners such as Plataforma psychoanalyst Marie Langer, went into exile, especially to Venezuela, Mexico, and Cuba. By the end of the decade, state terrorism against leftist mental health professionals, including the nullification of the FAP, which was officially closed in 1983, had all but crushed the revolutionary, anti-imperial dreams that had inspired leftist psychiatrists at the turn of the 1970s.[97]

Concluding Thoughts

Cold War psychiatry in Argentina reflected and reinforced a vast array of anti-imperial visions of the Third World. Although shared anticolonial sentiment brought actors together from all parts of the globe—Cooper and Pavlovsky in Buenos Aires, Bassin and Langer in Moscow, and Caparrós and Castro in Cuba—these encounters, I argue, were just as frequently desencuentros. Cooper's "anticolonial" vision of the Third World as a politico-medical laboratory clashed with Argentine psychiatrists' suspicions of First World hippismo and U.S. capitalist penetration. While Argentine psychiatrists found the Soviet promise of a successful mental health system under socialism intriguing, they also saw problems with Soviet anti-Semitism, international imperialism, and lack of solidarity with anticolonial movements in Latin America. Finally, with the rise of leftist Peronism in the 1970s, a "national, popular" vision of Third World psychiatry emerged that attempted to ground mental health in the history and culture of the Argentine nation.

Given this uneven and complex trajectory, it is tempting to conclude that anti-imperial discourse was little more than inflated, if often powerful, rhetoric. Practically anything or anyone could be labeled "anticolonial," and the Third World was a vague concept at best. Psychiatrists circulating around the globe used the language of anti-imperialism pragmatically and tactically: Cooper to fulfill his antipsychiatry dreams; Kesselman to bring international attention to the Plataforma movement; Caparrós to visit Che Guevara in Cuba; and Langer to see a postrevolutionary mental health system in the Soviet Union. Despite the initial promise and optimism of anti-imperial discourse in the early 1970s, transnational encounters were more often than not desencuentros.

But this deflationary reading misses something important about the legacy of anti-imperial thought in Argentine psychiatry and psychology following the violence of the late Cold War. During the 1980s and 1990s, psychiatrists facing state repression in Latin America revived much of the earlier anti-imperial work in efforts to seek human rights justice in the face of U.S.-sponsored terror. An illustrative case is that of the famous Spanish-born psychologist Ignacio Martín-Baro, who worked for years under politically repressive conditions in El Salvador until he was assassinated by a right-wing military group in 1989. In 1983, the year that the dictatorship fell in Argentina, Martín-Baro attended a "Mental Health and Human Rights" conference in Buenos Aires that focused on the theme of the psychological effects of political repression.[98] At the conference, Martín-Baro stated that the mental health community in El Salvador was "overwhelmed by the demands of hundreds of people suffering the consequences of state repression."[99] Initially, he relayed, mental health professionals had "inadequate means and few ideas in seeking responses to such urgent, demanding problems."[100] There was little knowledge of how to treat "tortured persons or the children of the disappeared," and psychologists and psychiatrists in El Salvador, he continued, had difficulty finding relevant literature on state violence beyond Fanon's *The Wretched of the Earth*.

However, as Latin American nations "transitioned" from authoritarianism to democracy, Martín-Baro began networking with other mental health professionals across Latin America who had faced similar experiences of state violence. Through meetings with Argentine psychoanalysts, for example, he learned about the work of Antonio and Nicolas Caparrós, whose 1974 book mentioned above, *Psicología de la Liberación* (Psychology of Liberation), would inspire the publication of Martín-Baro's similarly titled and extremely influential article "Hacia una Psicología de la Liberación" (Toward a Psychology of Liberation) over ten years later.[101] Martín-Baro also met Argentine psychoanalysts in the Equipo de Asistencia Psicológica, a team providing psychological support to the famous Madres de la Plaza de Mayo, an activist organization of Argentine mothers who demanded the return of their children disappeared by the state. Furthermore, Martín-Baro discovered the work of Chilean psychiatrist Elizabeth Lira, who would co-author the influential monograph *Psychotherapy and Political Repression* in 1984.[102] At the conference, Martín-Baro stated that his encounters with other Latin American mental health practitioners were productive, but also frightening, as they revealed a disturbing truth: "Structures of repression," he claimed, were largely "identical across countries, even where there are large cultural differences." Martín-Baro argued that the systematic nature of state terror in Latin America was due to the imperial influence of the United States, the "country that organizes repression in Latin America."[103] He concluded that a formalized transnational network of mental health providers would allow increased cooperation that would benefit both victims and human rights movements throughout the region.

Without a doubt, there are clear differences between the revolutionary mobilization of Caparrós and Langer from the early 1970s and the later human rights work of mental health practitioners, like Martín-Baro and Elizabeth Lira, in the 1980s and 1990s. Marxism and a forward-looking vision of a future (and potentially violent) revolution often guided the former, while the latter was driven by the trauma of the recent past and a desire for justice for crimes against humanity. But it might also be postulated that a historical strand woven through these diverse forms of psychiatric militancy in Latin America during the late Cold War was the commitment to an anti-imperial ethos that was—however vaguely articulated and translated into practice—nevertheless aspirational and enduring. As Martín-Baro wrote in his 1986 article "Toward a Psychology of Liberation" concerning the "slavery" of Latin American psychology (in language that mirrors closely Moffatt's writing on the "servile" nature of Argentine psychoanalysis in *Psychotherapy of the Oppressed*): "The misery of Latin American Psychology has its roots in a history of colonial dependence that does not coincide with the history of the Iberoamerican colony, but with the neocolonialism of the 'stick and carrot' that has been imposed on us for a century. The 'cultural stick'... finds in Psychology one instrument among others to mold minds and pacify consciousness to explain the undoubted advantages of the modernist and technological 'carrot.'"[104]

At the end of this article, Martín-Baro reached the same conclusion as Antonio Caparrós in a piece titled "The Illness Is Capitalism" published over a decade earlier, in 1972. The only way to "decolonize" psychology and psychiatry from the "neocolonial metropole," Caparrós argued, was to ground the discipline in the "specific conditions and historical period" of Latin American nations. According to Caparrós, only a truly Latin American psychology—tied to the concrete realities of Third World peoples—could provide a platform for "liberation" from dependency in all its forms, from the economic and cultural to the psychological.

Notes

1   David Cooper, *Psychiatry and Anti-Psychiatry*.

2   Kesselman, "Salud Mental y Neocolonialismo."

3   Alejandro Dagfal discusses transnational connections between psychologists in Buenos Aires and Paris in *Entre París y Buenos Aires*. For the significance of Kleinianism prior to the late 1960s in Buenos Aires, see Plotkin, *Freud in the Pampas*, 2. The major study of Lacanianism in Argentina is Izaguirre, *Jacques Lacan*. For the influence of Soviet psychology and Communism in Argentina, see Vezzetti, "Psicoanálisis y Revolución," and especially García's unpublished dissertation, "Recepción de la Psicología Soviética en la Argentina."

4   Hornstein, "Paseíto por Villa Freud."

5   Bruno Bosteels discusses the significance of Guevara and Mao's thought among leftists in Latin America in the 1970s in *Marx and Freud in Latin America*, 167.

6   A full transcription of the recorded exchange can be found in Golder and González, *Freud en Vigotsky*, 147–63.

7   See the introduction to this volume; Gordin, Hall, and Kojevnikov, "Intelligentsia Science"; Krementsov, *Stalinist Science*.

8   There are notable and significant exceptions, particularly in Cold War science, including Medina's study of revolutionary cybernetics in Chile, *Cybernetic Revolutionaries*; and Mitchell, *Constellations of Inequality*.

9   "Declaración del Grupo Plataforma."

10   Vezzetti, "Psicoanálisis y Revolución," 1.

11   "Información del Grupo Plataforma."

12   On the interplay between politics and the psychiatric profession, see also Lambe's chapter in this volume.

13   Langer, *Cuestionamos*, 17.

14   Langer, *Cuestionamos*, 17.

15   Ramos, "Psychiatry, Authoritarianism, and Revolution," 259.

16   Carpintero and Vainer, *Huellas de la Memoria*, 281.

17   David Cooper, *Psychiatry and Anti-Psychiatry*, 105.

18   David Cooper, *Psychiatry and Anti-Psychiatry*, 106.

19   "Huellas de la Antipsiquiatría," 32–33.

20   "Huellas de la Antipsiquiatría," 32.

21   Carpintero and Vainer, *Huellas*, 172.

22   Grimson, *Sociedad de Locos*, 247.

23   Grimson, *Sociedad de Locos*, 247.

24   Totton, *Politics of Psychotherapy*, 117.

25   "Psicoanálisis y Antiimperalismo."

26   "Psicoanálisis y Antiimperalismo."

27   "Psicoanálisis y Antiimperalismo."

28   "Psicoanálisis y Antiimperalismo."

29   David Cooper, "Comuna Política-Terapéutica."

30 McMahon, *Cold War in the Third World*, 213.

31 Galeano, *Venas Abiertas de América Latina*. See also Cardoso and Faletto, *Dependency and Development in Latin America*.

32 Ballvé and Prashad, *Dispatches from Latin America*, 16.

33 "Fanon Group," 1969, Salud Mental box, Centro de Documentación e Investigación de la Cultura de Izquierdas en la Argentina, Buenos Aires.

34 Carpintero and Vainer, *Huellas*, 67.

35 Carpintero and Vainer, *Huellas*, 70.

36 Vezzetti and Pecheny, "Standard Electric," 3–6.

37 Vezzetti and Pecheny, "Standard Electric," 4.

38 Vezzetti and Pecheny, "Standard Electric," 5.

39 Vezzetti and Pecheny, "Standard Electric," 7.

40 Carpintero and Vainer, *Huellas*, 68.

41 David Cooper, *Grammar of Living*.

42 "David Cooper o la Contestación Permanente."

43 David Cooper, *Psychiatry and Anti-Psychiatry*, 106.

44 Grimson, *Sociedad de Locos*, 247. On related pilot health projects in the community, see also Pieper Mooney's chapter in this volume.

45 Cooper's concept of "μ-shift" was an appropriation of the "μ" used to describe mutation rate in the field of genetics. In Cooper's work, μ referred to the bidirectional "mutation" of politics from the micro to macro, from the interpersonal to the societal. See "David Cooper o la Contestación Permanente."

46 See interview with Eduardo Pavlovsky in Carpintero and Vainer, *Huellas*, 172.

47 Kesselman, "Salud Mental y Neocolonialismo."

48 Nicolás Caparrós and Caparrós, *Psicología de la Liberación*. For the development of Liberation Psychology in Latin America, see Burton and Vázquez Ortega, "Psicología de la Liberación"; Hollander, *Love in a Time of Hate*.

49 "Antipsiquiatría y Colonización Cultural."

50 "Antipsiquiatría y Colonización Cultural."

51 David Cooper, "Use of LSD," 3.

52 Carpintero and Vainer, *Huellas*, 175.

53 See Marcuse, "Political Preface 1966," in *Eros and Civilization*, xxv.

54 Manzano, *Age of Youth in Argentina*, 163.

55 Zolov, "Expanding our Conceptual Horizons."

56 Manzano, *Age of Youth in Argentina*, 206.

57 Sigal, *Intelectuales y Poder en Argentina*, 81–84.

58 Carpintero and Vainer, *Huellas*, 106.

59 Lenin, *Imperialism*.

60 See Marie Langer's "Prólogo," in Bassin, *Problema del Inconsciente* (1972), 14.

61 Emiliano Galende, interview with the author, July 21, 2010, Buenos Aires.

62 Golder, *Reportajes Contemporáneos a la Psicología Soviética*, 16.

63 Historian Luciano García describes the meeting between Langer and Bassin in "Recepción de la Psicología Soviética," 269–72.

64 Luciano García, "Recepción de la Psicología Soviética," 270.

65 The translation of Bassin's book on the unconscious was published in 1972 with a prologue by Marie Langer. See Bassin, *Problema del Inconsciente* (1972).

66 A full transcription of the recorded exchange can be found in Golder and González, *Freud en Vigotsky*, 147–63.

67 Luciano García, "Recepción de la Psicología Soviética," 245.

68 Plotkin, "José Bleger."

69 The theme of "anti-Judaism" was specifically chosen over "anti-Semitism" for the conference, and as Plotkin notes, Argentine psychoanalyst Marie Langer later commented that the choice reflected an unconscious desire for "distance from the political and social reality" of anti-Semitism. See Plotkin, "José Bleger," 198.

70 Plotkin, "José Bleger," 199.

71 See José Bleger, "La Crisis del Medio Oriente," and José Itzigsohn, "La Alienación Recíproca," in Verbitzky et al., *Israel*.

72 Plotkin, "José Bleger," 200. See also Luciano García, "Recepción de la Psicología Soviética," 245.

73 Ernesto Guevara, "Socialismo y el Hombre en Cuba"; Mao, *Obras Escogidas I*.

74 Anguita and Caparrós, *Voluntad*, 90.

75 Ernesto Guevara, "At the Afro-Asian Conference in Algeria."

76 González Canosa, "Antecedentes de las 'Fuerzas Armadas Revolucionarias.'"

77 Elena, *Dignifying Argentina*, 15.

78 Consider, for example, the expulsion of psychoanalyst Enrique Pichon-Rivière from his post at the Hospicio de las Mercedes in Buenos Aires in 1947 because of pressure from a Peronist group. See Lema, *Conversaciones con Enrique Pichon-Rivière*, 49.

79 See Dagfal's discussion of Peronism, anti-Peronism, and psychoanalysis in the 1940s and 1950s in "Psychoanalysis in Argentina under Peronism and Anti-Peronism."

80 The Montoneros, for example, were a violent guerrilla group composed of leftist Peronists that attempted to destabilize military governments in Argentina throughout the 1970s. Montoneros were extremely influential in politics in the early 1970s in Argentina, and several Montoneros held seats in Congress, ministerial positions, and provincial governorships. See McSherry, *Incomplete Transition*, 70.

81 See, for example, "Fanon Group."

82 Anguita and Caparrós, *Voluntad*, 571–72; Luciano García, "Recepción de la Psicología Soviética," 243.

83 Caparrós himself joined the leftist Peronist group Fuerzas Armadas Revolucionarias.

84 Antonio Caparrós, "Hacia una Psicología Nacional y Popular."

85 Antonio Caparrós, "Hacia una Psicología Nacional y Popular."

86 Luciano García, "Recepción de la Psicología Soviética," 284.

87 Antonio Caparrós and Caparrós, "Problema de la Interpretación," 399.

88 Moffatt, *Psicoterapia*, 16.

89 Moffatt, *Psicoterapia*, 15. On October 17, 1945, a massive labor demonstration in the Plaza de Mayo resulted in the release of Juan Domingo Perón from captivity. The day now commemorates the founding of Peronism in Argentina.

90 Moffatt, *Psicoterapia*, 63–64.

91 Moffatt, *Psicoterapia*, 113.

92 A "peña" refers to a popular gathering or party. This one was a recurring event, named after the most famous Argentine tango singer.

93 Carpintero and Vainer, *Huellas*, 154.

94 Carpintero and Vainer, *Huellas*, 192.

95 Patient protests were not uncommon in Buenos Aires in the 1970s. The patient uprising and subsequent clash with police at the therapeutic community of Hospital Estévez in Buenos Aires is another example. See Golcman, "Experiment of the Therapeutic Communities in Argentina." See also chapter three in Armus, *Ailing City*.

96 "Psicoanálisis en la Picota," 6.

97 Ramos, "Psychiatry, Authoritarianism, and Revolution," 259.

98 "Primer Encuentro sobre Salud Mental y Derechos Humanos—Cono Sur," 12, Archive of the Centro de Estudios Legales y Sociales, Buenos Aires, Salud Mental Box.

99 "Primer Encuentro," 12.

100 "Primer Encuentro," 12.

101 Martín-Baro, "Hacia una Psicología de la Liberación."

102 Lira and Weinstein, *Psicoterapia y Represión Política*.

103 "Primer Encuentro," 12.

104 Martín-Baro, "Hacia una Psicología de la Liberación."

9

South–South Cooperation as a Cold War Tonic

*Cuban Medical Diplomacy to
Sandinista Nicaragua, 1979–1990*

CHEASTY ANDERSON

In 1979, when the Sandinista National Liberation Front (FSLN) won its struggle to oust the Somoza dictatorship from Nicaragua, the victorious revolutionaries inherited a nation ravaged not only by war, but also by decades of neglect. In addition to problems engendered by economic devastation and a literacy rate of approximately 35 percent, Nicaragua possessed some of the Western Hemisphere's most appalling health statistics. The number-one cause of death was diarrhea, and the official infant mortality rate, which was grossly underreported, was eighty-seven out of every one thousand live births. Almost one-half of the population did not have even a latrine, and health services were completely unavailable to 72 percent of the population.[1] The new Sandinista government quickly declared that providing comprehensive health care would be one of its key obligations to the Nicaraguan people. To implement this ambitious social reform, however, they would need assistance. The new government found an able and willing ally in Fidel Castro, a staunch supporter of the Nicaraguan revolution. Within a week of the Sandinista victory, the Cubans were on their way to Nicaragua.

Opposition groups have long critiqued the Sandinista regime for ineffectively managing agrarian reform, mishandling the economy, and suppressing dissent. Indeed, the time is ripe for an academic debate about the causes and nature of these shortcomings, including the role of U.S. interference. A monocular focus on these problems, however, obscures the Sandinista government's signal triumph: its health care program. From 1979 until 1990, Nicaragua's Ministry of Health (MINSA), with help from Cuba and other donor nations, built up its hospital network and expanded a nationwide, free, primary health care system that relied on a distribution of power to the regions, community organization, popular health education, and high levels of popular participation. This system, not coincidentally, was a near-replica of the world-renowned health care program in Cuba.[2] The Sandinistas' efforts were so successful that by 1983 Nicaragua was added to the World Health Organization's short list of countries that provided full-coverage health care to its population.[3] Through systematic, well-planned vaccination and sanitation campaigns, MINSA eradicated polio while greatly reducing levels of measles, whooping cough, diarrhea, respiratory disease, leishmaniasis, malaria, and dengue, all of which were previously endemic, especially in rural areas. That the Sandinista government managed all this is remarkable, considering the simultaneous rise of a counterrevolutionary movement (known as the "Contras"), backed by U.S. funds and intelligence, that aimed to destabilize and overthrow a regime perceived to be friendly toward communism.[4]

Nicaragua could not have done this without Cuba's technical, material, and advisory support. At the height of the Sandinista Revolution (1974–1979), Somoza's National Guard bombed most of the nation's hospitals. In the aftermath, some 30–40 percent of Nicaragua's doctors left the country, even as Somoza himself emptied the national treasury of all but $3 million on his way out of the country. To further complicate the problems engendered by this lack of personnel and the financial crisis, the erstwhile guerrillas who undertook governance of the Nicaraguan state were young and inexperienced. The oldest member of the FSLN directorate in 1979, Tomás Borge, was only thirty-nine years old, and he was almost a decade senior to many other leaders. Some had attended college; few had finished their degrees. Many had dropped out of medical or law school to devote themselves entirely to the revolution. As a result, the new government was, almost from the moment it took power, in crisis. Given its almost total lack of resources in 1979, and the deteriorating economic conditions Nicaragua faced as the 1980s wore on, several of Nicaragua's government ministries relied upon foreign assistance programs to maintain services. For example, MINSA depended heavily upon Cuban cooperation.

Among people interested in Nicaragua's recent history, it is commonly understood that during the Sandinista regime, Cuba assisted the fledgling MINSA in its efforts to build a nationwide, socialist health care system.[5] It is not, however, broadly realized just exactly how critical that cooperation was, or how pervasive the Cuban presence in Nicaragua was during the 1980s. Among Nicaraguans, on the other hand, there is a strong cultural memory of Cuba's role during the Sandinista government. As one Managua taxi driver put it, "Señorita, those Cuban doctors were everywhere. In every hospital, in every clinic, in the cities, and in the most rural communities in the country. In those days you couldn't get up to use the restroom without tripping over a Cuban."[6] This Cuban presence meant different things to different people; to Sandinista loyalists, it was a positive presence, and the work they did was laudatory in the extreme. Opponents of the revolution or of the Sandinista government felt quite the opposite.

Nonetheless, my fieldwork conducted in Managua, Matagalpa, and the rural mountainous North from 2008 to 2010 confirmed that a wide swath of Nicaraguans consider health care reform one of the Sandinista government's finest achievements. What's more, Nicaraguans freely acknowledge the importance of foreign assistance to that success, and—whether willingly or grudgingly—they point to Cuban contributions as particularly indispensable. To be sure, there are vocal detractors of Sandinista policies and Cuba's involvement, but the vast majority of more than one hundred oral history informants concur with contemporary newspaper accounts and government documentation that without Cuban cooperation, MINSA would have been unable to achieve even a fraction of what it accomplished.

What was the nature of this aid? In the fraught political climate of the Cold War, this health care program was vested with meanings, both sinister and noble, by capitalist and communist camps, respectively. Was Cuban activity in Nicaragua, as the United States claimed, an attempt to convert Nicaragua into another beachhead for communism in the Western Hemisphere? In particular, were Cuba's permanent medical brigades and policy advisers merely a clever disguise for political propagandists to penetrate the government bureaucracy? Further, were doctors and nurses inculcating a communist fervor in the deepest rural reaches of the Nicaraguan countryside? Or, as the Cuban medical professionals themselves saw the project, were they simply acting on a commitment to humanitarianism and a sense of moral obligation, rooted in the desire to build a postrevolutionary, socially just society?

As historians digest events of the recent past and attempt to understand the geopolitical context of foreign policy activities, all too often the "lived reality" of these efforts goes understudied. This chapter examines the impact of Cuban health diplomacy on the development of a socialist health care system in Sandinista Nicaragua. By focusing on the local and the personal as well as the global, this study explores not only what Cuban cooperation to Nicaragua meant vis-à-vis the Cold War and U.S.–Latin American relations, but also how Cuban medical support to Sandinista Nicaragua shaped the lives of Nicaraguan citizens and participating Cuban health workers.

A careful reading of oral histories, newspaper accounts, MINSA documentation, and secondary sources allows for a comprehensive reconstruction of the general themes and quotidian realities of the ongoing Cuban medical mission to Nicaragua, and points to several conclusions about this notable experience of South–South health cooperation within Latin America during the Cold War.[7] First, in spite of the broad perception that Cuba was an altruistic donor nation, the relationship between Cuba and Nicaragua was a mutually beneficial one. Though Nicaragua unquestionably received the lion's share of benefits in the relationship, Cuba perceived both practical and nontangible advantages in maintaining a permanent medical mission to Nicaragua. In practical terms, Cuba saw its support of the Sandinista government as part of its global mission to promote its health care policy and counter the hegemony of the capitalist United States in Latin America. As such, Cuba helped the socialist Sandinista government succeed by building and maintaining social services throughout Nicaragua. Nontangible benefits the Cuban government perceived included the continuing education Cuban medical workers received as they worked in abysmal Third World health conditions. Cuba had long since eradicated such conditions at home. In theory, then, an ancillary benefit of this exposure was to sustain revolutionary fervor among its own medical workers. The Castro government encouraged its health brigades to reflect upon the advantages of life in communist Cuba relative to the public health disaster that "capitalist" Nicaragua had become under the Somoza dictatorship.

Second, despite U.S. and international fears that Cuba was using its medical missions as a propaganda tool, humanitarian aid was the primary purpose of Cuba's medical diplomacy. The Cuban government structured its medical workers' experiences in ways that—as much as possible—curtailed their lives to the professional domain and restricted the extent to which they could engage in politics or form personal relationships with Nicaraguans in order to encourage them to return to Cuba. These efforts, by and large, were successful. However, as this chapter argues, there were significant gaps in enforcement. Therefore, though Cuba's broad geopolitical agenda included promoting communism and supporting anticapitalist revolution, the manner in which it managed its deployed medical brigades limited their ability to promote communist ideology.

Moreover, the Nicaraguan government itself reinforced Cuba's efforts to keep its medical workers from full social and cultural integration with the communities they served. Despite being modeled and reliant on the Cuban Ministry of Public Health, MINSA was at pains to maintain the illusion of autonomy and, if not self-sufficiency, at least self-determination. Although by all accounts the Cuban presence was considerable in the realm of health care, especially in some rural areas and small towns, government reports consistently elided the existence of large numbers of Cubans in Nicaragua. With a few exceptions, a researcher using only Nicaraguan government documentation would be hard-pressed to conclude that Cuba did more than minimally support health developments in in Sandinista Nicaragua. While newspaper accounts and oral histories praise the numerous brigades of Cuban doctors and nurses to the point of tribute, the official Nicaraguan position to minimize the role of Cuban medical workers was in line with the Castro government's attempt to impede its workers from integrating into Nicaraguan society.

Thus, although a traditional Cold War interpretive lens would cast Cuba as the tireless promoter of communism in the struggle against capitalism, in the realm of health care, the reality was vastly more complex.[8] Without a doubt, the Castro government saw its role in Nicaragua as critical to beating back U.S. capitalist hegemony. Without Cuba's military, material, and financial support, the Sandinista government might have toppled during the U.S.-backed Contra War in short order.[9] Medical aid was critical to ensure the Sandinistas' ability to follow through on their revolutionary promises but, in practice, it did not develop into a central aspect of the Cold War struggle against capitalism. On an advisory level, the Cubans certainly advocated building a system modeled upon their own, but the Sandinistas were not passive recipients of Cuban approaches, and the Cubans were remarkably cautious in the delegation of medical brigades throughout the country. Although the Reagan administration cast a broad accusation of communist propaganda across any and all Cuban activity in Nicaragua, neither Cuba nor Nicaragua saw health activities as an intrinsic part of ideological indoctrination in the global Cold War. In the words of one Cuban doctor, "Propaganda? That's funny. We didn't even have enough time to grab a bite to eat between treating patients. Talking politics was the last thing on my mind."[10]

The Global and Regional Reach of Cuban Cooperation during the Cold War

As the lone Communist government in the Western Hemisphere, post-1959 Cuba was repeatedly pitted against the United States during the Cold War period. After the 1962 Missile Crisis, Cuba avoided direct military confrontation with the United States, but it continued working in subtler ways to undercut the power of the capitalist hegemon to the north. A major objective was to support revolutionary movements spreading throughout Latin America and Africa in the second half of the twentieth century and, through that support, to reinforce the potential benefits of communism as an alternative to capitalism.[11] Funding, arming, training, and advising revolutionary groups in various parts of the Third World were ways to achieve this objective. Providing disaster relief, medical assistance, training for doctors, educational resources, and teachers, as well as negotiating international accords with other governments, also exemplified Cuba's approach to Cold War geopolitics.

In the 1970s and 1980s, Cuba's policy of international medical cooperation was meant to promote revolutionary objectives in Latin America and undermine U.S. hegemony in the region. Cuba's well-established tradition of supporting health care in underdeveloped nations was not, principally, a challenge to U.S. foreign policy, though in some cases that was certainly a side effect.[12] In Nicaragua the Cubans provided assistance to the Sandinista regime at the same time as the United States was funding, training, and organizing the Contras. Thus, although outright war was never declared between the United States and Cuba, they were nonetheless positioned on opposite sides of a war in which both had a vested interest. This sort of jockeying for influence and power was in line with key geopolitical aspects of the Cold War, which didn't always include direct military confrontation.[13]

In addition to reflecting a political position diametrically opposed to that of the United States, the Cuban presence in Nicaragua represented a more specific rebuke of U.S.-backed health programs in Nicaragua. With few exceptions, U.S. programs limited their investment in social services.[14] In his foreword to Julie Feinsilver's *Healing the Masses*, David Apter writes that in Cuba, "health care as a form of political outreach became one of the dominant narratives of the Cuban revolution. . . . Indeed, good medical practice [was] part of the 'historic and inversionary struggle' against imperialism in general and American instances of such imperialism in particular."[15] In the case of Nicaragua, increasing the accessibility and quality of health care became, as one expert writes, "symbolic of the contrast between socialism and capitalism, with aspects of U.S. society (and dependent capitalist societies) symbolic of capitalism's inherent inequality and failure to provide [José] Martí's goal, . . . a life of dignity."[16] In keeping with this sociopolitical orientation and a deep-seated belief in the superior virtues of socialism and communism, Cuba maintained a steady flow of personnel, administrators, advisers, medical supplies, and technical assistance to Nicaragua's MINSA throughout the eleven years of Sandinista rule.

However, in spite of the strong arguments for viewing Cuban aid to Nicaragua within the traditional concept of a Cold War framework—one in which the Capitalist West and the Communist Bloc battle for supremacy—this is far from the only, or even the most important, lens through which we can examine the relationship between Cuba and Nicaragua during the 1980s.[17] To date, few have examined the power dynamics within the Latin American and Caribbean Basin states—that is to say, the forces of power at work when the United States is not involved—or the ways in which Latin American states align and group themselves to either attract or rebuff U.S. involvement in regional issues. Yet these are precisely the most important dimensions of Cuba's medical assistance in Nicaragua. Understanding the relationship between these two leftist governments—one well established, one emergent—in a hemisphere whose recent history had been shaped and dominated by the United States is critical to grasping the full scope of Cold War geopolitics in Latin America.

Examining the power dynamics within Latin America and Caribbean states is therefore key to understanding the intraregional considerations of the Cold War in Latin America. Looking at the ways Latin American states aligned and grouped themselves to either attract or rebuff U.S. involvement in regional issues opens up a different lens for understanding Latin American geopolitics. For example, throughout the Cold War period, postrevolutionary Cuba tried to position itself to assume a mantle of authority and responsibility within the Latin American and Caribbean region. As the sole Communist state in the Western Hemisphere, Cuba was the first government many Latin American revolutionary groups contacted for help. Central and South American leftist factions from formal Communist parties to smaller revolutionary bands kept open lines of communication with Castro's Cuba, often soliciting advice, financing, military training, and public support.[18]

In this way, Cuba became, if not a global power, certainly a somewhat effective counterweight to U.S. regional hegemony. Most visibly, Cuba exercised its authority through its medical cooperation programs, which by the 1980s were well organized and internationally well regarded. In becoming the bearer of aid, the seat of technical know-how, and the provider of substantial sums of money, material, and personnel, Cuba took on an almost paternalist role vis-à-vis regional revolutionary and communist movements, a role it took very seriously.

Cuban Medical Diplomacy to Nicaragua: National and Regional

Cuba's quasi-paternalism is evident in the case of its involvement in 1980s Nicaragua. Although there was much talk of Cuban *brigadistas* (brigade members) being *compañeros de salud* (health partners), in reality, there was little doubt that Cuba was in charge. In every aspect of the arrangement between the two countries, Cuba was the leader, the teacher, and the donor. Nicaragua, though it took pains to present an image of autonomy and downplayed the importance of Cuban support in MINSA's official documentation and language, was the recipient of Cuba's largesse.

Cuban assistance to MINSA consisted of several components: a ministry-level advisory role; the provisioning of materials, equipment, and financing for health care; training and education for medical professionals; and the staffing of hospitals and health posts with nurses, doctors, specialists, and support personnel. Even a cursory glance reveals the extent to which Nicaragua's MINSA mirrored Cuba's Ministerio de Salud Pública (Ministry of Public Health). Just like Cuba, Sandinista Nicaragua built a hierarchical structure of rural health posts, urban health centers, polyclinics, and regional hospitals. This system functioned like a funnel: hundreds of small units (the health posts) stationed in rural areas and urban neighborhoods took care of preventive, primary, and triage care. Usually staffed by nurses and volunteers, health posts referred cases beyond their capacity to the bigger health centers. Health centers, usually staffed by at least one doctor, were located in towns and larger sections of cities. They took care of more serious illnesses, minor operations, and so forth. Anything a health center could not handle went to the small hospitals, of which there was one in each medium-sized city, and from there, to regional hospitals, of which there were seven nationwide. There were several even larger hospitals in Managua, some of which had a specialty, such as obstetrics, ophthalmology, and pediatrics.

In Cuba, the structured reorganization of clinical medicine began in the 1960s with the institution of a sectorized system that integrated clinical medicine and public health outreach by making local nurse-physician teams responsible for the health of a bureaucratically designated community sector (usually based on population).[19] In Nicaragua, the same principles of sectorizing and regionalizing were the basis of the Sandinista attempt to build a national primary-care-based health network. Though Nicaragua lacked the resources to fully staff the nurse-doctor teams employed in Cuba, MINSA nonetheless did its best to assign nurses and doctors to specific sectorized areas of cities, towns, and rural enclaves.

Following the Cuban model, MINSA inserted doctors into rural communities via compulsory social service assignments. The ministry also recruited and trained local health volunteers to educate and monitor local populations. Prior to 1979, in any given region, one privately owned hospital had been the only health resource for hundreds of thousands of people. Within a short period after the revolution, the Sandinistas, with help from Cuban and other international donors, had made health care accessible not only to the urban elite, but also to the urban and rural poor for the first time. The system was far from flawless, but given the almost total absence of health care nationwide prior to the revolution, the change was remarkable for its breadth, its depth, and the speed with which the network was built.

Dora María Téllez, Nicaragua's minister of health from 1984 to 1990, frankly acknowledged the extent to which her ministry relied upon the Cuban example: "Whenever we didn't know what to do, or how to resolve a problem, we looked for the most simple and effective solution. Many times—not always, but often—the example of the Cuban Ministry of Public Health gave us a good example to follow."[20] The permanent seat occupied by a "Cuban Adviser" in MINSA's main advisory council reflects the extent of Cuba's integration into Nicaragua's health bureaucracy.[21] By the mid-1980s the seat was usually vacant at monthly meetings, but, Dr. Téllez noted in an interview, "By then we didn't need him there every time, but earlier on, the adviser was always there."[22]

Many of Nicaragua's national health priorities mimicked contemporary health projects in Cuba. For example, beginning in 1981, Minister of Health Lea Guido launched a maternal-child (*materno-infantil*) health program that was closely modeled on the successful program that Cuba promoted in 1977. Nicaragua's project mandated the implementation of related health care initiatives, among them "early detection of pregnancy; early consultation with the obstetrical health team, provision of at least nine prenatal examinations and consultations for women in urban areas and six for women in rural areas; education about hygiene, health during pregnancy, childbirth, and childcare, among other topics; special prenatal attention to women considered at high obstetrical risk; psychological counseling with regard to childbirth; instruction in birth exercises; and finally, provision that all childbirth take place in hospitals."[23] Given personnel shortages, infrastructure problems, difficulties accessing the rural interior, and the worsening Contra War, MINSA could not enforce all of these norms effectively. Large numbers of women still gave birth at home with midwives, and in war zones few women could avail themselves of the prescribed six prenatal visits with a doctor.[24] Nonetheless, in most urban zones and in many rural areas, Guido oversaw a radical transformation in both maternal and infant health and a steep decline in these respective mortality rates.[25]

This Cuban-inspired program became the capstone of Guido's tenure in the ministry, and its effects were long-lasting. Even in 2008, at the time of the research conducted for this chapter, women's health cooperatives and local midwives still relied on many of the educational materials and methods emphasized in the early 1980s. For example, the MINSA-promoted oral rehydration solutions were so effective at preventing infant deaths from dehydration that women began mixing them at home. For decades, infant mortality rates due to dehydration and diarrhea have remained far below the statistical high-water mark of the 1970s.[26] In addition, many midwives interviewed still used the training manuals and mimeographed information sheets they were given during the 1980s.[27]

On a regional level, the Cuban advisory role was more limited. Dr. Orlando Rizo Espinosa, former regional director for Matagalpa and the mountainous North, indicated that only in Managua did MINSA offices have a Cuban adviser. In Matagalpa and in other regions, he said that the Cubans had the capacity to shape health policy, but only at a local level. For example, a Cuban surgeon at the regional hospital might share ideas about resource allocation, or another serving at a local health post could point out a place where people were not getting equal access to health resources.[28] Thus, at a national level, the advisory role of the Cuban medical presence was more clearly defined and formalized, and on the regional and local levels, more informal.

Nationally, Cuba not only provided an important advisory role, it was also an abundant source of much-needed medicines and medical equipment throughout the 1980s. The commitment of dispatching a medical mission was not just to send doctors and nurses. Cuba also undertook to fully equip the teams with everything they needed—from food and clothing to medicines, syringes, surgical equipment, bandages, and the like. By ship and by plane, reliable consignments arrived on a daily, weekly, and monthly basis for more than a decade. Sister Sandra Price, a U.S. citizen working in the remote mountain town of Siuna, remembers the Cuban ship that came once a month to Puerto Cabezas with medicines, vaccines, and medical supplies for the Atlantic Coast and mountainous Interior. "That Cuban shipment was the only thing that kept us in any kind of health" during the hardest years of the Contra War, Sister Price said. "You know, the Sandinistas did a good job, and they really did the best they could, but because of the war, they just couldn't get to us all the time. The Cuban shipment kept us going."[29] Without invoices or inventories of shipments, it is challenging to estimate exact quantities of aid, but oral histories indicate that Cuba was committed to a substantial level of material donation for the duration of the Sandinista regime.

To combat equipment shortages and to provide health care services for which Nicaragua was unequipped, Cuba also committed to bringing Nicaraguans in dire need of complicated surgical procedures to Cuban hospitals. Many interviewees spoke about this service, noting that a plane would leave for Cuba once a week with Nicaraguans in need of intensive treatment. The Cuban government would provide room, board, health care, and transportation free of cost. "That was one of the only good things, how they would take care of the sick and wounded like that," said Gabriel Pérez Rosales, a Matagalpan teacher and health volunteer who in all other respects was highly critical of Cubans as a people and of Cuban involvement in Nicaragua.[30]

Cubans on medical missions served not only as doctors and nurses, but also as educators and administrators. Cubans staffed positions at the medical schools and at training academies for nurses and nurse assistants. One of the first orders of business MINSA undertook was increasing the size of medical student cohorts. To do so, MINSA first expanded the class size at the medical faculty in León. By December 1979, it had enrolled a class of five hundred students, a tenfold increase over earlier class sizes.[31] The ministry subsequently founded a second medical college in Managua in 1982. Many Cuban doctors and administrators served long missions teaching at Nicaraguan medical schools in order to ensure that there were enough instructors for these larger classes, as well as to expand the number of specialties the schools offered, increase the quality of education, and administer an efficient degree program.[32]

The bulk of Cuban medical cooperation took the form most commonly imagined: doctors, nurses, and technical support staff were posted in hospitals, health centers, and rural health units, working directly with the Nicaraguan people. These Cuban doctors were not, according to the Cuban-Nicaraguan agreement, technically allowed to supervise Nicaraguan doctors, but outside of Managua, this stricture was widely ignored in practice. Dr. Félix Sosa Mas recalled working as a medical resident in the hospital at Jinotega, a position that was subordinate to the attending Nicaraguan physician. Dr. Sosa Mas found, however, that his attending physician often deferred to him, the Cuban medical resident, in matters of significance.[33] Miguel Angel Estupiñán, a Cuban nurse, commented that upon arriving at his post in Matagalpa, he immediately found the need to take charge of the ward in which he worked to ensure that medical best practices were followed.[34]

Despite the embedded nature of Cuban medical work in Nicaragua, the Cuban government shaped the experience of its health workers to emphasize their separateness from the Nicaraguan people, at the same time that the workers participated in creating social change at a local, personal level. Though the doctors and nurses working in Nicaragua lived in and engaged with the communities at health posts, teaching facilities, and in hospitals, they lived in separate quarters.[35] The doctors had almost nothing in the way of spending money; the Cuban government provided everything for them from food to clothing to equipment.[36] The brigadistas came and left on a fixed schedule—they worked in Nicaragua for a two-year period and then returned to Cuba.

The mission chiefs discouraged fraternization, and often required Cuban doctors to travel in pairs at all times.

This "together but separate" ethos enforced a paradigm in which the Cuban government tried to hold its workers both apart from and above the Nicaraguan state while at the same time standing in solidarity with the Sandinistas against hostile U.S. and counterrevolutionary actions. This position reflected Cuba's confidence in what by the 1980s was a well-organized mechanism of providing international medical assistance. As highly coordinated professional teams, Cuban medical workers arrived with the understanding that they were to work rigorously, serving a lofty revolutionary goal. Socializing with locals was subordinate to the task at hand.[37] The restrictive lifestyle conditions, however, also addressed Cuban fears of their medical workers defecting during their time serving abroad. These doctors were being temporarily deployed, not permanently relocated, so acculturation had to be curtailed.[38]

Cuba sent medical missions to Nicaragua and other nations out of a sense of revolutionary duty and to cement their regional position as an alternative to the United States for foreign aid. Nonetheless, Cuba did perceive obvious benefits from these medical missions. The service Cuban medical workers rendered during their missions was invaluable both to MINSA and to the health and well-being of the Nicaraguan people, but, as Feinsilver writes, "There is little doubt that the chance to do internationalist service and to see firsthand what colonialism, imperialism, and capitalism mean for Third World peoples, tends to increase the revolutionary zeal of Cuban youth, whose relative apathy worries Cuban leaders. . . . In medicine, internationalism has provided Cuban doctors with experience in tropical medicine and diseases of poverty long since eradicated in Cuba and has given them even greater pride in Cuba's own medical accomplishments."[39]

Cuban medical professionals who served in Nicaragua repeatedly maintained that they benefited from the educational opportunities presented by foreign service. For example, the medical conditions Cuban doctors witnessed in Nicaragua, especially in rural zones, were educational in the extreme and, for many doctors, a reminder of just how well cared for—in health terms—the Cuban population was. As Dr. Sosa Mas put it, "Look, in Cuba we didn't always understand how bad it was for people in other places. But when you arrive to your clinic at six in the morning and there are 150 people lined up for treatment, not just one day, but day after day for months and months and months, and you don't stop seeing patients even once to rest until late in the night, well, then you start to understand."[40] The end result for Cuban medical workers was an appreciation of a well-run and comprehensive health care system such as Cuba's, and—it was hoped—an increased loyalty to the homeland that provided such care for its people.

Cuban Experiences Providing Health Care, Up Close and Personal

When the first field hospital opened in Matagalpa, the Cuban brigade running it found "hundreds of patients queued up for treatment day and night."[41] Within one month the team had used up medicines they expected to last for three. Many of the Cuban doctors and nurses were shocked by what they saw. Patients suffered from diseases that had disappeared from Cuba, such as polio and neonatal tetanus. Malnutrition made the symptoms of measles so severe that the Cubans had difficulty recognizing this as the same disease that, in their country, had been controlled through mass immunization and improved nutrition. Nurse Estupiñán, who arrived in Nicaragua in 1981, said, "Seeing diseases like tetanus and measles, a ton of illnesses that you never see in Cuba, well, it was a shock. Some were so bad they didn't even look like the pictures I'd seen. But it was really good for my experience. And beginning to cure them, well, that was excellent."[42]

For some, however, the experience was not only educational, but also somewhat traumatic. Several doctors have particularly vivid recollections of treating leishmaniasis, a flesh-eating disease also called "mountain leprosy" that was endemic to the mountainous North. For many others, the memory of treating the war wounded, in particular women and children lacerated by bombs and grenades, remained painful years after deployment. "It was all-consuming work," commented Dr. Victor Pérez, a sentiment echoed by other Cubans interviewed for this project. "We saw patients, some in horrible conditions, at every hour of every day in twelve-hour shifts, twenty-four hours a day. It was work, work, work with no rest, and some of it was so hard, especially the war wounds. It still causes me pain to remember some of the most serious cases."[43] Nicaraguans also recall the intensity and dedication Cuban medical professionals brought to their work. "I tell you, those Cuban doctors and nurses," commented Dr. Rizo Espinosa, "the work they did was extraordinary. They did the sort of work that Nicaraguans wouldn't do, and in places Nicaraguans wouldn't go, like right into the war zones."[44]

Health workers on Cuban medical missions had disparate experiences depending on where they were stationed in Nicaragua. Cuban teams in urban areas tended to be large, with predictable work schedules, and a resident brigade chief who controlled their social interactions with the community. Smaller teams and individual doctors and nurses were deployed into the Interior and in war zones, where work habits tended to be more itinerant and situationally responsive than in larger towns, and where daily life was much more integrated with the local community. The brigade stationed in Matagalpa, the central city of the mountainous North, a two-hour drive northeast of Managua, offers a good example of what life was like within an urban Cuban medical mission. The first Cuban brigade arrived in Nicaragua on July 24, 1979, armed with a three-month supply of medicine and a fully equipped field hospital. Within twenty-four hours they had set up an open-air clinic next to the bombed-out hospital in Matagalpa and began treating patients the next day. To house the sixty-person team, the local Sandinista command center requisitioned a mansion that had belonged to Nacho Araúz, a Somocista who had fled Nicaragua when the revolution gained momentum.[45] For the duration of the Sandinista period, a team of health workers rotated out every two years. About half of those sixty workers were sent to other cities or Interior communities, and from 1979 until 1990 Matagalpa housed a contingent of thirty to forty Cuban health workers at all times.[46]

After Trinidad Guevara, the old hospital in Matagalpa, was rebuilt, medical treatment moved inside the building, and in 1984 when the new regional hospital opened on a hillside on Matagalpa's outskirts, the brigade split between "El Regional" and Trinidad Guevara, which became a twenty-four-hour health center.[47] Cuban doctors were also stationed around the city in each neighborhood's health clinic. They participated in sanitation and vaccination campaigns, going door-to-door in communities with Nicaraguan health workers. The Cuban medics also operated biannual continuing education programs for doctors and nurses, often supervising their Nicaraguan peers despite governmental prohibition of such informal hierarchies. Of the thirty specialties offered at the regional hospital, twenty-six of the positions were filled by Cubans, and Cuban nurses were often put in charge of entire wards when Nicaragua could provide a staff of only auxiliary nurses.[48]

This cooperation had an immediate impact on the lives of Nicaraguans, in very personal ways. Norma Ochoa, a domestic worker from Matagalpa, stated that before the revolution, she gave birth with a *partera empírica* (traditional midwife), just like every other woman she knew. When asked if she had noticed a change in health care during the 1980s, she responded, "Yes, well of course, I began to give birth in the hospital because then the medical attention was better there. Because the Cubans had come, the Cuban doctors, there were so many of them and they were very good, and the medicines [they brought] were free. They helped us out so much, and . . . a lot of Nicaraguan doctors went to Cuba to receive better training."[49] While many health care workers spoke about the Cuban medical brigades in positive terms, that a non-formally-educated, apolitical woman from a rural area also regarded the Cuban presence as beneficial demonstrates how much these medical missions shaped not only the development of the primary health care system, but also the life experiences of ordinary Nicaraguans. Although there were and still are vocal critics of the Cuban medical missions, the overwhelming response among informants was positive.

Cuban medical workers were not the only foreign health workers volunteering their services in support of the Sandinista government, but the Cuban experience differed dramatically from that of other *internacionalistas*. Volunteers from North America, Europe, and Latin American nations arrived either alone or in small brigades and stayed for periods ranging from two weeks to eleven years.[50] Bearing letters of introduction, they were relatively free to come and go in Nicaragua. They could leave the country at short notice or extend their service indefinitely, but while in the country they were subject to the dictates of the Nicaraguan state and were assigned roles within the auspices of the Ministries of Health, Agriculture, and Education.[51]

The Cuban brigade experience, by contrast, was organized in a quasi-military fashion, though participation was voluntary. According to Dr. Sosa Mas, "It was like this. Sometimes you wanted to do something—study a specialty, or see the world, or learn a new skill, so you signed up for these brigades, because good *compañeros* were rewarded for volunteering for service."[52] Others spoke of volunteering purely to serve those in need, like nurse Estupiñán, who came to Nicaragua at age seventeen.[53] Once on a brigade, however, the medical professionals surrendered all autonomy, a situation they were well trained to accept. As Katherine Hirschfeld notes in her book *Health, Politics, and Revolution in Cuba since 1898*, "Cuban doctors receive years of military training as part of their medical education—training that emphasizes hierarchy, rank, and unquestioning obedience to authorities."[54] The Cuban government sought to control every aspect of its brigadistas' lives abroad, from the time of deployment: the nature of their work, their location, the provision of supplies for daily life (food, clothing, spending money, and so on), and even when and with whom they were allowed to consort—an effort that met with greater success in urban areas than in rural placements.

Medical brigades were composed not just of doctors, but of workers of all ages and experience levels: general practitioners, surgeons, medical specialists, dentists, nurses, equipment technicians, and medical educators. Each health worker was subject to the command of a brigade chief, and the entire brigade typically lived in one house, homes that are still known in communities around

Nicaragua as *las casas de los cubanos* (Cuban homes). Ochoa, quoted earlier about her appreciation for the Cuban medical workers, was still rather dismissive of their reluctance to become part of the community: "Yes, they were good workers, but you know, they always stayed within their own circle, lived in their house, had their own lives there, and just went to work and then back home."[55]

The rather cloistered existence of the Cuban medical brigades was partly due to their brutal work schedule but also reflected a strategic move by the Cuban government, which had two purposes in mind. First, the restrictions were designed to protect the health workers from being attacked by anti-Sandinistas who were unfriendly to the Cuban presence in Nicaragua. Though the popular mythology of selfless Cuban doctors is that they served, in the words of former regional health director Rizo Espinosa, "in the most rural and most dangerous places, where no Nicaraguan doctor would even go," the reality is that the Cuban government kept its health workers from great personal danger by designating both where they were permitted to work and how their lives were structured. It is true that Cuban doctors worked in the war zones and in the Interior, but when the Contra War heated up and medical workers started dying in bombings and kidnappings, the terms of Nicaragua's agreement with Cuba allowed them to be stationed only at well-guarded military hospital installations or in urban areas. For example, in Siuna, an extremely dangerous conflict zone in the Interior, Sister Price said Cuban doctors as well as Nicaraguans worked in the town, and at least in the early years, they also went beyond its bounds: "[But then,] because of the war, the doctors were forbidden to go out into the campo, it would've been too dangerous. And we did have a few instances where doctors who did go out were kidnapped by the Contra and some of them were killed . . . so the doctors were forbidden to go outside of the town."[56]

Second, the rules were in place to prevent Cuban personnel from permanently defecting to capitalist or mixed-economy nations. Dr. Pérez explained,

> We had a lot of restrictions. It was prohibited to walk alone, or with a non-Cuban that wasn't part of our mission. This was because it was wartime, and we could have been kidnapped. That was the theory. In reality, it was because they didn't want us to get too comfortable living in another country—they didn't want to lose the investment they put in us, so they didn't want us to fall in love or stay here. But many of us did anyway.[57]

This belief was expressed repeatedly by both Nicaraguans and Cubans, and in fact, a great number of Cuban doctors who served abroad did eventually defect from Cuba to another country. Dr. Sosa Mas estimated that of his brigade of forty Cubans, perhaps only fifteen or twenty still live in Cuba today.[58] Not all stayed in Nicaragua, but over time around 50 percent settled in or defected to other countries, which indicates that the Cuban government had good reason to fear losing its personnel.

In spite of the restrictions and their training, however, Cuban medical brigadistas often stepped outside their designated role and formed enduring relationships with individuals or the communities they served. It is revealing of a deeper humanitarian impulse that in interviews, many of these *militantes de salud* (health activists/warriors) talked about serving "with love in their hearts."[59] One doctor, Geraldo Pais, spoke with great conviction, saying, "I did [my service here] from my heart, to serve, out of my true commitment to humanitarian medicine."[60] Dr. Sosa Mas said that the only thing that kept him motivated in the most difficult days of epidemics, scarcity of resources, hunger, and shortage of personnel was a genuine care for the poor and sick: "Our work here in that time was tremendous, voluminous, and absolutely exhausting. We worked around the clock, with no rest, on call for whatever emergency might arise. It was twenty-four-hour-a-day kind of work. We did it because we cared."[61] Though confined to collective living arrangements, forbidden to walk about the towns and cities alone, and moved from station to station depending upon the needs of the health care system, some Cuban medical workers still managed to form affective ties and build personal relationships with Nicaraguans.

These relationships took different forms and evolved in different ways. Many Cubans fell in love and married Nicaraguan women whom they met in the course of their work. Dr. Sosa Mas married his surgical nurse, and Dr. Pérez married the daughter of one of his chronic patients. Nurse Estupiñán fell in love "at first sight" with a young woman who attended the school two doors down from the Cuban's house. "I used to see her walking past our house every afternoon," he recalled, "and one time I couldn't stop myself, I just called out to her. She stopped to talk, and we fell in love. Two years later we married right before I had to go home to Cuba, and she came with me."[62]

Less life-altering relationships took place in the exchanges of daily life and commerce. The owner of a small cafeteria near one of Matagalpa's medical clinics said that she always liked it when the Cubans came in for lunch, "mostly because their accents were so funny, and they were always good for laughing at themselves." A favorite story was of a time they came in for lunch and one of the doctors said, in a typical Cuban accent, "Señora, quiero una sopa de pesca'o." She asked him why they always contracted the end of their words, and the Cuban looked back at her, somewhat perplexed. "Oh, sí? Pues, no sé. No me había fija'o."[63] In these simple moments of cultural exchange, laughter, familiarity, and falling in love, Cubans and Nicaraguans managed to break down some of the barriers that the Cuban government placed in the way of those relationships.

Voices in Opposition

Though the majority of Nicaraguans interviewed generally approved of and appreciated the work of the Cuban medical brigades during the 1980s, it is worth noting the vocal minority that accused, criticized, and blamed Cubans for many of the problems that faced Nicaraguans during the Sandinista period. Besides believing that the Cubans deliberately isolated themselves from communities, some Nicaraguans felt that Cuban doctors were high-handed and considered themselves superior to their Nicaraguan counterparts. Others blamed the Cuban medical presence for inhibiting MINSA's ability to deliver health care in rural areas. More broadly, various believed the Cuban presence had instigated the Contra War; others held that their "medical work" was really a front for ideological indoctrination.

While some Nicaraguans—such as Ochoa, who tried to remain neutral—simply offered the observation that Cuban doctors kept to themselves, others attributed a more sinister purpose to the isolated living conditions of the Cuban medical brigades. "They thought they were better than everybody else, that they should automatically be the boss over Nicaraguans," commented Pérez Rosales, the Matagalpan teacher. "The trouble with the Cubans is that they are arrogant, and they made a lot of people mad." In fact, some Cuban doctors did feel frustrated with what they perceived as antiquated and inefficient practices in the Nicaraguan hospitals. "Well, we had to teach a lot of people a lot of new techniques and sometimes even educate them about how to cure diseases they didn't understand," argued Estupiñán. As in many cases in Nicaragua, political perspectives colored perceptions of Cubans' attempts to educate or improve.[64]

Some felt, especially in the hardest years of the Contra War, that the presence of Cuban doctors was a challenge to the effective delivery of health services to rural mountainous zones. One doctor, Virgilio Cisne, explained, "Look, at first I was okay with the Cuban doctors. Sometimes I'd have them over to my house for dinner because they were here, working hard, and the poor bastards didn't have even a few cents to spend on the basics." Then, he continued, as the Contra War got worse and the Sandinistas got more rigid and ideological, the Cubans grew bolder in talking about their politics. "And I wasn't all right with that, because health, in my opinion, ought to be separate from politics, and the Cubans can't see it that way." He explained that many Nicaraguans, trying to avoid taking sides in the conflict, would avoid going to a Cuban doctor, even if that was the only doctor around. "Because of fear, you understand? Especially out in the country, the thought was, if you go to a Cuban doctor, the Contra would come in the night and take you for a Sandinista."[65] Dr. Cisne was one of many who spoke about this concern and blamed the Cuban presence for actually restricting access to health care in rural zones.

The most die-hard anti-Sandinistas blamed the Cuban presence for the U.S.-backed Contra War. As a result, some ingenious (if decidedly inaccurate) rumors spread rapidly in the countryside to discourage the peasantry from interacting with the Sandinistas and their Cuban allies. "If the Cubans hadn't been here in the first place, the United States never would have attacked us," an anti-Sandinista peasant from Mulukukú asserted. "Or if they hadn't, the Sandinistas would have fallen a lot faster." In his view, one of the most malicious things the Cubans did was to spread communism. When asked how, exactly, they did so if the peasants wouldn't even talk to the Cubans, he stated matter-of-factly, "It was those 'vaccines.' They said they were curing polio or whatever, but we knew they were really injecting people with communism."[66] I heard similar comments from several other informants. Nicaraguan brigadista Rafael "Don Payo" Hernández shook his head sadly when I asked him about it. "It was ridiculous, they didn't even know what communism was, but they knew they didn't want any of it, and that it came with the Cubans."[67] Ochoa, the domestic worker quoted earlier, also confirmed the story, though she giggled. "Yes, that's what some of us thought." When asked to define communism, she responded, "Well, I don't really know. I think it's that little pain you feel after you get an injection, right?"[68]

As evidenced by these anecdotes, Nicaraguan feelings of fear or anger toward Cubans were not always based on facts, or even a clear understanding of the issues at hand. Nonetheless, they were damaging not only to the work Cuban and Nicaraguan health care workers were attempting, but also to the reputation and legacy Cubans would leave in Nicaragua after the Sandinista years. Stories like these illustrate how social improvement programs continue to be captive to the politics of ideology.

Conclusion

Cuba's role in Nicaragua reflected the Castro government's commitment to ideologically motivated health cooperation during and beyond the Cold War. Over the years, Cuba has provided support, including military aid, disaster relief, and technical assistance, to over one hundred countries in the Global South—both to governments espousing communist aspirations, and to many others that formed part of the Non-Aligned Movement, of which Fidel Castro became de facto leader in the 1980s. Yet in no other country did Cuban support come close to the levels it reached in Nicaragua during the 1980s. There, in 1987 alone, Cuban doctors attended 856,000 patients, performed 7,163 major operations, and delivered 1,704 babies.[69]

Cuba's foreign policy of supporting health care initiatives (particularly primary health care delivery and medical training) in Third World nations has drawn much well-deserved praise over the years, but the effects of this policy are poorly understood. This chapter teaches us something about Cuba's geopolitical goals and logistical fears, but also about how these missions affected the lives of both the Cuban medical workers delivering care and the citizens of the country in which they served. Cuba's extraordinary support for the development of a socialist health care network in Nicaragua was part of its Cold War foreign policy, but supporting leftist governments against U.S. coercion and aggression was only one objective.

Concomitantly, Cuba attempted—with greater and lesser degrees of success—to constrain the lives of its medical workers and prevent their integration with Nicaraguan communities for two reasons: to assert its superiority over the emergent socialist Nicaraguan state, and to prevent Cuban medical workers from defecting to other countries. There is, then, a contradiction between the global and even intra-regional assumptions about Cuba's intent in deploying medical missions as a tool of foreign diplomacy, and what this medical cooperation actually represented and generated. Though the United States and much of the world assumed that the ulterior motive of these brigades was to use health personnel to spread communism, Cuba constrained the lives of its medical workers so strictly as to limit the potential for that outcome. In reality, Cuban medical professionals serving in Nicaragua had very little ability to encourage Nicaraguans to become communist. Writ large, the brigades were able "only" to proffer an example of how communism could provide a path to equality and opportunity for all. If their proximate purpose was simply to serve in their capacity as health care workers, the underlying South–South health solidarity role of Cuban-Nicaraguan cooperation in the 1980s may have ultimately been more influential than direct communist infiltration and overtures in the context of a proxy war fomented by the United States.

In the ongoing debates around transnationalism, internationalism, and regional hegemony, the case of Cuban medical missions to Nicaragua is an excellent lens through which to examine these questions. For instance, the nature of the work would seem to fit the definition of transnational, as medical workers mixed with the Nicaraguan communities in which they were stationed. However, because of the restrictions placed upon the Cuban brigadistas and the fear of Contra retributions among rural Nicaraguans, both the Cuban and Nicaraguan governments implemented a stopgap between the two cultures and populations, in order to hold them separate from each other outside of a health care delivery context. It was, in essence, internationalism more than transnationalism, as the governments attempted to interrupt the mixing of personal lives and experiences with regulations and restrictions.

The irony of this scenario is that the West's great fear of international communism was that it would result in breaking down national borders, offering communist ideology as a unifying principle and a palliative for all ills. Yet in Nicaragua, it was Cuba, the communist state, that worked to maintain the integrity of borders and national identity. Even with such constraints, however, the Cuban medical missions to Nicaragua had lasting implications for subsequent South–South solidarity, particularly within Latin America. For one, health internationalism *a la cubana* was tinged with a sense of shared responsibility to support other nations' broadest efforts to increase health equity and social justice.

This recognition of common aspirations increased the Cubans' ability to interact with various forms of (health) resistance to repressive regimes in the late Cold War period (e.g., welcoming health leftists in exile from South American dictatorships and rehabilitating militants from the Farabundo Martí National Liberation Front injured in the Salvadoran Civil War) and with the rising forces of progressive nationalism in Latin America in the decades following the Cold War.[70] Indeed, the Cuban-Nicaraguan missions served as a beacon for the South–South health cooperation that flourished during Latin America's post-2000 Pink Tide of elected left-leaning governments. In particular, Cuban-Venezuelan mutual aid in the form of the Castro-Chávez doctors-for-oil exchange—and its flagship Misión Barrio Adentro program of community health services—built upon the experiences in Nicaragua twenty years earlier.[71] These efforts also held multiple, and even contradictory, meanings around issues of dependency, bottom-up versus top-down directives, technical health services intertwined with political aims, and the role of training local health personnel to replace the Cubans, all in the context of a counter-hegemonic community health experiment with wide resonance. Above all, the Cuban-Nicaraguan "episode" helped solidify Cuban health solidarity within and beyond Latin America as a legitimate form of South–South social-justice-oriented health diplomacy.[72]

Notes

1   Donahue, *Nicaraguan Revolution in Health*, 11.
2   Feinsilver, *Healing the Masses*. See also Elizundia Ramírez, *Nicaragua, No Somos Dioses*; Prevost, "Cuba and Nicaragua."
3   María Hamlin Zúniga, interview with author, March 19, 2009. See also Bossert, "Health Care in Revolutionary Nicaragua"; Bossert, "Nicaraguan Health Policy"; Donahue, *Nicaraguan Revolution in Health*; Donahue, "International Organizations, Health Services, and Nation Building"; Garfield and Williams, *Health Care in Nicaragua*.
4   Booth, *End and the Beginning*; Timothy Brown, *Real Contra War*; Crawley, *Dictators Never Die*; Crawley, *Nicaragua in Perspective*; Heyck, *Life Stories of the Nicaraguan Revolution*; Kinzer, *Blood of Brothers*; Morris Morley, *Washington, Somoza, and the Sandinistas*; Paige, *Coffee and Power*; Christian Smith, *Resisting Reagan*; Zimmerman, *Sandinista*.
5   Cuba also sent brigades to assist with education, agriculture, and military programs, among others, and cooperated with other countries in these fields. See Hickling-Hudson, González, and Preston, *Capacity to Share*; Hatzky, *Cubans in Angola*.
6   Managua taxi driver, conversation with author, September 2008.
7   Lamentably, many of the statistics regarding Cuban medical support for the Sandinista government are unknown due to an absence of archival records in Nicaragua. Given the lack of archived budgets, invoices, signed accords, professional reports, proposals, or personal communications, it is impossible at this point to reconstruct a statistical portrait of the program. For example, we do not know the number of Cuban medical workers who served in Nicaragua from 1979 through 1990, nor can we know the quantities or monetary value of medicines and equipment donated by the Cuban government or the specific input of advisers and administrators working at the national and regional levels. Nonetheless, oral histories, published annual health plans, the scattered remnants of MINSA documents, newspaper accounts, and some statistics from secondary sources fill in many of these gaps.
8   See, for example, Kirk, *Healthcare without Borders*. On the nuances of medical cooperation sans the United States, see also Soto Laveaga's chapter in this volume and the epilogue.
9   Garfield and Williams, *Health Care in Nicaragua*; Feinsilver, *Healing the Masses*; Donahue, *Nicaraguan Revolution in Health*.
10 Dr. Geraldo Pais, interview with author, Matagalpa, March 7, 2009.
11 Feinsilver, *Healing the Masses*.
12 Here I distinguish between the Cuban government's political purposes and the medical brigades' professional and humanitarian goals. Cuba sent military assistance to Latin American and to Africa, but this chapter deals only with its medical brigades. For more information on Cuba's military campaigns in Africa, see Gleijeses, *Conflicting Missions*.

13   Fink, *Cold War*; Westad, *Global Cold War*.

14   Consider the Rockefeller Foundation's campaign to combat hookworm in the 1940s or the aid programs that emerged out of John F. Kennedy's Alliance for Progress in the 1960s. Although the latter did encourage improvements in social services such as health care and education, the Somoza regime appropriated much of the Alliance for Progress funds and employed the remainder to combat dissident movements in the mountains. As a result, this U.S. policy was short-lived, corrupt, and unequally implemented within the Nicaraguan nation. In the minds of most Nicaraguans, the balance of U.S. influence over the years has been overwhelmingly negative. See Ligia Peña, "Salud Pública"; Ligia Peña and Palmer, "Rockefeller Foundation Health Primer"; Rodolfo Peña et al., "Fertility and Infant Mortality Trends."

15   David Apter, foreword to Feinsilver, *Healing the Masses*, xiii.

16   Cited in Feinsilver, *Healing the Masses*, 17.

17   A fine example of engaging scholarship on transnationalism, internationalism, and hegemony in the Western Hemisphere is Joseph, LeGrand, and Salvatore, *Close Encounters of Empire*. Still, it is one that privileges historical analyses almost entirely along a North–South axis. More recent works offer an excellent starting point for an exploration of intraregional hegemonic and transnational relationships in the Caribbean and Latin America. See Joseph and Spenser, *In from the Cold*; Steve Stern, *Battling for Hearts and Minds*; Seigel, "Beyond Compare."

18   See, for example, Metzi, *Por los Caminos de Chaletenango con la Salud en la Mochila*; Terry and Turiano, "Brigadistas and Revolutionaries."

19   Feinsilver, *Healing the Masses*, 214.

20   Dr. Dora María Téllez, interview with author, Managua, December 3, 2008.

21   Actas Ministeriales, Dora María Téllez personal papers.

22   Téllez interview.

23   Garfield and Williams, *Health Care in Nicaragua*, 48.

24   Dr. Orlando Rizo Espinosa, interview with author, Matagalpa, March 21, 2009.

25   On the imperative to improve health conditions in rural areas, see also Bliss's and Hochman and Paiva's chapters in this volume.

26   Dr. Francisco Gutiérrez, interview with author, Managua, October 24, 2008.

27   Midwife Lucia Mantila, interview with author, Matagalpa, February 3, 2009.

28   Rizo Espinosa interview.

29   Sister Sandra Price, interview with author, Matagalpa, March 5, 2009.

30   Gabriel Pérez Rosales, interview with author, Managua, September 24, 2008.

31   "500 Estudiantes en Facultad de Medicina."

32   Gutierrez interview.

33   Dr. Félix Sosa Mas, interview with author, Matagalpa, March 11, 2009.

34   Miguel Angel Estupiñán, interview with author, Matagalpa, March 13, 2009.

35   Sosa Mas interview; Estupiñán interview; Mario Zúniga, interviews with author, Matagalpa, February 4, 2009, March 13, 2009.

36   Dr. Victor Pérez, interview with author, March 10, 2009.

37 Pais interview.

38 Pérez interview; Estupiñán interview.

39 Feinsilver, *Healing the Masses*, 13.

40 Sosa Mas interview.

41 J. M. C. Cruz, "La Salud en la Revolución," *El Nuevo Diario*, November 27, 1980, quoted in Garfield and Williams, *Health Care in Nicaragua*, 20.

42 Estupiñán interview.

43 Pérez interview.

44 Rizo Espinosa interview.

45 Mario Zúniga interview; Dr. Noe García, interview with author, Matagalpa, February 6, 2009.

46 García interview; Dr. Virgilio Cisne, interview with author, Matagalpa, February 11, 2009.

47 García interview.

48 Estupiñán interview.

49 Norma Ochoa, interview with author, Matagalpa, February 3, 2009.

50 See, for example, Braveman, "Find the Best People and Support Them."

51 As broad and varied a group as the *internacionalistas* were, it is difficult to describe the work they did in any brief way. In the city of Matagalpa, for example, people came from all over and for varied time periods to volunteer in any number of capacities, from education to agriculture to health care. In the arena of public health, for example, a group of East Germans arrived in the mid-1980s and stayed for six months to build a water treatment plant. A Peruvian military doctor became a Sandinista military trainer at the behest of Tomás Borge, the minister of the interior, and subsequently worked at Trinidad Guevara in Matagalpa as a doctor. A Spanish midwife came to conduct a two-week training for local midwives and ended up staying for the rest of her life. The most famous of all internacionalistas is perhaps a young American, Benjamin Linder, who volunteered in any capacity he could find, whether it was juggling to entertain children or riding his unicycle through town to promote an upcoming vaccination campaign. He was killed in a Contra attack while inspecting a dam for possible repair work. Though many volunteers came and went rather quickly, for those who stayed, the opportunity for internacionalistas to embed themselves in the communities in which they lived and worked was profound.

52 Sosa Mas interview.

53 Estupiñán interview.

54 Hirschfeld, *Health, Politics, Revolution in Cuba Since 1898*, 217.

55 Ochoa interview.

56 Dr. Freddy Meynard, interview with author, Managua, October 8, 2008; Gutiérrez interview; Rizo Espinosa interview; Price interview.

57 Pérez interview.

58 Sosa Mas interview.

59 Pais interview.

60 Pais interview.

61 Pérez interview.

62 Estupiñán interview.

63 Anonymous, interview with author, Matagalpa, February 3, 2009.

64 Pérez Rosales interview; Estupiñán interview.

65 Cisne interview.

66 Anonymous rural Nicaraguan, interview with author, Mulukukú, February 24, 2009.

67 Don Rafael Hernández, interview with author, Matagalpa, February 18, 2009.

68 Ochoa interview.

69 Feinsilver, *Healing the Masses*, 162.

70 A parallel, earlier process is noticeable in the case of the peaceful coexistence strategy launched by Soviet leaders post-Stalin that smoothed their interactions with the newly established regime of Fidel Castro. See Pettinà, "Shadows of Cold War."

71 Amy Cooper, "Doctor's Political Body."

72 Birn, Muntaner, and Afzal, "South–South Cooperation in Health."

A Lingering Cold (War)?

*Reflections for the Present and an
Agenda for Further Research*

ANNE-EMANUELLE BIRN
AND RAÚL NECOCHEA LÓPEZ

In September 2009, Venezuelan president Hugo Chávez made his eighth trip to Russia, where he gave an animated lecture at Peoples' Friendship University, some twenty years after U.S. President Ronald Reagan addressed a prior generation of university students in Moscow.[1] In his speech, Chávez decried the unremitting and dangerous U.S. political and military role: "In all history, there was never a government that perpetrated more terrorism than that of the U.S. empire."[2] Chávez expressed gratitude for Russia's support on the international stage and discussed Venezuela's social policy advances, highlighting its markedly improved access to health care, enabled by a large-scale Cuba-Venezuela doctors-for-oil swap to staff and train health personnel in low-income areas across the country via the Misión Barrio Adentro program (providing much-needed energy resources to Cuba). Just a few months later, while North America and Europe were still reeling from the 2008 global financial crisis, Venezuela and Russia deepened their economic ties during Putin's 2010 visit to Venezuela, even as the largest share (almost 40 percent) of Venezuela's petroleum exports continued going to the United States.[3] When Chávez was diagnosed with cancer the following year, he chose to pursue treatment in Havana (traveling back and forth until his death in 2013), where he was under the care of Cuba's acclaimed oncology specialists and near his political mentor, emblematic Latin American health internationalist Fidel Castro.[4]

On one level, these vignettes seem a vestige of Cold War–era Latin America: a strongman "games" the two superpowers, aligning with one in geopolitical and rhetorical terms, while relying on the other economically. Yet on another level, Chávez's signature health and social well-being program, Misión Barrio Adentro—and indeed his own cancer therapy—involved a purely Latin American exchange, suggesting that notwithstanding the larger global context, the region did not need the patronage of either the United States or Russia nor would it accede to the double-edged sword of outside aid and economic agreements. Of course, the sovereign destiny-forging efforts of Latin American countries, as we have seen, were apparent from early on in—and in many ways enabled by—the Cold War.

Here in the epilogue we revisit this and other themes and imaginaries that emerge from this volume, contemplate lingering aspects of the Cold War in Latin America in the health and medical arenas, and propose a future research agenda.

Themes

Just as the introduction showed that the Cold War's onset in Latin America—and the relationships it engendered—fed on earlier, vibrant intellectual and political exchanges within and beyond the region, the Cold War's unleashing of alliances, interchange of powerful ideas, and sometimes bitter rivalries survived the formal end of the conflict between the Communist and Capitalist Blocs. As such, it remains essential to ground early twenty-first-century phenomena, such as the Pink Tide of leftist Latin American governments and the region's renewed economic and political ties with China and Russia, in the longer historical processes of the Cold War.[5]

More immediately connected to the health care arena are critical ongoing debates about South–South health cooperation, and the establishment and expansion of more inclusive medical care systems (in terms of race/ethnicity/Indigeneity, class, and geographic location). For example, Evo Morales, a farmer of Aymara background who rose to prominence as a *cocalero* leader in the 1980s protesting the United States–led War on Drugs in Bolivia before being elected Bolivia's president in 2006, strongly advocated intercultural approaches to health, giving official legitimacy to traditional medicine, and overseeing the constitution's incorporation of the Andean Indigenous "buen vivir" philosophy of ecological harmony (though like his ally Chávez, Morales was unable to break from economic reliance on extractive industries). Into the present, these issues are informed—if not deeply marked—by Cold War struggles. Thus, the themes that have emerged from the preceding chapters remain salient for a (medical) history of the present as well as the Cold War past.

A central theme that this volume's contributors have emphasized again and again is that Latin American health and medical actors navigated the Cold War context while constrained by larger geopolitical forces, even as they deftly pursued domestic and institutional interests. This flexibility was enabled both by long-standing professional ties and by the cleverly portrayed "neutral nature" of the health and medical arenas. The fierce and often paranoid rivalry between the U.S. and Soviet blocs was reflected in pointed and sometimes unexpected efforts to court key constituencies in Latin America and shape health policy, medical training and research institutions, and overall health and development approaches in individual countries. At the same time, postwar state-building and professionalization efforts within and across Latin American countries played the superpowers against one another. Both the United States and the Soviet Union frequently found themselves responding to Latin American demands for domestically driven development efforts rather than able to compel Latin American acquiescence to their respective imperatives.[6] This was certainly the case for Mexico's pharmaceutical sector and Chile's health policy experiments. Latin American health leaders also readily turned to Soviet cooperation, especially as bilateral agreements with countries across the Third World proliferated in the 1960s as alternate avenues for commercial relations, training, and medical infrastructure support. These agreements not only involved Cuba, and later Sandinista Nicaragua, but also countries that were not socialist-leaning, such as Mexico (in the realm of medical equipment), Peru (medicines), Argentina, and Brazil.[7]

Amplifying domestic aspirations to grow medical research and training and expand the reach of public health was a defiant set of antihegemonic health and medical solidarities both within and beyond Latin America that, for example, motivated a Communist Brazilian parasitologist to wield his international clout as part of an international commission investigating the U.S. use of bacterial warfare in the Korean War; led the Mexican government to shelter a dissident U.S. nurse; witnessed Argentine psychiatrists struggle across borders to define their mode of practice in a context of political repression; and saw the rise of Cuban-Nicaraguan health cooperation amid a brutal antileftist insurgency. Sometimes skirting controversy, health and medical realms often distinguished themselves from other cultural and political arenas through their ability to "pass" as technical and humanitarian endeavors even as they pitted donors and supporters against each other.

To be sure, alternative solidarities were not merely aspirational—they evolved by necessity. This was true for revolutionary regimes shut out from Pan-American and international venues and resources under U.S. pressure (e.g., Cuba was expelled from the Organization of American States [OAS], and the U.S. Agency for International Development, the Inter-American Development Bank, the World Bank, and the International Monetary Fund [IMF] pulled out of 1980s Sandinista Nicaragua). Under repressive regimes, meanwhile, cross-border civil society solidarities abetted some health leftists to flee, hide, survive, and even thrive for years on end in locales as distinct as Sweden, Oaxaca, the Bronx, East Germany, and Havana, yet many others were imprisoned, assassinated, or left with broken spirits.[8]

Indeed, a significant factor enabling Cold War Latin American solidarities was travel, both within and beyond the continent, in its multiple forms—including long and short stints back and forth, conference attendance, extended periods of study and work abroad, and even forced exile. The circumstances propelling travel by scientists and health workers, together with their actual experiences and the multifarious consequences of their travels, augment existing theorization about the production and circulation of scientific knowledge, health practices, and professional norms, which for Latin America is particularly rich for the eighteenth and nineteenth centuries.[9] In pulling the topic of circulating knowledge, practices, and norms into the mid-twentieth century—together with the related concepts of *histoire croisée*, or entangled (interconnected) history and mobilities—we call attention to new configurations of power ushered in by the Cold War, with Latin American experts poised to chart, reinforce, reroute, and challenge emerging ideas as simultaneously circumscribed and facilitated by the larger geopolitical context.[10]

Travel not only spread knowledge about medical novelties and systems, but also affirmed the preexisting, and still seductive, notion that linguistic and historical similarities abounded—despite the region's astoundingly diverse human geography—that could bind Latin America toward a modernity and future of its own making, as envisioned by the Buenos Aires psychiatrists Marco Ramos discusses. Even when travel became a necessity, rather than a choice, as Katherine E. Bliss illustrates through the career of Lini de Vries, the persecution and surveillance of exiles could foment, perhaps unwittingly, a lifelong identification with Mexico and its health challenges. Travel also allowed Latin American experts to meet, learn from, and network with partners in the United States, Canada, and Western Europe as well as the USSR, Eastern Europe, and China in the context of what became a tripolar Cold War by the 1960s. The powerful visions about national health care principles and organization articulated by travelers such as Chilean Benjamín Viel or Brazilian Samuel Pessoa were—at least in part—the result of such travels. Likewise, their willingness and skill to resist the wholesale imposition of U.S. norms in health research and policy matters undoubtedly stemmed from having been exposed to alternatives abroad either in person or through publications and epistolary contacts.

Given the variegated health and medicine contexts, political circumstances, and actors to be found in Cold War Latin America, it should not be surprising that both the United States and the USSR at times failed to comprehend the forces that animated local changes and continuities. The U.S. researchers who advanced the Puerto Rico Family Life Study, for example, were oblivious to their dependence on local patrons and subordinate assistants, and were blindsided by nationalist critics on the island. Nicole L. Pacino's chapter highlights how the fear of U.S. government censure led the Rockefeller Foundation to pull back from supporting medical education in Bolivia, despite the fact that the governing regime was not a communist one and that the U.S. State Department justified supporting leftists precisely because of communist presence in Bolivia. Soviets, too, could fail to read fluently the Latin American context. Soviet psychiatrists and their Cuban followers, as laid out by Jennifer Lynn Lambe, imagined Pavlovian experimentalism would rapidly displace the Freudian tradition after the 1959 revolution, only to see it endure, adapt, and hold its own, for a while at least, at the hands of Cuban specialists accustomed to eclectically combining research and treatment approaches.

Alongside Pastor and Long, then, we argue for the influential role of Latin Americans in shaping the Cold War, expanding on the diverse manifestations of their agency to encompass actors in the fields of health and medicine.[11] As this volume has revealed, during the Cold War era the Latin American experience offered instances of imposition, adaptation, exploration, resistance, and even rejection, producing societal laboratories for implanting and maneuvering around the period's contrasting health ideologies. At the same time, Latin Americans created autochthonous countercurrents that were chronologically autonomous and only tangentially in dialogue with the dominant contours and models presented by the two superpowers.

Lingerings and Echoes

In 1996, the government of Alberto Fujimori in Peru launched an involuntary sterilization plan the likes of which had never been seen before in Latin America, either in scope or in cruelty. In alignment with international credit agencies' demands to reduce the size of the population and thereby reduce spending on social programs, the so-called voluntary surgical sterilizations primarily affected Indigenous women in rural areas—those already disproportionately burdened by poverty, a sustained trajectory of political corruption that jeopardized rural social programs more than urban counterparts, and the violence wrought by the Shining Path and the armed forces' reaction against it.

Fujimori's Peru also echoed Cold War exigencies in other ways. While miserable conditions had long plagued vast swaths of Peru and much of the Andes, they worsened in the late Cold War with the 1980s debt crisis and the international financial sector's rollout of neoliberal policies aimed at slashing government spending and unraveling regulatory protections.

Under pressures stretching well into the 1990s, Fujimori's health reforms included the deregulation of medical education and the privatization of social security benefits. Fujimori's successful control of Peru's inflation and subduing of Shining Path emboldened his regime, which became increasingly authoritarian and unwilling to police its own (health) technocrats, particularly after Fujimori's 1995 reelection. With the Ministry of Health's self-monitoring function diminished, its ability to investigate complaints was hampered, compounding the human suffering caused by the involuntary sterilization program, which went on for nearly two years. The repercussions on much-needed family planning services continue to the present, even as assignment of medicopolitical responsibility for the program's implementation remains unresolved.[12]

The shadow of the involuntary sterilization program comes into sharper focus when considered alongside Latin American health-related initiatives that took place during the Cold War, such as those explored in this volume. Especially salient are those efforts that sought to adapt U.S. and Soviet ideas to Latin American realities linking health and development writ large, as well as particular medical approaches in realms ranging from psychiatry to health policy and medical education. In the Peruvian case, the government borrowed a page from the U.S. Cold War population policy playbook, which since the 1940s emphasized the economic advantages of technologically driven limitation of rapid population growth in the Third World, as Raúl Necochea López shows in his chapter, and built upon prior prejudices motivating eugenic policies determining who was fit to reproduce.[13] Fujimori's sterilization program makes plain that the 1990s did not translate into a wholesale rebooting of health philosophies and proposals in Latin America, instead hosting a mingling of the old and the new—a post–Cold War admixture that did not shed its Cold War outerwear—that this epilogue seeks to underscore as we strive to formulate multidisciplinary and collaborative research agendas into the future.[14]

Another way in which the Cold War history of Latin America strengthens our understanding of present-day health and medical features of this diverse region is by encouraging us to appreciate the deep roots of a range of health solidarities that have reappeared in recent years. As detailed in Anne-Emanuelle Birn's introduction, these "alternative" health solidarities and agendas (that is, alternative to more dominant North American and Western European North–South interventions) existed well before the Cold War, flourishing in the 1950s. They became increasingly constrained (or isolated) in the later Cold War period (mid-1970s through the 1980s), when the heavy hand of U.S. foreign and economic policy generated, backed, and coincided with harsh dictatorial regimes across much of Latin America, severe economic crises, and brutal civil wars in Central America, Peru, and Colombia. Yet, as civil wars and dictatorships gave way to peace and rising citizen expectations into the 1990s, new manifestations of health solidarity have (re)surfaced, especially concerning the rebuilding of medical systems and infrastructure and the crafting of innovative health policies.

Patent remnants from the late Cold War with particularly vivid expression in Latin America were the neoliberal social and health policy reforms that emerged in the context of the West's geo-economic onslaught against the Third World's vocal 1960s/1970s stance for a new international order, responsive United Nations system, and end to unfair trade conditions and prejudicial commodity pricing. On the heels of oil shocks and an orchestrated debt crisis unleashed first in Latin America, the 1980s structural adjustment demands by the World Bank and the IMF for deregulation, privatization, public spending cuts, and expanded protections for investors built on the brutal prototype tested out under the Pinochet regime. These policies, and their health effects, extended into the post–Cold War period, resulting in reductions in access to and quality of health care and other social services and in an overall worsening of occupational, economic, and living conditions.[15]

In some settings, reforms were implemented with relish by domestic elites who recognized the benefits of growing inequality for their own gain. Continuities of this agenda into the 1990s were made visible by a panoply of health reforms across the region.[16] These drew directly from the 1993 World Bank health reform model (in conjunction with the conditionalities accompanying its structural adjustment loans) at a time when the bank surpassed the World Health Organization (WHO) in playing a role in global health.[17] Through this period, country after country from the Southern Cone to Central America/Mexico and the Caribbean saw long-standing, already extremely segmented health care arrangements (by particular industry, degree of rurality or urbanity, level of formality or informality, etc.) become further fragmented, underfunded, reoriented via market incentives, and opened up to investment by foreign (typically U.S.) insurance companies.[18]

As such—with the notable exceptions of Costa Rica and Cuba—much of the region saw deepening inequities in access to care, in comprehensiveness, and in health status. The large informal workforce, the indigent, and Indigenous groups were increasingly relegated to receiving care in underfunded public facilities or forced to pay out of pocket for private health care. For example, by 2000 over half of Mexico's population, especially poor, Indigenous, and rural residents, had no health insurance coverage and relied on public clinics of uneven quality, insufficient distribution and accessibility, and inadequate staffing.[19] Meanwhile over half of health care expenditures occurred in the private sector, mostly covering a small elite.

And yet, even in the wake of the debt crisis, capital flight, structural adjustment policies, and extreme austerity, a new approach appeared in Brazil out of Cold War antidictatorship resistance, shadow health policymaking, and pent-up demands articulated by social movements, portending a wave of progressive health and social reforms of the Pink Tide starting in the late 1990s. Brazil's postdictatorship 1988 constitution, enshrining health care as a universal right, established a tax-funded, "unified" socialist-inspired health care system (SUS), providing "free" services for the entire population just as the Cold War was waning.[20] Brazil's reform, though not eliminating the private sector, attempted to rectify inequities in health care access and fragmentation of services via a publicly financed, decentralized, and integrated system involving federal, state, and municipal governments.[21] For a time, Brazil was even a world leader in defying World Trade Organization (WTO) patent rules to produce and provide generic AIDS drugs to all in need of them.[22] While funding shortfalls, a deficit of primary care doctors in the poorest and most rural areas (compelling the Brazilian government in 2014 to contract over fourteen thousand doctors, mostly through South–South cooperation from Cuba), and most significantly political turmoil since 2016 are accelerating SUS's privatization and generating clawbacks in the right to health care under a right-wing government elected in 2018, the founding and endurance of SUS is a testament to health care struggles "against the grain" that emerged in the late Cold War period and survived well past it.

Perhaps the most dynamic dimension of a Cold War–tinged view of Latin America's health and medical recent history is the Pink Tide of progressive and social democratic parties elected on social redistribution, welfare regime-building, and social rights platforms.[23] These governments came into power across the region starting circa 2000, beginning with Hugo Chávez's Bolivarian revolution in Venezuela, and continuing to Brazil, Argentina, Uruguay, Bolivia, Ecuador, Paraguay, and El Salvador. By the late 1990s, Latin American countries were emboldened to "go it alone" both in terms of promoting more inclusive and equitable domestic health and social policies that challenged fiscal austerity models, *and* in terms of fashioning bilateral and regional health policies not supported or sanctioned by the United States. This assertion of power was motivated at least in part by the absurd situation of Cuba being excluded from the OAS but remaining a member of UN agencies such as the Pan American Health Organization (PAHO) and WHO (with U.S. representatives reportedly walking out of meetings whenever a Cuban spoke).

If such maneuvering also flourished at certain moments during the Cold War, when Latin American countries became particularly adept at reading the possibilities for gaming the superpowers (as in Mexico's courting of the Soviets in pharmacultural realms, presented in Gabriela Soto Laveaga's chapter), post–Cold War power politics were enabled by the soaring prices of commodities, including Venezuela's oil (the world's largest reserves), Brazil's oil and soy, and Bolivia's minerals and natural gas. As such, even as the United States was pursuing the Free Trade Agreement of the Americas, the Bolivarian Alternative (now Alliance) for the Peoples of Our America (ALBA) was created in 2004, involving Bolivia, Venezuela, Ecuador, Cuba, Nicaragua, and several Caribbean islands, to boost cooperative activities while maintaining its own virtual currency, the sucre, instead of the U.S. dollar.[24] Among the most prominent cooperative efforts has been the long-term financing of Cuban medical brigades in remote areas of Haiti and, following the 2010 earthquake, construction of health centers and community hospitals via solidarity financing and "reciprocal exchange."[25]

Exemplary of these Latin American nations' mutual investment and antipathy toward the Northern financial establishment was the creation of the "Bank of the South" (Banco del Sur) in 2009. Led by Venezuela, and supported by Brazil, Argentina, Bolivia, Ecuador, Uruguay, and Paraguay, it was founded after Chávez paid off Venezuela's debt to the IMF and World Bank and pulled out of both institutions, with the new Banco del Sur pointedly emphasizing social development, including health activities, and rejecting international financial institutions' privatization pressures. Although this endeavor has been slow to launch,[26] other efforts have been more successful and illustrative of the centrality of health to South–South cooperation efforts in Latin America, if not necessarily with the same ideological lilt. For example, the 1971 agreement between the health ministries of Bolivia, Colombia, Chile, Ecuador, Peru, and Venezuela, later known as the Hipólito Unanue Treaty, has been vital to the Pacto Andino trade bloc (now the Andean Community of Nations, CAN), which to this day urges governments to support epidemiologic surveillance, the good management of health human resources, and community participation in health campaigns.[27]

The treaty's goal of using health policymaking as a means of fostering regional integration was shared by Mercosur (the economic bloc comprising Brazil, Argentina, Uruguay, and Paraguay), which bolstered regional governance in health and the right to health care upon its formation in 1991. Established with a progressive guiding agenda, the Union of South American Countries (UNASUR, launched in 2008 by countries of Mercosur and the CAN but disintegrating by 2019) set up a South American Health Council aimed at regional health care integration, with an institute to oversee research and common policymaking around universal access to health care and medicines, equity, social determinants of health, disease surveillance, and unified regional positions vis-à-vis WHO.[28]

Notwithstanding its hobbled influence due to the recent exodus of most members, UNASUR powerfully illustrates the persistence of the ties established among many progressive South American health professionals who actively or quietly contested authoritarian regimes during the Cold War.[29] Various experts traveled to or studied in the Soviet Union and Eastern Bloc countries, including during the period of turmoil preceding the collapse of the Soviet Union. For instance, a study group whose participants included Paulo Buss of Brazil (at the time director of Brazil's National School of Public Health, later head of the country's national institutes of health, Fiocruz, and director of its Center for International Relations) and Miguel Malo of Ecuador (who held a range of international health posts and rose to become Ecuador's vice minister of health governance) went so far as to recommend that Latin American countries increase their technical cooperation to the Soviet Bloc, since their long experience and "strong theoretical base" in decentralized and pluralistic health care systems could offer a "valuable contribution" to contentious health policy deliberations in the USSR.[30] This was a notable twist on the North–South directionality of how most cooperative efforts involving either Western or Eastern blocs transpired, foreshadowing Latin American global health and cooperation leadership in subsequent decades.

Some recent initiatives, such as ALBA and the Community of Latin American and Caribbean States (CELAC, an alternative to the OAS without the United States, explicitly aiming to reduce U.S. influence in the region though not parting from U.S.-style disease control pragmatism), have, like their Cold War predecessors, sought to sidestep or even challenge U.S. geoeconomic power with more symmetrical and democratic arrangements. Other alliances that many Latin American countries have made with the grouping known as BRICS (Brazil, Russia, India, China, and South Africa), most notably China and Russia—and with powerful domestic corporate players—have left some observers arguing that these efforts represent not so much an alternative to but a reconfiguration of imperial capitalism with a strong backing of the state.[31]

Just as during the Cold War, when extensive "cross-Curtain" medical collaboration took place around vaccine testing and development, space medicine, cancer therapeutics, and cardiac surgical techniques, among other areas,[32] similarly "strange bedfellows" reemerged in response to a post–Cold War outbreak. When Cuba experienced an epidemic of optic and peripheral neuropathy in the early 1990s, for example, the U.S. Centers for Disease Control's epidemiologic intelligence unit—despite renewed U.S.-Cuban ideological tensions—became an important cooperating party, helping Cuba identify the lead role of nutritional deficiencies. According to epidemiological consensus, the epidemic was generated by a combination of the loss of Soviet subsidies and an intensification of the U.S. embargo.[33] But the afterlife of this story is also a Cold War artifact, with charges made by Cuban exiles of an "ideological epidemic" stage-managed by the Castro regime.[34]

Moreover, Cold War echoes are evident in terms of Latin America's engagement with broader global health efforts. The 1978 WHO-UNICEF International Conference on Primary Health Care (PHC), held in Alma-Ata, Kazakhstan, Soviet Union, and celebrated for questioning asymmetrical power structures and biomedical reductionism, experienced a mixed reception in Latin America. Partially heeded by authoritarian regimes across the region, the Alma-Ata vision was critiqued from the left for offering "primitive care" or health care for the poor.[35] Nonetheless, in some countries, including Peru, initiatives such as China's "barefoot doctors" caught health policymakers' attention as an inexpensive way of delivering primary care to rural areas at a time when Chinese bilateral cooperation in health was blossoming not only through formal diplomatic ties, but also through organizations such as the Instituto Cultural Peruano-Chino, launched in 1968.[36]

Significantly, it was after the Cold War that the PHC agenda saw a dynamic and far more radical rebirth under Pink Tide governments.[37] The 2005 PAHO Declaration of Montevideo consciously rejected "poor health care for the poor," instead emphasizing social inclusion; family and community participation; equity in health and health care access; intersectoral approaches; comprehensive, integrated, and appropriate health care; social solidarity; accountability; and the infusion of PHC principles throughout the health care system.[38] Such progressive regional responses did not materialize in a vacuum but built upon past social justice ties. As with Brazil's dictatorship-era collective health movement, ABRASCO, which engaged in shadow progressive health planning as a form of resistance, region-wide social medicine efforts forged during the Cold War through civil society solidarity efforts, to provide clandestine protection and, sometimes, rehabilitation of health revolutionaries, gave way to many "health leftists" who found themselves in government positions during the Pink Tide and were eager to work together through formal channels.[39]

Indeed, an enduring, albeit changing, element of a lingering Cold War relates to Latin America's social-justice-oriented South–South health cooperation (SJSSC). Although it has involved, at one point or another, almost all countries in the region, the prime protagonist—during and after the Cold War—is undoubtedly Cuba.[40] On one level, Cuba's SJSSC seems a Cold War relic, born of necessity in the context of regional isolation following its 1959 revolution. Heeding, but independent from, the burgeoning Eastern Bloc cooperation that started in the 1950s, Cuba began its efforts pragmatically, sending a team of medics to earthquake-struck Valdivia, Chile in 1960. In 1963, Cuban "disaster humanitarianism" embraced a new approach, providing medical cadres to sister Third World nations that had supported the Cuban Revolution, such as Algeria following its brutal liberation struggle from France. Cuban cooperation both complemented contemporary Soviet Bloc health aid (which offered big-ticket infrastructure as well as both primary and specialized care) and at times competed with the Soviet Bloc counterpart, with Cubans establishing over a dozen Third World medical schools and training tens of thousands of doctors in Vietnam, Yemen, Mali, Congo, Guinea, and many more settings. Over time, however, Cuba's unique, no-quid-pro-quo health diplomacy expanded well beyond socialist countries and those that supported its revolutionary efforts, cementing its leadership role in South–South medical cooperation.[41]

Despite unrelenting U.S. attempts to squeeze the Castro regime out of existence, Cuba's health cooperation efforts accelerated after the end of the Cold War, especially within Latin America, from millions of cataract surgeries performed through "Operación Milagro," to 35 million medical consultations provided in Guatemala over fifteen years, to a door-to-door project in Bolivia that identified and addressed the health and social needs of almost one hundred thousand persons with disabilities. Most notable was the establishment of a model medical school in 1999. The Latin American School of Medicine (ELAM) welcomes students from all nations, favoring candidates from low-income backgrounds, and offers world-class medical training with low fees (no fees, originally), while instilling in all graduates an ethic and expectation of serving the most disadvantaged populations in the students' home communities. Thus far, ELAM has trained more than twenty-eight thousand physicians from over one hundred countries and as many racial and ethnic backgrounds, with tens of thousands more currently studying across Cuba.[42] In a nod to Cold War–era professional training as a form of influence across the "Iron Curtain," some two hundred U.S. students are ELAM alumni and have returned home as practicing physicians and researchers.

Perhaps the most striking illustration of Cold War–like antihegemonic solidarity is Cuba's cooperation with Venezuela through Misión Barrio Adentro (Inside the Neighborhood). Established through an agreement between the late presidents Fidel Castro and Hugo Chávez to fulfill reciprocal needs (Cuba's need for oil in exchange for Venezuela's need for doctors to provide primary health care in low-income, medically underserved communities), Barrio Adentro spans multiple domains, including housing, education, employment, sports, and neighborhood improvement, in addition to health care. When Castro and Chávez inaugurated it in 2003, they invoked socialist principles of solidarity (at a popular level) and equitable cooperation (at the level of the state) instead of patronizing aid, and emphasized symmetrical agenda-setting and the shared imperative of resisting neoliberal capitalism.[43]

Beyond the political optics, the community-driven nature of Barrio Adentro reflects constituents' power to shape health and social programs. Such power stems from a long experience of collective and resourceful popular mobilization that resurfaced in response to the late–Cold War neoliberal retrenchment from social welfare provision. Barrio Adentro—arising out of frustration that the state and physicians alike were neglecting basic health needs—combines state-driven initiatives and local *auto-gestión*, self-governance efforts grounded in and aiming for popular self-sufficiency.[44] The twenty thousand Cuban doctors who have participated in Barrio Adentro (now being replaced by recently trained Venezuelan doctors from low-income backgrounds), while sharing the same spirit and lack of privilege (i.e., not the high-paid consultants typical of North–South aid) as those who served in 1980s Sandinista Nicaragua, are not kept separate from the local population, as Cheasty Anderson's chapter recounts, but rather live with families in the same neighborhoods where they practice. Misión Barrio Adentro's "bottom-up" approach emphasizes mutual understanding between providers and patients, as well as the inclusion of local residents in decision-making around the activities that affect them most directly. However, Barrio Adentro has not been integrated with the existing state public health system (the two still operate mostly in parallel), much like the 1960s Quinta Normal experiment in Chile discussed in Jadwiga E. Pieper Mooney's chapter. Although Venezuela has been beleaguered by political and economic turbulence in recent years, the government and the populace have remained committed to the program.[45]

In sum, a range of health and medical activities and phenomena in post–Cold War Latin America, from equity-oriented health policies, to alternative intergovernmental configurations, to socialist-style health cooperation, are inspired (or revived) by Cold War–era solidarity and made possible by the many ties and forms of resistance shared by health professionals during decades of repression. In that sense, they offer, at least in part, Cold War lenses to interpret, and offer innovative answers to, post–Cold War issues. Simultaneously, as evidenced throughout this section, a host of powerful socioeconomic forces let loose during the Cold War continue to hold sway within Latin America and warrant greater examination. Such deepening of our understanding of the Cold War's entwining with health and medicine in Latin America is a much-needed and sizable scholarly task.

A Research Agenda

As the cases in this volume show, a further and ample research agenda around health, medicine, and the Cold War in Latin America is justified and much needed. Indeed, to date, health and medicine have been overlooked by emerging historical scholarship about the Cold War in Latin America.[46] What is more, on the rare occasions when medical historians have invoked the Cold War, they have privileged analyses of the interactions between local actors and the United States without addressing the USSR's (or China's) role or have fallen back on stereotypes of Latin American leftist dalliances with rigid and authoritarian Soviet approaches, shortchanging the actual give-and-take of medical actors with counterparts in the Soviet Bloc.[47] We hope that this volume, in its demonstration of nerve and audacity in the periphery, will forestall such tendencies and entice historians to make the already multifaceted arena of Cold War Latin American health and medicine into an even more vibrant, inclusive, and evidentiary-thorough field.

There are, of course, important professional and institutional constraints to overcome in seeking to bring about the changes we envision. As mentioned in the introduction, broadening of language training for historians in current and future generations and adequate access to archival materials in Russia and, especially, China—as well as funding opportunities to carry out this research—are crucial. Moreover, just as with the spirited historical actors covered in this collection, collaboration and reciprocal research exchanges among scholars across disciplines and national and regional boundaries might draw and energize Latin Americanists to the health and medical aspects of the Cold War scholarly agenda.

Where to begin? International institutions are a central place for examining how the range of Cold War health and medical interactions unfolded on public, global stages, and through backroom (including domestic) channels. Much study is needed, for example, on how the Soviet Union's almost decade-long withdrawal from WHO, starting in 1949 (followed by other members of the Soviet Bloc), was understood and addressed by Latin American countries.[48] These nations shared the USSR's concerns that WHO dues (not to mention mounting UN obligations) outstripped the amount of cooperation received, that WHO's technical missions were only marginally useful, and that most health professionals hired by WHO headquarters were Western Europeans or North Americans, or had personal and/or professional ties to U.S. organizations.[49]

A notable if partial exception to the pattern of privileging high-income country representation was longtime WHO director-general Marcolino Candau (1953–1973), who, although Brazilian, nonetheless had close U.S. ties, having worked under Rockefeller Foundation (RF) strongman Fred Soper both in Brazil and at PAHO. Once at WHO's helm, he remained under enormous pressure from U.S. players as the organization's RF-style, global antimalaria campaign was dually marshalled as an anticommunist effort. Candau also had to navigate the return of the Soviet Bloc in the late 1950s and the surge of newly decolonized WHO members, expanding Third World presence well beyond Latin America and South Asia.

How did potential misgivings, day-to-day negotiations, and sometimes fraught ties shape Latin American dealings with the Soviet Bloc and other Third World countries then and two decades later, in the context of the Alma-Ata conference and declaration, when much of Latin America was governed by authoritarian regimes? Thus far, we have only hints.[50] Developments at PAHO, again covered principally by institutional histories, also deserve more attention in terms of Cold War politics: PAHO was certainly a creature in the U.S. orbit, yet it was also a conduit for alternative interactions and ties between Latin American nations and with the Eastern Bloc, typically via Cuba.[51]

Beyond formal health agencies, UN venues such as UNICEF, UNFPA, UNDP, and others offer promising avenues for research on international institutions. To begin with, UNICEF was not only highly active in Latin America, but even sought to upstage regional organizations such as the Montevideo-based International Institute for the Protection of Childhood. Meanwhile, Latin American countries played an active role in UNESCO and its ventures in the health realm. The second director-general of UNESCO was Mexican diplomat and professor Jaime Torres Bodet (who succeeded the far better-known British zoologist Julian Huxley). Torres Bodet's call for greater equity in access to science and education seems to have spelled his downfall.[52] What Cold War battles was he waging? Given Latin America's enormous racial and ethnic diversity (including Indigenous peoples and successive waves of forced laborers and migrants from every continent), its participation in UNESCO's statements on race and the deep involvement of Brazilian specialists and research similarly hint at larger Cold War politics.[53] Relations between "Southern" actors and agencies offer fodder for additional work on the intertwining of the Cold War with Latin American health and medicine themes. As alluded to in the introduction, although Latin American countries were not founders of the Non-Aligned Movement, Cuba became a beacon in this effort by the late 1970s, and many of the region's countries participated in G-77 meetings, even under dictatorships. What health discussions were held in these venues? How did Latin America's long trajectory and diversity of health care systems get taken up? Which Latin American specialists, other than Cubans, interacted with counterparts in Africa and Asia? And what did U.S., Soviet, and international players make of these dialogues?

Moving from the largely institutional to the imbricated institutional-individual expert level—and building on accounts of various forms of travel peppered throughout this volume—a fruitful line of research comprises Latin American fellowships and exchanges to the Soviet Bloc (and vice versa). While Tobias Rupprecht's magisterial work examines the question of mutual learning between Latin America and the countries behind the "Iron Curtain" in cultural and political terms, it barely touches upon the medical dimensions of these relations, except as a curiosity or in terms of health tourism (as in the case of Diego Rivera seeking treatment in the USSR).[54] Student visitors to the Soviet Union and Eastern Europe were already apparent in the interwar period and early Cold War, but their numbers burgeoned in the 1960s when the Soviet Bloc enhanced its role beyond bilateral cooperation as a hub for professional training of Third World youth—in concerted competition with the efforts of philanthropies and the U.S. government. Starting in the 1960s, the famed Moscow Peoples' Friendship University (soon renamed Patrice Lumumba University after the assassinated Congolese liberation leader), together with numerous other universities, trained tens of thousands of doctors, engineers, social scientists, agrispecialists, and other experts from across the Third World (with roughly one-third from Latin America).[55]

Upon returning home, these graduates served as important interlocutors, enabling support for socialism (if not necessarily the Soviet variant) to thrive in distinct milieus.[56] We know much less about Latin American student and professional visitors to China, despite wide interest in its revolutionary transformations, as attested to by visits of prominent leftist health leaders, such as Salvador Allende in 1954 and Javier Torres-Goitia in 1959. The latter headed a delegation of physicians of the Bolivian Confederación Médica Sindical on a monthlong tour of health facilities in Shanghai and Beijing; the visitors were especially struck by their encounters with barefoot doctors and by the continued role of traditional Chinese medicine.[57] For decades thereafter, activism at Latin American faculties of medicine and universities more generally included Maoist factions, with left-wing students often organized according to their affiliation as "rusos" or "chinos."

Studying these varied interchanges from new angles, such as via Afro–Latin Americans, also portends the opening of novel windows on the Cold War and the dynamics of race, racism, and (medical) professionalism within and beyond Latin America.[58] Here an ever-more complex hybridity of Afro-Latino consciousness might be infused with ideological and healing dimensions heretofore unseen.[59]

The role of the Western Bloc's interplay with Latin American health experts and authorities also has ongoing resonance and merits revisiting. This includes augmenting scholarship on the ways in which U.S. World War II health cooperation through the State Department's Institute of Inter-American Affairs was amplified into the 1950s with an extensive program of hospital- and clinic-building across the region, which then branched into Alliance for Progress efforts to curry further favor and support in health quarters.[60] While most European countries were tied up in the ideological maelstrom of postwar decolonizing and neocolonial (health) relations in Africa, Asia, and the Caribbean, West Germany made a space for itself through hospital investment in Brazil, Bolivia, Chile, Peru, and Mexico.[61] Likewise, the dominant U.S. philanthropies in health sciences training and institutional investment, such as the Rockefeller, Carnegie, Kellogg, and Ford Foundations, have been examined in terms of U.S. health activities (fellowships, in-country programs, etc.) but warrant deeper exploration under Cold War exigencies and from the perspective of Latin American players.[62] The same due diligence is needed to better understand the training and travel support the U.S. State Department provided through the Fulbright Fellowship program as well as analogous opportunities offered by Western European foreign affairs and education agencies, along with philanthropies based in Europe.[63]

Time is on researchers' side—for now—should we reach out to these travelers and former trainees and strive to build and disseminate oral history collections about how their experiences abroad shaped their careers and outlooks during and after the Cold War. A range of those who came of age during the Cold War still have a commanding share of influence over Latin American medical and health policy matters; indeed, in recent years various of these have shepherded equitable health approaches from government perches. The most prominent of this cohort include leaders such as two-time Chilean president Michelle Bachelet, detained and tortured by Augusto Pinochet's CIA-backed regime, who then studied medicine in exile in East Germany (a degree she had to re-earn, since the local academy did not accept her foreign credentials), and who, like Salvador Allende, served as minister of health preceding her first term as president. Bachelet, in 2018 appointed the UN's high commissioner for human rights, is among the most visible members of an enormously influential generation of government officers, public health researchers, and academic administrators born between the 1940s and 1970s who cut their teeth focusing on local manifestations of corruption and abuse while refusing to align with U.S.- or Soviet-linked entreaties, and whose professional trajectory is inseparable from the context of the Cold War.

Interestingly, although these experts denounced and resisted imperialist impositions, they sometimes looked favorably on expressions of international solidarity beyond the two superpowers per se. For example, in the 1980s, the Sandinistas welcomed East German cooperation; unlike Cuba, East Germany could contribute little in terms of primary health care cooperation. Instead, the country helped build Nicaragua's Carlos Marx Hospital; in parallel, ordinary citizens donated tens of thousands of used eyeglasses (provided biannually by the government).[64] To date, very little is known about these exchanges and their impact on either side, but anecdotally we are aware of countless cases.[65]

Solidarity was also cultivated internally, through programs that sent medical workers to rural areas in Bolivia and Peru in the 1970s and 1980s. The Bolivian Programa Integral de Atención de Areas de Salud (PIAAS), for instance, was the brainchild of syndicalist physicians who led the Ministry of Health in 1970. Ousted and exiled by General Hugo Banzer, who accused them of fomenting left-wing radicalism, they returned to the ministry in 1982 to implement their vision of physician and nurse cadres who would cooperate with community-based Comités Populares de Salud in rural areas.[66] How did the shifting winds of the Cold War influence the establishment of this program and the decisions of health workers to join it? PIAAS personnel played a key role in the eradication of measles and goiter in Bolivia, but similar programs faced diverse and, to date, underexplained forms of resistance. To illustrate, Peru's Servicio Civil de Graduandos (SECIGRA, inspired by Mexico's program begun in the mid-1930s), launched in 1975, deployed medical graduates to practice in rural areas for yearly stints before receiving their degrees. Until its revocation in 1981, SECIGRA was hotly contested by left-wing medical students, who condemned this poorly planned policy for advancing the interests of an authoritarian military government that placed populism ahead of appropriate work conditions for health professionals.[67] These efforts expose the perils and promise of Cold War engineering of solidarity with the neediest populations, which has been the subject of autobiographical accounts but has received scant historical consideration.[68]

Attention to rural environments, especially in countries with sizable Indigenous populations, helps pivot our proposed agenda away from health policymakers in national and international institutions and from medical experts as travelers, learners, and caregivers toward a set of subaltern actors whose struggles for better health could inspire fresh approaches to the study of the Cold War for years to come. Indigenous peoples in Latin America have been persistent interlocutors, critics, and users of allopathic medicine, as well as originators of healing traditions that hybridized with those of early currents of European colonizers and African enslaved and "free" migrants.[69] Such ingenuity has not abated in the present, but those most often studying contemporary Indigenous accounts of medical problems and resources have been engineers, social scientists, and even the clergy, rather than historians.[70] Yet phenomena exacerbated by or originating during the Cold War, such as the denunciation of Indigenous repression, the (unequal) availability of new pharmaceuticals, medical devices, and diagnostic tests, and the rolling out of disease control campaigns, have altered health conditions and expectations in Indigenous Latin America, just as they have reverberated throughout Latin American society at large.[71] The challenge to historians is twofold: finding and preserving sources that pinpoint Indigenous agency in these matters (including across the continent into the United States and Canada), a difficult but ethically indispensable task; and historicizing the work of experts who claimed to accurately represent Indigenous views, interests, and even physiologies during the Cold War.[72]

Another subaltern form of mobilization decisively shaped by the Cold War—and perennially intersecting with health and well-being issues—is the Latin American women's movement. A multilevel effort, the women's movement has involved leaders in global institutions as much as in grassroots organizing, and we still have much to learn about how the movement took up health-related causes. A signal event on the global stage was the pathbreaking 1979 UN Convention on the Elimination of All Forms of Discrimination against Women (CEDAW), which invokes the importance of equal rights to health care for men and women.[73] Whereas the USSR ratified the treaty in the 1980s, as did most Latin American nations, the United States never did. How did the Latin American women's movement interpret the contrasting U.S. defiance and Soviet support? We also know very little about the political negotiations that took place in late 1970s Latin America to ratify CEDAW, particularly under military dictatorships, or about the role of women who laid the groundwork for CEDAW, such as Mexican ambassador Aída González Martínez, also responsible for the organization of the first UN World Conference on Women, celebrated in Mexico in 1975.[74]

At the local level, we must also pay more attention to the women's collectives that arose in the mid-1970s and their connections to the health field. Not only did these groups denounce institutions such as beauty pageants, but they also, at great personal cost, decried the exercise and reproduction of patriarchal power in Cold War militaristic and anti-insurgency Latin American governments alike. Yet, even as women's collectives joined forces with other opposition currents deploring socioeconomic and political oppression, they did not always receive the reciprocal support of the Latin American male-dominated left, which often ridiculed and subordinated women's demands—including health-related ones such as birth control, maternity benefits, and an end to the physical and mental abuse of women—to the abolition of class inequalities.[75] At the same time, the Latin American maternalist tradition still held sway for many conservative and working-class women of the 1970s, for whom childbearing and domesticity constituted important aspirations and provided positions of household authority from which to claim political rights.[76]

In the early 1980s, however, a more capacious women's movement began to blossom in Latin America, thanks to the Encuentros Feministas that began to be celebrated in 1981 (first in Bogotá) and to the Comité de América Latina y el Caribe para la Defensa de los Derechos de las Mujeres (CLADEM), which nurtured an inclusive brand of feminism that, while left-leaning, supported women's equality initiatives across the political spectrum. Much historical work remains to be done concerning the health-related causes (besides sexual and reproductive rights) that the women's movement embraced in the 1980s, amid the democratic transitions of the late Cold War, such as their stance decrying discrimination against female health workers, favoring more research on women's health, and nurturing women leaders in the health professions.[77] (How) did, for instance, these objectives regard or interact with women's power and position in socialist countries? Were transnational venues also sites for contesting Cold War constraints, from the right and the left, on women's (health) agency?

Beyond exploring these diverse actors and experiences, future analyses of health and the Cold War in Latin America could also offer new perspectives on the conflict and health nexus. How did the Vietnam War, for example, echo through Latin American society? The exposure to Agent Orange and the deaths and debilitating injuries suffered by Puerto Rican soldiers may well have reverberated in distinct ways among the Latin American "allies" (though not combatants per se) of the United States in the war.[78] And with Cuba on the other side of the conflict, how did Latin Americans view Cuban involvement? It would also be valuable to take stock of the remarkable 1967 Treaty of Tlatelolco, which made Latin America the first (and, to date, only) subcontinent committed to remaining free of nuclear arms—a cherished dream since the 1950s of Latin American health activists such as Samuel Pessoa, as Gilberto Hochman and Carlos Henrique Assunção Paiva showed.[79] Signed at the cusp of a wave of repressive regimes supported by U.S. authorities (part of a proxy Cold War that unfolded even as the United States and Soviet Union enjoyed heightened scientific cooperation under a period of détente), the treaty is part of an underexamined and extraordinary story of preventing ultimate destruction as the definitive public health act, decades before the group International Physicians for the Prevention of Nuclear War won the Nobel Peace Prize.

Still, the peace the Treaty of Tlatelolco contrasted with the lived reality of many during the Cold War. The guerrilla movements that had crisscrossed the region starting in the 1950s spawned violent counterreactions by Latin American political and military leaders under the tutelage of a quintessential U.S. Cold War institution—the "counterinsurgency" torture training center (located in the U.S. state of Georgia) known as the School of the Americas.[80] To the extent that state-run killing machines outlasted the Cold War and continue to echo in the massacre of hundreds of thousands by paramilitaries, drug cartels, and gang members across the region, the Cold War origins of state-sanctioned killing sprees also represented a troubling connection to the imperial "conquest" of Latin America in the sixteenth and seventeenth centuries, with its concomitant population debacle. The massive death toll in

Latin America under repressive regimes provides a tragic health history in itself, far worse proportionately, in terms of political prisoners, torture, and execution of dissenters, than that experienced in the Soviet Union once Stalin's gulags were dismantled in the 1960s. In Central America alone, over three hundred thousand people died in civil wars between 1975 and 1991, with over one million fleeing as refugees.[81] And yet, in the 1980s, a pathbreaking Latin American approach would offer a small silver lining amid numbing everyday violence, showing how health could be at least partially privileged above war, through PAHO's "health as a bridge to peace" effort, which sponsored cease-fires for child vaccine days during civil wars in El Salvador and Nicaragua, an initiative that was later emulated in conflict situations in Sri Lanka and elsewhere.[82]

Another dimension of health and the Cold War in Latin America meriting attention revolves around the interaction of health with trade and investment agreements, for decades a lively topic among economists, policy analysts, and activists, but not yet broached in a concerted manner by historians. The General Agreement on Tariffs and Trade (GATT), particularly the Uruguay Round that traversed the mid-1980s until the founding of the WTO in 1994, pushed for previously excluded domains, such as agriculture, intellectual property, and foreign investment, to be included in trade liberalization. With much of Latin America serving as an incubator for such neoliberal globalization, the direct and indirect health effects have been enormous. Canadian megainvesting in mining in Latin America has resulted in large-scale environmental contamination, the assassination of dozens of resisters, and widespread land dispossession, with perhaps no country as deleteriously affected as Honduras.[83] Likewise, competition from U.S. and Canadian agribusiness under the 1994 North American Free Trade Agreement (NAFTA) displaced and disrupted the lives of millions of Mexican agrarian workers, who were forced to migrate internally and northward. The simultaneous influx of Big Food and Big Soda, and Mexico's perennial failure to invest adequately in clean water access, transformed the nutritionally ideal Nahuatl diet into a junk food nightmare, by 2000 turning Mexico into the first country with diabetes as the leading cause of death.[84]

Development, of course, neither started nor was contained within the Cold War, but Latin America played a central, often experimental, role during this time, such as through the Green Revolution (albeit only now being studied in its South–South dimensions) and the Alliance for Progress, both of which have just seen the surface scratched by medical historians.[85] Historians' perspectives on trade and development nodes, for example, would enrich general understanding of how the Cold War's waning has affected health in uncharted ways. Latin America's health and development agenda was neither passive, even if some dimensions were emulative (e.g., Cuba looking to Czechoslovakia as it was designing its revolutionary health system, as discussed in the introduction), nor innocent, given the multiple shades of complicity evidenced in this volume.

In all, then, this collection begins to address a vital period that sheds light on—as per José Martí's rallying call—Nuestra América's present-day health and medical landscape while acknowledging just how much further we could go. Landmark works, notably Leslie Bethell and Ian Roxborough's *Latin America between the Second World War and the Cold War*, emphasize the pivotal role the Cold War played in constructing the idea of Latin America, especially from the standpoint of the United States and Western Europe, as a region with common features, problems, opportunities, and political leanings.[86] The history of medicine and public health offers a rejoinder to this claim, showing the extent to which a variety of health experts constructed their own visions of Latin American distinctiveness as early as the nineteenth century, reflected in the deep scientific and professional engagement that proliferated among regional neighbors.[87] Rather than restraining these relations, the Cold War expanded them to include the Soviet Union and its Eastern Bloc allies plus China, multiplying the fields in which such interchanges took place—population research, bacteriology, psychiatry, and public health, to name a few of the topics this collection addresses—as well as adding to the number of stakeholders whose ideas and interests must be represented in the new stories we will tell. No full account of Latin America's health trajectory can be provided while ignoring the diverse political forces that arose via the opportunities, conflicts, and vacuums the Cold War created.

At the risk of posing a romanticized vision of the historiographic task ahead, we close with the figure of Argentine (health) radical Ernesto "Che" Guevara. In addition to his iconic status as a revolutionary leader, Guevara was a physician, a fact that is barely addressed in the Cold War health and medicine literature.[88] Since this dimension of his story has yet to be told, we end with an evocative snapshot. Coming of age at the beginning of the Cold War, troubled both by a physical ailment (asthma) and soulful ideological questioning, Guevara and his fellow medical student Alberto Granado traveled the continent yearning for philosophical social justice. Their 1952 trip to Peru included stints at the Portada de Guía Leprosy Hospital in Lima and the San Pablo Leprosy Colony near Iquitos, both arranged by Dr. Hugo Pesce, Peru's foremost leprosy investigator and the architect of the country's national antileprosy campaign. These stays provoked not just a medical awakening but a political one for Guevara: the dedicated Dr. Pesce was a steadfast member of the Communist Party who inspired in his students a passion for understanding and combating the social injustices that cause and worsen disease.[89]

Although Guevara himself was never moved to return to medical practice, this experience changed him in other critical ways. At Fidel Castro's side in the 1959 Cuban Revolution, Guevara argued: "Integrating the doctor or any other health worker into the revolutionary movement [is crucial], because . . . the work of educating and feeding the children . . . and . . . of redistributing the land from its former absentee landlords to those who sweat every day on that very land without reaping its fruits—is the grandest social medicine effort that has been done in Cuba."[90]

Guevara also championed social medicine across borders, accompanying the first Cuban medical mission to postliberation Algeria and involving several dozen physicians, nurses, technicians, and dentists in the provision of health assistance to rebuild the war-torn country. This early instance of Cuba's hallmark social-justice-oriented cooperation was at one and the same time a symbol and the realization of Latin American efforts to forge alternative medical solidarities amid, despite, and transcending the Cold War. Such nerve in the health and medical arenas, evinced in this episode and so many others brought to light throughout the volume, surely warrants corresponding pluck and resolve of a new generation of scholars committed to countering this region's relegation to the periphery of historical accounts of the Cold War.

Notes

1 Reagan, "Remarks and a Question-and-Answer Session."
2 "Hugo Chavez Kicks Off Russia Visit."
3 Observatory of Economic Complexity, "Venezuela."
4 Acosta-Alzuru, "No News Is Bad News"; Anderson, "Chávez, Cancer, and Cuba."
5 See, for example, León-Manríquez, "Power Vacuum or Hegemonic Continuity?"
6 Adelman, "Epilogue."
7 Berríos, "Relaciones Económicas"; Shchepin, *Problemy Zdrabookhraneniia Razvivai-ushchikhsia Stran*; Shchepin, *Aktual'nye Problemy Zarubezhnogo Zdravookhranenniia*; Varas, *Documento de Trabajo Programa*; Venediktov, *Mezhdunarodnye Problemy Zdravookhraneniia*.
8 Waitzkin et al., "Social Medicine in Latin America."
9 See, for example, Lack, *Alexander von Humboldt*; Cañizares-Esguerra, *How to Write the History of the New World*; Gerbi, *Dispute of the New World*; Cunha, *Amazon*; Weaver, *Medical Revolutionaries*.

10 Raj, *Relocating Modern Science*. Examples deploying this sort of analytic include Marcos Cueto, "Asymmetrical Network"; Suárez-Díaz, "Indigenous Populations in Mexico"; Soto Laveaga, "*Largo Dislocare.*"

11 Pastor and Long, "Cold War and Its Aftermath in the Americas."

12 A recent twist has been a lawsuit against Fujimori and three of his former ministers of health. See "Fiscal Ordena Acusar a Fujimori y Tres Exministros por Caso de Esterilizaciones." In 2016, the Ministry of Justice set up a registry of victims of this program (https://www.minjus.gob.pe/defensapublica/interna.php?comando =1036). For the fullest account thus far of Peru's sterilization program, see Ballón, *Memorias del Caso Peruano de Esterilización Forzada*.

13 See the introduction to Necochea López, *History of Family Planning*; Laura Briggs, *Reproducing Empire*. On the use of sterilization as a component of eugenics policies in the early twentieth century, see Alexandra Stern, *Eugenic Nation*.

14 The coeditors of this volume published a 2011 piece in the *Hispanic American Historical Review* that did something similar for Latin American medical history generally. See Birn and Necochea López, "Footprints on the Future."

15 Birn, Nervi, and Siqueira, "Neoliberalism Redux."

16 Armada, Muntaner, and Navarro, "Health and Social Security Reforms in Latin America"; Franco, "Entre los Negocios y los Derechos"; Laurell, "Health System Reform in Mexico."

17 World Bank, *World Development Report 1993*; Laurell and Lopez Arellano, "Market Commodities and Poor Relief."

18 Iriart, Merhy, and Waitzkin, "Managed Care in Latin America."

19 Knaul et al., *Preventing Impoverishment*.

20 Paim et al., "Brazilian Health System."

21 Elias and Cohn, "Health Reform in Brazil"; Lima et al., *Saúde e Democracia*.

22 Biehl, "Pharmaceutical Governance."

23 Fleury, "What Kind of Social Protection for What Kind of Democracy?"; Mahmood and Muntaner, "Politics, Class Actors, and Health Sector Reform in Brazil and Venezuela."

24 De la Torre, "A Populist International?"

25 Baranyi, Feldmann, and Bernier, "Solidarity Forever?"

26 Gabriel Garcia, "Rise of the Global South."

27 Núñez et al., "Política Andina de Planificación y Gestión de Recursos Humanos en Salud."

28 Herrero and Tussie, "UNASUR Health"; Riggirozzi and Grugel, "Políticas de Salud en UNASUR."

29 Paraguassu, "Six South American Nations Suspend Membership of Anti-U.S. Bloc."

30 J. R. Ferreira and M. H. Malo, "Final Report: Traveling Seminar on the Training and Utilization of Feldshers for Primary Health Care in the Soviet Union," May 8–23, 1991, WHO Archives, Washington, DC, PAHO-AMRO, box R.0915, file E3-440-61, jacket no. 2, p. 23.

31 "Cuban President Inaugurates International Health Convention"; DeHart, "Remodelling the Global Development Landscape"; Twigg, *Russia's Emerging Global*

Health Leadership*; Larionova, Rakhmangulov, and Berenson, "Russia"; Fontes and Garcia, "Brazil's New Imperial Capitalism."

32 See, for example, Krementsov and Birn, "Hall of Distorting Mirrors"; Nicogossian, *Apollo-Soyuz Test Project Medical Report*; *U.S.-Soviet Cooperation in Space*; Raymond, "US-USSR Cooperation in Medicine and Health"; Vargha, *Polio across the Iron Curtain*.

33 Garfield and Santana, "Impact of the Economic Crisis"; "U.S.-Cuba Health and Science Cooperation."

34 See Coutin-Churchman, "Cuban Epidemic Neuropathy," 84.

35 Birn, "Back to Alma-Ata."

36 Carbone and Palomino, "Atención Primaria en Salud"; Tamagno and Velásquez, "Dinámicas de las Asociaciones Chinas en Perú."

37 Barten, Rovere, and Espinoza, *Salud para Todos*; People's Health Movement et al., *Global Health Watch 4*.

38 Nervi, "Alma Ata y la Renovación de la Atención Primaria de la Salud"; PAHO, *Renewing Primary Health Care in the Americas*.

39 Lima and Santana, *Saúde Coletiva como Compromisso*; Birn and Muntaner, "Latin American Social Medicine across Borders"; Granda, "Algunas Reflexiones a los Veinticuatro Años de la ALAMES"; Iriart et al., "Medicina Social Latinoamericana."

40 Benzi and Zapata, "Good-Bye Che?"; Birn et al., "Is There a Social Justice Variant of South–South Health Cooperation?"

41 Kirk, *Healthcare without Borders*; Birn, Muntaner, and Afzal, "South–South Cooperation in Health."

42 Gorry, "Your Primary Care Doctor May Have an MD from Cuba."

43 Armada et al., "Barrio Adentro and the Reduction of Health Inequalities in Venezuela."

44 Kingsbury, *Only the People Can Save the People*.

45 Amy Cooper, "What Does Health Activism Mean in Venezuela's Barrio Adentro Program?"; Mahmood et al., "Popular Participation in Venezuela's Barrio Adentro Health Reform"; Timothy Gill, "Possibilities and Pitfalls."

46 See, for example, Adelman and Fajardo, "Between Capitalism and Democracy"; Engerman, "Development Politics and the Cold War"; Harmer, "Cold War in Latin America"; Macekura and Manela, *Development Century*; Pastor and Long, "Cold War and Its Aftermath"; Coatsworth, "Cold War in Central America."

47 Marcos Cueto and Palmer, *Medicine and Public Health*; Suárez-Díaz, "Molecular Basis of Evolution and Disease." This is also the case for most works on medical history and the Cold War at the global level. See, for example, Manela, "Pox on Your Narrative."

48 Vargha, "Forgotten Episode." Hints about this are revealed in Beigbeder, *Organisation Mondiale*; Siddiqi, *World Health and World Politics*.

49 See Birn, "Backstage"; Marcos Cueto, *Cold War, Deadly Fevers*; Hochman, "From Autonomy to Partial Alignment"; Stepan, *Eradication*; Marcos Cueto, Brown, and Fee, *World Health Organization*.

50 The first historical analyses taking into account Soviet perspectives of the famed Alma-Ata conference are appearing only now, forty years later. Birn and Krementsov, "'Socialising' Primary Care?"

51 Marcos Cueto, *Valor de la Salud*; Delgado García and Pichardo Díaz, *Representación OPS/OMS en Cuba*; Hernández and Obregón, *OPS y el Estado Colombiano*; Organización Panamericana de la Salud, *Cien Años de Cooperación*.

52 "Torres Bodet in Warning," 8.

53 Abarzúa Cutroni, "Intersticios de Poder de América Latina en la UNESCO"; Maio, "Projeto Unesco e a Agenda das Ciências Sociais no Brasil dos Anos 40 e 50"; Maio and Ventura Santos, "Antiracism and the Uses of Science"; Petitjean and Domingues, "Paulo Carneiro"; Gil-Riaño, "Relocating Anti-Racist Science."

54 Rupprecht, *Soviet Internationalism after Stalin*, 155–56.

55 Katsakioris, "Lumumba University in Moscow."

56 For example, Brazilian medical student Leôncio Basbaum studied in Yugoslavia in the early 1960s, publishing his observations in a book-length treatise, *No Estranho País dos Iugoslavos*. See also Kirillova, "Soviet Internationalism."

57 Ruilova, *China Popular en America Latina*; Torres-Goitia Torres, "Visión Médica y Sanitaria de China."

58 On these issues, mostly focused on African Americans, see Carew, "Black in the USSR."

59 Gilroy, *Black Atlantic*.

60 Marcos Cueto, "International Health, the Early Cold War and Latin America"; Campos, "Institute of Inter-American Affairs"; Pacino, "Stimulating a Cooperative Spirit?"

61 Donzé, "Siemens and the Construction of Hospitals in Latin America."

62 Krige and Rausch, *American Foundations*; Parmar, *Foundations of the American Century*; Sharpless, "Population Science, Private Foundations, and Development Aid."

63 A few hints are in Oreskes and Krige, *Science and Technology in the Global Cold War*; Tournès and Scott-Smith, *Global Exchanges*.

64 Borowy, "East German Medical Aid to Nicaragua."

65 One of the coeditors has a Russian partner and on family travels around Latin America inevitably stumbles into Russian speakers—medical, engineering, agricultural, and other graduates. Moreover, our research assistant (re)discovered that in the 1980s her uncle went on scholarship from Nicaragua to study at the Instituto de Zooveterinaria N. M. Borissenko in Jarkov, Ukraine.

66 Torres-Goitia Torres, Torres-Goitia Caballero, and Lagrava Burgoa, *Salud como Derecho*.

67 Agüero Jurado, *Experiencias del Programa del Servicio Civil*.

68 See, for example, Maguiña, *Ser Médico en el Perú*.

69 See, for example, Crandon-Malamud, *From the Fat of Our Souls*; Few, *Women Who Live Evil Lives*; Pablo Gómez, *Experiential Caribbean*.

70 Acero and Dalle Rive, *Medicina Indígena*; Asociación Chuyma de Apoyo Rural, *Así Nomás Nos Curamos*; Charles Briggs et al., *Enfermedad Monstruo*.

71 See, for example, Marcos Cueto, *Cold War, Deadly Fevers*, chapter 4.

72 See, for example, Dent and Ventura Santos, "Unusual and Fast Disappearing Opportunity"; Suárez-Díaz, "Indigenous Populations in Mexico."

73 See UN General Assembly, Convention on the Elimination of All Forms of Discrimination against Women, December 18, 1979, UNTS 1249, articles 10h, 12, 14b, 16e.

74 Schöpp-Schilling and Flinterman, *Circle of Empowerment*.

75 Sternbach et al., "Feminisms in Latin America"; Francesca Miller, *Latin American Women*; Virginia Vargas, "Feminismos Peruanos."

76 Portugal, "Retorno de las Brujas"; Power, *Right-Wing Women in Chile*.

77 See, for example, Córdova Cayo, *Mujer y Liderazgo en Salud*.

78 See Avilés-Santiago, "War! What Is It Good For?"

79 Musto, "Desire So Close to the Hearts"; UN General Assembly, "Treaty on the Prohibition of Nuclear Weapons."

80 Lesley Gill, *School of the Americas*.

81 Coatsworth, "Cold War in Central America."

82 Quadros and Epstein, "Health as a Bridge for Peace."

83 North, Clark, and Patroni, *Community Rights and Corporate Responsibility*; Gordon and Webber, *Blood of Extraction*.

84 Barquera et al., "Diabetes in Mexico"; Otero, "Neoliberal Globalization."

85 Kumar et al., "Roundtable"; Gorsky and Sirrs, "World Health by Place"; Pires-Alves and Maio, "Health at the Dawn of Development"; Taffet, *Foreign Aid as Foreign Policy*.

86 Bethell and Roxborough, *Latin America between the Second World War and the Cold War*. Others, most prominently Michel Gobat, trace Latin America's political and epistemological origins to the mid-nineteenth century anti-imperialist struggle. See "Invention of Latin America."

87 Hochman, di Liscia, and Palmer, *Patologías de la Patria*.

88 Drinot, "Awaiting the Blood"; Zulawski, "National Revolution and Bolivia." For a pair of classic biographies, see Castañeda, *Compañero*; Anderson, *Che*.

89 Burstein, "Hugo Pesce Pesceto."

90 Ernesto Guevara, "Discurso," 119.

Abarzúa Cutroni, Anabella. "Los Intersticios de Poder de América Latina en la UNESCO (1945-1984)." *Horizontes Sociológicos* 8 (2016): 34-56.

Abel, Christopher. "External Philanthropy and Domestic Change in Colombian Health Care: The Role of the Rockefeller Foundation, ca. 1920-1950." *Hispanic American Historical Review* 75, 3 (1995): 339-76.

Acero, Gloria, and María Dalle Rive. *Medicina Indígena: Cacha, Chimborazo*. Quito, Ecuador: Abya Yala, 1992.

Ackerknecht, Erwin. *Rudolf Virchow: Doctor, Statesman, Anthropologist*. Madison: University of Wisconsin Press, 1953.

Acosta, Ivonne. *La Mordaza: Puerto Rico, 1948-1957*. Río Piedras, PR: Edil, 1989.

Acosta-Alzuru, Carolina. "No News Is Bad News: Examining the Discourse around Hugo Chávez's Illness." In *Health Communication in the Changing Media Landscape: Perspectives from Developing Countries*, edited by Ravindra Kumar Vemula and SubbaRao M. Gavaravarapu, 135-57. Cham, Switzerland: Palgrave Macmillan, 2016.

"Acta No. 26, Sesiones del Consejo de Dirección." *Revista del Hospital Psiquiátrico de la Habana* 5, 3 (1964): 524.

"Acta No. 78, Sesiones del Consejo de Dirección." *Revista del Hospital Psiquiátrico de la Habana* 9, 1 (1968): 189.

"Actas de la Sociedad Cubana de Neurología y Psiquiatría." *Revista Archivos de Neurología y Psiquiatría* 5, 1 (1950): 107-8.

Adelman, Jeremy. "Epilogue: Development Dreams." In *The Development Century: A Global History*, edited by Stephen Macekura and Erez Manela, 326-38. Cambridge: Cambridge University Press, 2018.

Adelman, Jeremy, and Margarita Fajardo. "Between Capitalism and Democracy: A Study in the Political Economy of Ideas in Latin America, 1968-1980." *Latin American Research Review* 51, 3 (2016): 3-22.

Agostoni, Claudia. "Médicos Rurales y Medicina Social en el México Posrevolucionario (1920-1940)." *Historia Mexicana* 63, 2 (2013): 745-801.

Agostoni, Claudia. "Las Mensajeras de la Salud: Enfermeras Visitadoras en la Ciudad de México durante la Década de los 20." *Estudios de Historia Moderna y Contemporánea de México* 33 (2007): 89-120.

Agüero Jurado, Gottardo. *Experiencias del Programa del Servicio Civil de Graduandos de las Ciencias de la Salud Humana en el Perú*. Lima, Peru: Ministerio de Salud, 1982.

Aguirre Beltrán, Gonzalo. "The Interpretation of Health Programs in Cross-Cultural Situations." Paper presented at the VIII World Health Assembly, May 10-June 3, 1955.

Alexander, Robert J. *The Bolivian National Revolution*. New Brunswick, NJ: Rutgers University Press, 1958.

Alexander, Robert J. *Communism in Latin America*. New Brunswick, NJ: Rutgers University Press, 1957.

Alexander, Robert J., and Eldon M. Parker. *A History of Organized Labor in Bolivia*. Westport, CT: Praeger, 2005.

Allende, Salvador. "Chile's Medical-Social Reality." *Social Medicine* 1, 3 (2006): 151–55.

Allende Gossens, Salvador. *La Realidad Médico-Social Chilena*. Santiago, Chile: Ministerio de Salubridad, Previsión y Asistencia Social, 1939.

Allende Gossens, Salvador. *Salvador Allende Reader: Chile's Voice of Democracy*. Edited by James Cockcroft and Jane Canning. Melbourne, Australia: Ocean Press, 2000.

"Al Margen de Rusia por Dentro." *El Día* (Montevideo), July 20, 1946.

Almeida, Marta de. "Circuito Aberto: Idéias e Intercâmbios Médico-Científicos na América Latina nos Primórdios do Século XX." *História, Ciências, Saúde-Manguinhos* 13 (2006): 733–57.

Amrith, Sunil S. "Internationalising Health in the Twentieth Century." In *Internationalisms: A Twentieth Century History*, edited by Glenda Sluga and Patricia Clavin, 245–64. Cambridge: Cambridge University Press, 2017.

Anderson, Jon Lee. "Chávez, Cancer, and Cuba." *New Yorker*, July 18, 2011.

Anderson, Jon Lee. *Che: A Revolutionary Life*. Rev. ed. New York: Grove, 2010.

Andrade, Ana Maria R. de. *Físicos, Mésons e Política: A Dinâmica da Ciência na Sociedade*. São Paulo, Brazil: Hucitec-Mast/Cnpq, 1998.

Andrade Galindo, Jorge, and Martín González Solano. "La Ex-Comisión del Papaloapan y la Recuperación de Su Memoria Histórica." *Boletín del Archivo Histórico del Agua* 8 (2003): 42–50.

Angelini, Alberto. "History of the Unconscious in Soviet Russia: From Its Origins to the Fall of the Soviet Union." *International Journal of Psychoanalysis* 89, 2 (2008): 369–88.

Angell, Alan. "The Left in Latin America since c. 1920." In *The Cambridge History of Latin America*, vol. 6, part 2, edited by Leslie Bethell, 163–232. Cambridge: Cambridge University Press, 1995.

Anguita, Eduardo, and Martín Caparrós. *La Voluntad: Una Historia de la Militancia Revolucionaria en la Argentina 1966–1978*. Vol. 1. Buenos Aires, Argentina: Planeta/Booket, 2006.

Anhalt, Diana. *A Gathering of Fugitives: American Political Expatriates in Mexico, 1948–1965*. Santa Maria, CA: Archer, 2001.

Antic, Ana. "Therapeutic Fascism: Re-educating Communists in Nazi-Occupied Serbia, 1942–44." *History of Psychiatry* 25, 1 (2014): 35–56.

Antic, Ana, Johanna Conterio, and Dóra Vargha. "Conclusion: Beyond Liberal Internationalism." *Contemporary European History* 25, 2 (2016): 359–71.

"Antipsiquiatría y Colonización Cultural." *Acta Psiquiátrica y Psicológica de América Latina* 19, 2 (1973): 126.

Aramburú, Carlos. "Is Population Policy Necessary? Latin America and the Andean Countries." *Population and Development Review* 20 (1994): 159–78.

Arechiga, Ernesto. "Historia de la Salud y el (Re)descubrimiento de Nuestra América." *Canadian Journal of Latin America and Caribbean Studies* 35, 69 (2010): 155–70.

Armada, Francisco, Carles Muntaner, Haejoo Chung, Leslie Williams-Brennan, and Joan Benach. "Barrio Adentro and the Reduction of Health Inequalities in Venezuela: An Appraisal of the First Years." *International Journal of Health Services* 39, 1 (2009): 161–87.

Armada, Francisco, Carles Muntaner, and Vicente Navarro. "Health and Social Security Reforms in Latin America: The Convergence of the World Health Organization, the World Bank, and Transnational Corporations." *International Journal of Health Services* 31, 4 (2001): 729–68.

Armijo, Rolando, and Tegualda Monreal. "Epidemiology of Provoked Abortion in Santiago." *Eugenics Review* 55 (1963): 32–33.

Armijo, Rolando, and Tegualda Monreal. "Factores Asociados a las Complicaciones del Aborto Provocado." *Revista Chilena de Obstetricia y Ginecología* 29 (1964): 175–78.

Armijo, Rolando, Tegualda Monreal, R. Puffer, Mariano Requena, and Christopher Tietze. "The Problem of Induced Abortion in Chile." *Milbank Memorial Fund Quarterly* 43, 4 (1965): 263–80.

Armus, Diego. *The Ailing City: Health, Tuberculosis and Culture in Buenos Aires, 1870–1950.* Durham, NC: Duke University Press, 2011.

Armus, Diego. "Disease in the Historiography of Modern Latin America." In *Disease in the History of Modern Latin America: From Malaria to AIDS*, edited by Diego Armus, 1–24. Durham, NC: Duke University Press, 2003.

Ashby, Eric. *Scientist in Russia.* New York: Penguin, 1947.

Asociación Chuyma de Apoyo Rural. *Así Nomás Nos Curamos.* Puno, Peru: Chuyma, 1997.

Attolini, José. "La Ganadería en la Cuenca del Papaloapan." *Investigación Económica* 8, 4 (1948): 375–417.

Avendaño, Onofre. *Desarrollo Histórico de la Planificación de la Familia en Chile y en el Mundo.* Santiago, Chile: APROFA, 1975.

Avilés-Santiago, Manuel. "War! What Is It Good For? Absolutely Nothing: Testimonios de Soldados sobre la Guerra de Vietnam." In *Tiempos Binarios la Guerra Fría en Puerto Rico y el Caribe*, edited by Manuel R. Rodríguez and Silvia Álvarez Curbelo, 335–76. San Juan, PR: Ediciones Callejón, 2017.

Ayala, César, and Rafael Bernabe. *Puerto Rico in the American Century: A History since 1898.* Chapel Hill: University of North Carolina Press, 2007.

Ayllón Morgan, Julio. "Algunos Casos de Neurosis en Adolescentes Cubanos (Experiencias de la Escuela 'Manuel Ascunce Domenech')." *Servicio Médico Rural* 1 (1963): 15–25.

Babiracki, Patryk, and Austin Jersild, eds. *Socialist Internationalism in the Cold War: Exploring the Second World.* Cham, Switzerland: Palgrave Macmillan, 2016.

Balcázar, Juan Manuel. *Historia de la Medicina en Bolivia.* La Paz, Bolivia: Ediciones Juventud, 1956.

Ballón, Alejandra. *Memorias del Caso Peruano de Esterilización Forzada.* Lima, Peru: Biblioteca Nacional, 2014.

Ballvé, Teo, and Vijay Prashad, eds. *Dispatches from Latin America: On the Frontlines against Neoliberalism*. Cambridge, MA: South End, 2008.

Baranyi, Stephen, Andreas E. Feldmann, and Lydia Bernier. "Solidarity Forever? ABC, ALBA and South–South Cooperation in Haiti." *Third World Quarterly* 36, 1 (2015): 162–78.

Barney, Timothy. "Diagnosing the Third World: The 'Map Doctor' and the Spatialized Discourses of Disease and Development in the Cold War." *Quarterly Journal of Speech* 100, 1 (2014): 1–30.

Barquera, Simon, Ismael Campos-Nonato, Carlos Aguilar-Salinas, Ruy Lopez-Ridaura, Armando Arredondo, and Juan Rivera-Dommarco. "Diabetes in Mexico: Cost and Management of Diabetes and Its Complications and Challenges for Health Policy." *Globalization and Health* 9, 3 (2013).

Barten, Françoise, Mario Rovere, and Eduardo Espinoza. *Salud para Todos: Una Meta Posible*. Pueblos Movilizados y Gobiernos Comprometidos en un Nuevo Contexto Global. Buenos Aires, Argentina: IIED, 2009.

Bartley, Russell H. "The Cold War and Latin American Area Studies in the Former USSR: Reflections and Reminiscences." *Latin American Perspectives* 45, 4 (2018): 115–40.

Basbaum, Leôncio. *No Estranho País dos Iugoslavos*. São Paulo, Brazil: Editora Edaglit, 1963.

"Basin Becomes Test Tube for Studying People." *Science News-Letter* 60, 22 (1951): 342–43.

Bassin, F. V. *El Problema del Inconsciente*. Buenos Aires, Argentina: Granica, 1972.

Bassin, F. V. *El Problema del Inconsciente*. Havana: Ministerio de Salud Pública, Hospital Psiquiátrico de la Habana, 1980.

Beamish, Rob, and Ian Ritchie. "The Spectre of Steroids: Nazi Propaganda, Cold War Anxiety and Patriarchal Paternalism." *International Journal of the History of Sport* 22, 5 (2006): 777–95.

Beigbeder, Yves. *L'Organisation Mondiale de la Santé*. Paris: Presses Universitaires de France, 1995.

Beltrán, Enrique. *Los Recursos Naturales de México y el Crecimiento Demográfico*. Mexico City: Ediciones del Instituto Mexicano de Recursos Naturales, 1967.

Benítez, Jaime. *Junto a la Torre: Jornadas de un Programa Universitario*. Río Piedras: Universidad de Puerto Rico, 1962.

Benzi, Daniele, and Ximena Zapata. "Good-Bye Che? Scope, Identity, and Change in Cuba's South–South Cooperation." In *South-South Cooperation beyond the Myths: Rising Donors, New Aid Practices?*, edited by Isaline Bergamaschi, Phoebe Moore, and Arlene B. Tickner, 79–106. London: Palgrave Macmillan, 2017.

Bentley, Elizabeth. *Out of Bondage: KGB Target: Washington, D.C.* New York: Ballantine, 1988.

Bernal, Guillermo. "Dr. Alfonso Bernal del Riesgo: Cronología." Accessed February 27, 2019. http://www.bernaldelriesgo.com/p/cronologia.html.

Berríos, Rubén. "Relaciones Económicas entre la Unión Soviética y América Latina." *Comercio Exterior* 40, 5 (1990): 425–36.

Bethell, Leslie, and Ian Roxborough, eds. *Latin America between the Second World War and the Cold War: Crisis and Containment, 1944-1948*. Cambridge: Cambridge University Press, 1993.

Beveridge, William. *Social Insurance and Allied Services: Report*. New York: Macmillan, 1942.

Bhattacharya, Sanjoy. "Global and Local Histories of Medicine: Interpretive Challenges and Future Possibilities." In *A Global History of Medicine*, edited by Mark Jackson, 243-62. Oxford: Oxford University Press, 2018.

Biehl, João. "Pharmaceutical Governance." In *Global Pharmaceuticals: Ethics, Markets, Practices*, edited by Adriana Petryna, Andrew Lakoff, and Arthur Kleinman, 206-39. Durham, NC: Duke University Press, 2006.

Birn, Anne-Emanuelle. "Backstage: The Relationship between the Rockefeller Foundation and the World Health Organization, Part I: 1940s-1960s." *Public Health* 128, 2 (2014): 129-40.

Birn, Anne-Emanuelle. "Back to Alma-Ata, from 1978 to 2018 and Beyond." *American Journal of Public Health* 108, 9 (2018): 1153-55.

Birn, Anne-Emanuelle. "Little Agenda-Setters: Uruguay's International American Institute for the Protection of Childhood and Rights Approaches to Child Health, 1920s-1940s." *Journal of Social History of Medicine and Health* [in Chinese] 2, 2 (2017): 3-38.

Birn, Anne-Emanuelle. *Marriage of Convenience: Rockefeller International Health and Revolutionary Mexico*. Rochester, NY: University of Rochester Press, 2006.

Birn, Anne-Emanuelle. "O Nexo Nacional-Internacional na Saúde Pública: O Uruguai e a Circulação das Políticas e Ideologias de Saúde Infantil, 1890–1940." *História, Ciências, Saúde-Manguinhos* 13 (2006): 675–708.

Birn, Anne-Emanuelle. "Revolution, the Scatological Way: The Rockefeller Foundation's Hookworm Campaign in 1920s Mexico." In *Disease in the History of Modern Latin America: From Malaria to AIDS*, edited by Diego Armus, 158-82. Durham, NC: Duke University Press, 2003.

Birn, Anne-Emanuelle. "Las Unidades Sanitarias: La Fundación Rockefeller versus el Modelo Cárdenas en México." In *Salud, Cultura y Sociedad en América Latina*, edited by Marcos Cueto, 203-33. Washington, DC: Pan American Health Organization/Instituto de Estudios Peruanos, 1996.

Birn, Anne-Emanuelle. "Uruguay on the World Stage: How Child Health Became an International Priority." *American Journal of Public Health* 95, 9 (2005): 1506-17.

Birn, Anne-Emanuelle, and Theodore M. Brown. "The Making of Health Internationalists." In *Comrades in Health: U.S. Health Internationalists, Abroad and at Home*, edited by Anne-Emanuelle Birn and Theodore M. Brown, 15-42. New Brunswick, NJ: Rutgers University Press, 2013.

Birn, Anne-Emanuelle, and Nikolai Krementsov. "'Socialising' Primary Care? The Soviet Union, WHO, and the 1978 Alma-Ata Conference." *BMJ Global Health* 3 (2018). https://gh.bmj.com/content/bmjgh/3/Suppl_3/e000992.full.pdf.

Birn, Anne-Emanuelle, and Carles Muntaner. "Latin American Social Medicine Across Borders: South–South Cooperation and the Making of Health Solidarity." *Global Public Health* (2018). https://doi.org/10.1080/17441692.2018.1439517.

Birn, Anne-Emanuelle, Carles Muntaner, and Zabia Afzal. "South–South Cooperation in Health: Bringing in Theory, Politics, History, and Social Justice." *Cadernos de Saúde Pública 33* (2017): S37–S52.

Birn, Anne-Emanuelle, Carles Muntaner, Zabia Afzal, and Mariajosé Aguilera. "Is There a Social Justice Variant of South–South Health Cooperation?: A Scoping and Critical Literature Review." *Global Health Action 12*, 1 (2019): 1–20.

Birn, Anne-Emanuelle, and Raúl Necochea López. "Footprints on the Future: Looking Forward to Latin American Medical History in the Twenty-First Century." *Hispanic American Historical Review 91*, 3 (2011): 503–27.

Birn, Anne-Emanuelle, Laura Nervi, and Eduardo Siqueira. "Neoliberalism Redux: The Global Health Policy Agenda and the Politics of Cooptation in Latin America and Beyond." *Development and Change 47*, 4 (2016): 734–59.

Bizzo, Maria Letícia Galluzzi. "Agências Internacionais e Agenda Local: Atores e Idéias na Interlocução entre Nutrição e País (1932–1964)." PhD diss., Casa de Oswaldo Cruz/Fiocruz, 2012.

Blanes, José. "Bolivia, el Papel de la Universidad en el Desarrollo Científico y Tecnológico de la Región Amazónica." In *Universidade e Desenvolvimento Amazônico*, edited by Luis A. Aragón and Maria de Nazaré O. Imbiriba, 61–122. Belém, Brazil: Universidade Federal do Pará, 1988.

Blasier, Cole. *The Giant's Rival: The USSR and Latin America*. Rev. ed. Pittsburgh: University of Pittsburgh Press, 1987.

Blasier, Cole. *The Hovering Giant: U.S. Responses to Revolutionary Change in Latin America*. Pittsburgh: University of Pittsburgh Press, 1975.

Blasier, Cole. "The United States and the Revolution." In *Beyond the Revolution: Bolivia since 1952*, edited by James Malloy and Richard Thorn, 53–109. Pittsburgh: University of Pittsburgh Press, 1971.

Bliss, Katherine Elaine. *Compromised Positions: Prostitution, Public Health, and Gender Politics in Revolutionary Mexico City*. University Park: Pennsylvania State University Press, 2001.

Bliss, Katherine Elaine. "For the Health of the Nation: Gender and the Cultural Politics of Social Hygiene in Revolutionary Mexico." In *The Eagle and the Virgin: Nation and Cultural Revolution in Mexico*, edited by Mary Kay Vaughan and Steven Lewis, 196–220. Durham, NC: Duke University Press, 2006.

Bohoslavsky, Ernesto. "El Anticomunismo en Chile en el Siglo XX: Ideologemas Transnacionales y Usos." Paper presented at the meeting for the Proyecto de Investigación Científica y Tecnológica, Pensar lo Público: Los 'Saberes de Estado' y la Redefinición de las Fronteras entre lo Público y lo Privado, Argentina, 1890–1955, Buenos Aires, May 4, 2012.

"Bolivia: Chaos in the Clouds." *Time*, March 2, 1959.

"Bolivia: Diez Años de Revolución." *La Paz*, April 1962, 35.

Booth, John. *The End and the Beginning: The Nicaraguan Revolution*. Boulder, CO: Westview, 1985.

Borowy, Iris. *Coming to Terms with World Health: The League of Nations Health Organisation, 1921–1946*. Bern, Switzerland: Lang, 2009.

Borowy, Iris. "East German Medical Aid to Nicaragua: The Politics of Solidarity between Biomedicine and Primary Health Care." *História, Ciências, Saúde-Manguinhos* 24 (2017): 411–28.

Borowy, Iris. "Medical Aid, Repression, and International Relations: The East German Hospital at Metema." *Journal of the History of Medicine and Allied Sciences* 71, 1 (2016): 64–92.

Borowy, Iris. "Health-Related Activities of the German Democratic Republic in West Africa during the 1960s." In *Warsaw Pact Intervention in the Third World: Aid and Influence in the Cold War*, edited by Philip E. Muehlenbeck and Natalia Telepneva, 173–96. London: Tauris, 2018.

Bosque-Perez, Ramón, and José Colón Morera, eds. *Puerto Rico under Colonial Rule: Political Persecution and the Quest for Human Rights*. Albany: State University of New York Press, 2006.

Bossert, Thomas. "Health Care in Revolutionary Nicaragua." In *Nicaragua in Revolution*, edited by Thomas Walker, 259–72. New York: Praeger, 1982.

Bossert, Thomas. "Nicaraguan Health Policy: The Dilemma of Success." *Medical Anthropology Quarterly* 15, 3 (1984): 73–74.

Bosteels, Bruno. *Marx and Freud in Latin America: Politics, Psychoanalysis, and Religion in Times of Terror*. London: Verso, 2012.

Brands, Hal. *Latin America's Cold War*. Cambridge, MA: Harvard University Press, 2010.

Braveman, Paula. "Find the Best People and Support Them." In *Comrades in Health: U.S. Health Internationalists, Abroad and at Home,* edited by Anne-Emanuelle Birn and Theodore Brown, 168–83. New Brunswick, NJ: Rutgers University Press, 2013.

Brickman, Jane Pacht. "Medical McCarthyism and the Punishment of Internationalist Physicians in the United States." In *Comrades in Health: U.S. Health Internationalists, Abroad and at Home*, edited by Anne-Emanuelle Birn and Theodore M. Brown, 82–100. New Brunswick, NJ: Rutgers University Press, 2013.

Briggs, Charles, Norbelys Gómez, Tirso Gómez, Clara Mantini-Briggs, Conrado Moraleda, and Enrique Moraleda. *Una Enfermedad Monstruo: Indígenas Derribando el Cerco de la Discriminación en Salud*. Buenos Aires, Argentina: Lugar, 2015.

Briggs, Laura. *Reproducing Empire: Race, Sex, Science, and U.S. Imperialism in Puerto Rico*. Berkeley: University of California Press, 2002.

Brockington, C. Fraser. "Public Health in Russia." *The Lancet* 268, 6934 (1956): 138–41.

Brown, James C. *Printed Hearings of the House of Representatives Found among Its Committee Records in the National Archives of the United States, 1824–1958*. Washington, DC: National Archives and Records Service, General Services Administration, 1974.

Brown, Jonathan C. *Oil and Revolution in Mexico*. Berkeley: University of California Press, 1993.

Brown, Matthew, ed. *Informal Empire in Latin America: Culture, Commerce, and Capital*. Malden, MA: Blackwell, 2009.

Brown, Matthew, and Gabriel Paquette, eds. *Connections after Colonialism: Europe and Latin America in the 1820s*. Tuscaloosa: University of Alabama Press, 2013.

Brown, Timothy. *The Real Contra War: Highlander Peasant Resistance in Nicaragua*. Norman: University of Oklahoma Press, 2001.

Buchanan, Tom. "The Courage of Galileo: Joseph Needham and the 'Germ Warfare' Allegations in the Korean War." *History* 86, 284 (2001): 503–22.

Bueno, Silveira. *Visões da Rússia e do Mundo Comunista.* São Paulo, Brazil: Saraiva, 1961.

Buitrago, Carlos. "La Investigación Social y el Problema de los Investigadores Puertorriqueños en las Ciencias Sociales y Disciplinas Relacionadas en Puerto Rico." *Revista de Ciencias Sociales* 10, 1 (1966): 93–103.

Bulmer-Thomas, Victor. *The Economic History of Latin America since Independence.* Cambridge: Cambridge University Press, 2003.

Bunge, Augusto. *El Continente Rojo.* Buenos Aires, Argentina: Rosso, 1932.

Burawoy, Michael. "The Extended Case Method." *Sociological Theory* 16, 1 (1998): 4–33.

Burstein, Zuño. "Hugo Pesce Pesceto." *Revista Peruana de Medicina Experimental y Salud Pública* 20, 3 (2003): 172–73.

Burton, Mark, and José Joel Vázquez Ortega. "La Psicología de la Liberación: Aprendiendo de América Latina." *Revista Polis* 1 (2004): 101–24.

Bustamante, José Angel. *La Psiquiatría en Cuba en los Ultimos Cincuenta Años.* Havana: Modelo, 1958.

Bustamante, Miguel E., Carlos Viesca Treviño, Federico Villaseñor, C. Alfredo Vargas Flores, Roberto Castañon, and Xochitl Martínez B. *La Salud Pública en México, 1959–1982.* Mexico City: Secretaría de Salubridad y Asistencia, 1982.

Caballero, Manuel. *Latin America and the Comintern, 1919–1943.* Cambridge: Cambridge University Press, 1986.

Caballero Argáez, Carlos, Patricia Pinzón de Lewin, Eduardo Escallón Largacha, and María Natalia Marín Suárez. *Alberto Lleras Camargo y John F. Kennedy: Amistad y Política Internacional: Recuento de Episodios de la Guerra Fría, la Alianza para el Progreso y el Problema de Cuba.* Bogotá, Colombia: Universidad de Los Andes, Escuela de Gobierno Alberto Lleras Camargo, 2014.

Cabello González, Octavio. "Influencia de la Unidad Sanitaria de Quinta Normal en la Reducción de la Mortalidad Infantil de la Comuna." *Revista Chilena de Higiene y Medicina Preventiva* 8, 1–2 (1946): 15–27.

Cáceres, Virgen, María Teresa Ríos, Ruth Silva, Mayra Muñoz, and Nilsa Torres, eds. *La Violencia Nuestra de Cada Día: Manifestaciones de la Violencia contra las Mujeres.* Río Piedras, PR: CIS, 2002.

Calandra, Benedetta, and Marina Franco, eds. *La Guerra Fría Cultural en América Latina: Desafíos y Límites para una Nueva Mirada de las Relaciones Interamericanas.* Buenos Aires, Argentina: Biblos, 2012.

Campos, André Luiz Vieira de. *Políticas Internacionais de Saúde na Era Vargas: O Serviço Especial de Saúde Pública, 1942–1960.* Rio de Janeiro, Brazil: Editora Fiocruz, 2006.

Campos, André Luiz Vieira de. "The Institute of Inter-American Affairs and Its Health Policies in Brazil during World War II." *Presidential Studies Quarterly* 28, 3 (1998): 523–34.

Cañizares-Esguerra, Jorge. *How to Write the History of the New World: Histories, Epistemologies, and Identities in the Eighteenth-Century Atlantic World.* Stanford, CA: Stanford University Press, 2001.

Caparrós, Antonio. "La Enfermedad es el Capitalismo." *Primera Plana,* May 1972. http://www.elortiba.org/old/apa.html.

Caparrós, Antonio. "Hacia una Psicología Nacional y Popular." *Primera Plana,* May 1972. http://www.elortiba.org/old/apa.html.

Caparrós, Antonio, and Nicolás Caparrós. "El Problema de la Interpretación del Significado de la Conducta." *Acta Psiquiátrica y Psicológica de América Latina* 20, 6 (1974): 395-402.

Caparrós, Nicolás, and Antonio Caparrós. *Psicología de la Liberación.* Madrid: Fundamentos, 1976.

Carbone, Fernando, and Yely Palomino. "La Atención Primaria en Salud: La Experiencia Peruana." *Revista Peruana de Ginecología y Obstetricia* 64, 3 (2018): 367-73.

Cárdenas, Héctor. *Historia de las Relaciones entre México y Rusia.* Mexico City: Fondo de Cultura Económica, 1993.

Cardoso, Fernando Henrique, and Enzo Faletto. *Dependency and Development in Latin America.* Berkeley: University of California Press, 1979.

Carew, Joy Gleason. "Black in the USSR: African Diasporan Pilgrims, Expatriates and Students in Russia, from the 1920s to the First Decade of the Twenty-First Century." *African and Black Diaspora: An International Journal* 8, 2 (2015): 202-15.

Carpintero, Enrique, and Alejandro Vainer. *Huellas de La Memoria: Psicoanálisis y Salud Mental en la Argentina de los '60 y '70.* Vol. 1. Buenos Aires, Argentina: Topía, 2004.

Carr, Barry. "Pioneering Transnational Solidarity in the Americas: The Movement in Support of Augusto C. Sandino, 1927-1934." *Journal of Iberian and Latin American Research* 20, 2 (2014): 141-52.

Carrillo, Ana María. "From Badge of Pride to Cause of Stigma: Combatting Mal del Pinto in Mexico." *Endeavour* 37, 1 (2013): 13-20.

Carrillo, Ana María. "La Patología del Siglo XIX y los Institutos Nacionales de Investigación Médica en México." *LABORAT-acta* 13, 1 (2001): 23-31.

Carrillo, Ana María, and Anne-Emanuelle Birn. "Neighbours on Notice: National and Imperialist Interests in the American Public Health Association, 1872-1921." *Canadian Bulletin of Medical History* 25, 1 (2008): 83-112.

Carter, Eric. "Social Medicine and International Expert Networks in Latin America, 1930-1945." *Global Public Health* 14 (2019): 791-802.

Castañeda, Jorge. *Compañero: The Life and Death of Che Guevara.* New York: Vintage, 1997.

César, Osório. *A Medicina na União Soviética.* São Paulo, Brazil: Laboratorio Carrano, 1945.

César, Osório. *Onde o Proletariado Dirige: Visão Panoramica da U.R.S.S.* São Paulo, Brazil: Edição Brasileira, 1932.

César, Osório. "A Proteção da Saúde Pública na União Soviética no 16 Aniversário da Revolução de Outubro." *São Paulo Médico* 7, 2 (1934): 2.

César, Osório. *Que E o Estado Proletário?* São Paulo, Brazil: Edição Udar, 1933.

Chastain, Andra, and Timothy Lorek, eds. *Itineraries of Expertise: Science, Technology, and the Environment in Latin America's Long Cold War.* Pittsburgh: University of Pittsburgh Press, 2020.

Chilcote, Ronald. *Partido Comunista Brasileiro: Conflito e Integração, 1922-1972.* Rio de Janeiro, Brazil: Graal, 1982.

Chile. *Proyectos de Leyes de Reforma y Unificación de las Leyes de Previsión Social: Estructuración de los Servicios de Salubridad Nacional en Conformidad a los Acuerdos de la Convención de la Asociación Médica de Chile, celebrada en Constitución los días 7, 8 y 9 de abril de 1939*. Santiago: Departamento de Previsión Social, 1939.

Cifuentes, Oswaldo. "Etapas del Proceso Sanitario Chileno." *Revista Chilena de Higiene y Medicina Preventiva* 15, 1–2 (1953): 25–37.

Clark, Hal. "Lini Fuhr Is Back from Spain, Where Fascists Bomb Hospitals." *Daily Worker*, May 20, 1937.

Cleland, John. "A Critique of KAP Studies and Some Suggestions for Their Improvement." *Studies in Family Planning* 4, 2 (1973): 42–47.

Coatsworth, John. "The Cold War in Central America, 1975–1991." In *The Cambridge History of the Cold War*, edited by Melvyn Leffler and Odd Arne Westad, 201–21. Cambridge: Cambridge University Press, 2010.

Cohen, Robert. *When the Old Left Was Young: Student Radicals and America's First Mass Student Movement, 1929–1941*. New York: Oxford University Press, 1993.

Collier, Simon, and William Sater. *A History of Chile, 1808–2002*. New York: Cambridge University Press, 2004.

Cooper, Amy. "The Doctor's Political Body: Doctor-Patient Interactions and Political Belonging in Venezuelan Neighborhood Clinics." *American Ethnologist* 42, 3 (2015): 459–74.

Cooper, Amy. "What Does Health Activism Mean in Venezuela's Barrio Adentro Program? Understanding Community Health Work in Political and Cultural Context." *Annals of Anthropological Practice* 39, 1 (2015): 58–72.

Cooper, David. "La Comuna Política-Terapéutica." *La Opinión*, July 16, 1972.

Cooper, David. *The Grammar of Living*. New York: Pantheon, 1974.

Cooper, David. *Psychiatry and Anti-Psychiatry*. London: Tavistock, 1967.

Cooper, David. "The Use of LSD." *La Opinión*, November 5, 1972.

Córdova Cayo, Patricia, ed. *Mujer y Liderazgo en Salud: Los Profesionales ante los Nuevos Desafíos*. Lima, Peru: Asociación Yunta, 1997.

Corkill, David. "The Chilean Socialist Party and The Popular Front, 1933–41." *Journal of Contemporary History* 11, 2–3 (1976): 261–73.

"The Cortisone Shortage." *Fortune*, May 1951.

Cottam, Martha L. *Images and Intervention: U.S. Policies in Latin America*. Pittsburgh: University of Pittsburgh Press, 1994.

Cotter, Joseph. "The Rockefeller Foundation's Mexican Agricultural Project: A Cross-Cultural Encounter." In *Missionaries of Science: The Rockefeller Foundation in Latin America*, edited by Marcos Cueto, 97–125. Bloomington: Indiana University Press, 1994.

Cotter, Joseph, *Troubled Harvest: Agronomy and Revolution in Mexico, 1880–2002*. Westport, CT: Praeger, 2003.

Coutin-Churchman, Pedro. "The 'Cuban Epidemic Neuropathy' of the 1990s: A Glimpse from Inside a Totalitarian Disease." *Surgical Neurology International* 5, 84 (2014). doi: 10.4103/2152-7806.133888.

Cowan, Benjamin. *Securing Sex: Morality and Repression in the Making of Cold War Brazil*. Chapel Hill: University of North Carolina Press, 2016.

Crandon-Malamud, Libbet. *From the Fat of Our Souls: Social Change, Political Process, and Medical Pluralism in Bolivia.* Berkeley: University of California Press, 1993.

Crawley, Eduardo. *Dictators Never Die: A Portrait of Nicaragua and the Somoza Dynasty.* London: Hurst, 1979.

Crawley, Eduardo. *Nicaragua in Perspective: An Illuminating History of Nicaragua's Past, Its Domination by Two Generations of Somozas, and Its Current Sandinista Rule.* New York: St. Martin's, 1984.

Cruz Coke, Eduardo. "The Chilean Preventive Medicine Act." *International Labour Review* 38, 2 (1938): 161–89.

Cruz Coke, Eduardo. *Discursos: Política, Economía, Salubridad, Habitación, Relaciones Exteriores, Agricultura.* Santiago, Chile: Nascimento, 1946.

Cruz Goyenola, Lauro. *Rusia por Dentro, Apuntes.* 5th ed. Montevideo, Uruguay: Universo, 1946.

"Cuanto Vale la Mentira de Cruz Goyenola? Madre Rusia versus Rusia por Dentro." *Justicia, Órgano Central del Partido Comunista (Montevideo)*, May 24, 1946.

"Cuban President Inaugurates International Health Convention to Promote International Cooperation." *Xinhua*, April 24, 2018.

Cueto, Emilia. "Entrevista a Juan Carlos Volnovich (Segunda Parte)." *elSigma*, April 5, 2001. http://www.elsigma.com/entrevistas/entrevista-a-juan-carlos-volnovich -segunda-parte/697.

Cueto, Marcos. "An Asymmetrical Network: National and International Dimensions of the Development of Mexican Physiology." *Journal of the History of Medicine and Allied Sciences* 71, 1 (2016): 43–63.

Cueto, Marcos. *Cold War, Deadly Fevers: Malaria Eradication in Mexico, 1955–1975.* Baltimore, MD: Johns Hopkins University Press, 2007.

Cueto, Marcos. "International Health, the Early Cold War and Latin America." *Canadian Bulletin of Medical History* 25, 1 (2008): 17–41.

Cueto, Marcos. "Introduction." In *Missionaries of Science: The Rockefeller Foundation in Latin America*, edited by Marcos Cueto, ix–xx. Bloomington: Indiana University Press, 1994.

Cueto, Marcos, ed. *Missionaries of Science: The Rockefeller Foundation and Latin America.* Bloomington: Indiana University Press, 1994.

Cueto, Marcos. "The Rockefeller Foundation's Medical Policy and Scientific Research in Latin America: The Case of Physiology." In *Missionaries of Science: The Rockefeller Foundation in Latin America*, edited by Marcos Cueto, 126–48. Bloomington: Indiana University Press, 1994.

Cueto, Marcos. *La Salud Internacional y la Guerra Fría: Erradicación de la Malaria en México, 1956–1971.* Mexico City: UNAM, 2013.

Cueto, Marcos. *El Valor de la Salud: Historia de la Organización Panamericana de la Salud.* Washington, DC: Organización Panamericana de la Salud, 2004.

Cueto, Marcos. "Visions of Science and Development: The Rockefeller Foundation's Latin American Surveys of the 1920s." In *Missionaries of Science: The Rockefeller Foundation in Latin America*, edited by Marcos Cueto, 1–22. Bloomington: Indiana University Press, 1994.

Cueto, Marcos, Theodore M. Brown, and Elizabeth Fee. *The World Health Organization: A History*. Cambridge: Cambridge University Press, 2019.

Cueto, Marcos, and Steven Palmer. *Medicine and Public Health in Latin America: A History*. Cambridge: Cambridge University Press, 2015.

Cunha, Euclides da. *The Amazon: Land without History*. Translated by Ronald Sousa. Oxford: Oxford University Press, 2006.

Czeresnia, Dina, and Adriana Maria Ribeiro. "O Conceito de Espaço em Epidemiologia: Uma Interpretação Histórica e Epistemológica." *Cadernos de Saúde Pública* 16 (2000): 595–605.

Dagfal, Alejandro. *Entre París y Buenos Aires: La Invención del Psicólogo (1942–1966)*. Buenos Aires, Argentina: Paidos, 2009.

Dagfal, Alejandro. "Psychoanalysis in Argentina under Peronism and Anti-Peronism (1943–1963)." In *Psychoanalysis and Politics: Histories of Psychoanalysis under Conditions of Restricted Political Freedom*, edited by Joy Damousi and Mariano Ben Plotkin, 135–63. New York: Oxford University Press, 2012.

Dale, Iain. *Labour Party General Election Manifestos, 1900–1997*. London: Routledge, 2000.

Danielson, Ross. *Cuban Medicine*. New Brunswick, NJ: Transaction, 1979.

Darnton, Christopher. *Rivalry and Alliance Politics in Cold War Latin America*. Baltimore, MD: Johns Hopkins University Press, 2014.

"David Cooper o la Contestación Permanente." *La Opinión*, November 5, 1972.

David-Fox, Michael. *Showcasing the Great Experiment: Cultural Diplomacy and Western Visitors to the Soviet Union, 1921–1941*. New York: Oxford University Press, 2012.

Davis, Kingsley. "Latin America's Multiplying Peoples." *Foreign Affairs* 25 (1946–1947): 643–54.

de Cicco, Andrés. *Un Año en Moscú: Una Visión Objetiva y Real de la Vida en la Unión Soviética*. Buenos Aires, Argentina: Difusión, 1950.

"Declaración del Grupo Plataforma." *Los Libros* 25 (1972): 5.

DeHart, Monica. "Remodelling the Global Development Landscape: The China Model and South–South Cooperation in Latin America." *Third World Quarterly* 33 (2012): 1359–75.

de la Mora, Constancia. *In Place of Splendor: The Autobiography of a Spanish Woman*. New York: Harcourt, Brace, 1939.

de la Torre, Carlos. "A Populist International? ALBA's Democratic and Autocratic Promotion." *SAIS Review of International Affairs* 37, 1 (2017): 83–93.

de la Torre Molina, Carolina Luz. "Historia de la Psicología en Cuba: Cincuenta Años de Psicología-Cincuenta Años de Revolución." *Psicología para América Latina, Revista Electrónica Internacional de la Unión Latinoamericana de Entidades de Psicología* 17 (2009). http://psicolatina.org/17/cuba.html#notas.

Delgado García, Gregorio, and Marío Pichardo Díaz. *La Representación OPS/OMS en Cuba: Conmemorando 100 años de Salud*. Havana: OPS, 2002.

Demeny, Paul. "Social Science and Population Policy." *Population and Development Review* 14, 3 (1988): 451–79.

Dent, Rosanna, and Ricardo Ventura Santos. "'An Unusual and Fast Disappearing Opportunity': Infectious Disease, Indigenous Populations, and New Biomedical Knowledge in Amazonia, 1960-1970." *Perspectives on Science* 25, 5 (2017): 585-605.

de Ramón, Armando. *Santiago de Chile, 1541-1991: Historia de una Sociedad Urbana.* Santiago, Chile: Sudamericana, 2000.

Derickson, Alan. "The House of Falk: The Paranoid Style in American Health Politics." *American Journal of Public Health* 87 (1997): 1836-44.

DeShazo, Peter. *Urban Workers and Labor Unions in Chile, 1902-1927.* Madison: University of Wisconsin Press, 1983.

de Viado, Manuel. "The Aims and Achievements of the Chilean Preventive Medicine Act." *International Labour Review* 46, 2 (1942): 123-35.

de Vries, Lini. *España 1937 (Memorias).* Translated by Carlo Antonio Castro. Xalapa: Universidad Veracruzana, 1965.

de Vries, Lini. *Please, God, Take Care of the Mule.* Mexico City: Minutae Mexicana, 1969.

de Vries, Lini. *Up from the Cellar.* Minneapolis: Vanilla Press, 1979.

Díaz P., Salvador. *La Escuela de Salubridad de la Universidad de Chile: Ensayo Crítico.* Santiago, Chile: Impresora Cultura, 1957.

Dietz, James. *Economic History of Puerto Rico: Institutional Change and Capitalist Development.* Princeton, NJ: Princeton University Press, 1986.

"Discurso de Inauguração do Novo Prédio." *O Estado de São Paulo*, June 6, 1943.

Doboş, Corina. "Psychiatry and Ideology: The Emergence of 'Asthenic Neurosis' in Communist Romania." In *Psychiatry in Communist Europe*, edited by Mat Savelli and Sarah Marks, 93-117. London: Palgrave Macmillan, 2015.

Domingues, Heloisa Maria Bertol, and Patrick Petitjean. "International Science, Brazil and Diplomacy in UNESCO (1946-50)." *Science, Technology and Society* 9, 1 (2004): 29-50.

Domínguez, Jorge I., and Christopher N. Mitchell. "The Roads Not Taken: Institutionalization and Political Parties in Cuba and Bolivia." *Comparative Politics* 9, 2 (1977): 173-95.

Domínguez, Manuel W. "Conceptos Actuales de la Psiquiatría." *Revista del Hospital Psiquiátrico de la Habana* 14, 3 (1973): 521.

Donahue, John. "International Organizations, Health Services, and Nation Building." *Medical Anthropology Quarterly* 3, 3 (1989): 258-69.

Donahue, John. *The Nicaraguan Revolution in Health: From Somoza to the Sandinistas.* South Hadley, MA: Bergin and Garvey, 1986.

Donzé, Pierre-Yves. "Siemens and the Construction of Hospitals in Latin America, 1949-1964." *Business History Review* 89, 3 (2015): 475-502.

Dorn, Glenn J. *The Truman Administration and Bolivia: Making the World Safe for Liberal Constitutional Oligarchy.* University Park: Pennsylvania State University Press, 2011.

Dörnemann Maria, and Teresa Huhle. "Population Problems in Modernization and Development: Positions and Practices." In *Twentieth Century Population Thinking: A Critical Reader of Primary Sources*, edited by The Population Knowledge Network, 142-71. London: Routledge, 2016.

"El Dr. Allende nos Expone la Acción Desarrollada desde el Ministerio de Salubridad." *Acción Social* 12, 100 (1941): 28–31.

Drinot, Paulo. "Awaiting the Blood of a Truly Emancipating Revolution: Che Guevara in 1950s Peru." In *Che's Travels: The Making of a Revolutionary in 1950s Latin America*, edited by Paulo Drinot, 88–126. Durham, NC: Duke University Press, 2010.

Duany, Jorge. "¿Modernizar la Nación o Nacionalizar la Modernidad? Las Ciencias Sociales en la Universidad de Puerto Rico durante la Década de 1950." In *Frente a La Torre: Ensayos del Centenario de la Universidad de Puerto Rico, 1903–2003*, edited by Silvia Alvarez Curbelo and Carmen Raffucci, 176–207. San Juan: Universidad de Puerto Rico, 2005.

Dueñas Becerra, Jesús. "La Ciencia Psicológica Cubana. Antecedentes y Desarrollo." *Revista del Hospital Psiquiátrico de la Habana* 2, 2 (2005): n.p.

Dueñas Becerra, Jesús. "Profesor Carlos Acosta Nodal: Psicoanalista Ortodoxo hasta el Ultimo Aliento." *Revista del Hospital Psiquiátrico de la Habana* 8, 2 (2011): n.p.

Dugac, Željko. "'Like Yeast in Fermentation': Public Health in Interwar Yugoslavia." In *Health, Hygiene and Eugenics in Southeastern Europe to 1945*, edited by Christian Promitzer, Sevasti Trubeta, and Marius Turda, 193–233. Budapest, Hungary: Central European University Press, 2011.

Duncan, Ronald, and Edward Richardson, eds. *Social Research in Puerto Rico: Science, Humanism, and Society*. San Juan, PR: Interamerican University Press, 1983.

Dunkerley, James. *Rebellion in the Veins: Political Struggle in Bolivia, 1952–82*. London: Verso, 1984.

Ekbladh, David. *The Great American Mission: Modernization and the Construction of an American World Order*. Princeton, NJ: Princeton University Press, 2011.

Elena, Eduardo. *Dignifying Argentina: Peronism, Citizenship, and Mass Consumption*. Pittsburgh: University of Pittsburgh Press, 2011.

Elias, Paulo Eduardo M., and Amelia Cohn. "Health Reform in Brazil: Lessons to Consider." *American Journal of Public Health* 93, 1 (2003): 44–48.

Elizundia Ramírez, Alicia. *Nicaragua, No Somos Dioses: Colaboración Médica Cubana*. Havana: Pablo de la Torriente, 2001.

Ellenberger, Henri F. *The Discovery of the Unconscious: The History and Evolution of Dynamic Psychiatry*. New York: Basic Books, 1970.

Endicott, Stephen, and Edward Hagerman. *The United States and Biological Warfare*. Bloomington: Indiana University Press, 1998.

Engels, Friedrich. *The Condition of the Working Class in England*. Stanford: Stanford University Press, 1968.

Engerman, David. "Development Politics and the Cold War." *Diplomatic History* 41 (2017): 1–19.

Engerman, David. "The Second World's Third World." *Kritika: Explorations in Russian and Eurasian History* 12, 1 (2011): 183–211.

"Entrevista da Editoria da Revista Brasileira de Epidemiologia com a Dra. Maria Eneida de Almeida e com o Prof. Dr. Luiz Hildebrando Pereira da Silva." *Revista Brasileira de Epidemiologia* 9, 4 (2006): 527–32.

Espinosa, Mariola. *Epidemic Invasions: Yellow Fever and the Limits of Cuban Independence, 1878-1930*. Chicago: University of Chicago Press, 2009.

Espinosa, Mariola. "Globalizing the History of Disease, Medicine, and Public Health in Latin America." *Isis* 104, 4 (2014): 798-806.

Facultad de Medicina. *Ediciones Soviéticas de Medicina Exhibidas en la Facultad de Medicina de la Universidad de la República. Reseña de los Libros en Idioma Ruso*. Montevideo: Uruguaya, 1959.

Fagen, Patricia W. *Exiles and Citizens: Spanish Republicans in Mexico*. Austin: University of Texas Press, 1973.

"Falando Perante 2000 Representantes de 80 Países no Congresso de Viena, o Cientista Samuel Pessoa Denuncia o Emprego de Guerra Bacteriológica, por ele Mesmo Comprovada, na Coréia e na China." *A Voz Operária*, February 28, 1953.

Faria, Lina. *Saúde e Política: A Fundação Rockefeller e Seus Parceiros em São Paulo*. Rio de Janeiro, Brazil: Editora Fiocruz, 2007.

Farley, John. *Brock Chisholm, the World Health Organization, and the Cold War*. Vancouver: University of British Columbia Press, 2008.

Farley, John. *To Cast Out Disease: A History of the International Health Division of the Rockefeller Foundation (1913-1951)*. New York: Oxford University Press, 2004.

Fein, Seth. "Producing the Cold War in Mexico: The Public Limits of Covert Communications." In *In from the Cold: Latin America's New Encounters with the Cold War*, edited by Gilbert Joseph and Daniela Spenser, 171-213. Durham, NC: Duke University Press, 2008.

Feinsilver, Julie. "Fifty Years of Cuba's Medical Diplomacy: From Idealism to Pragmatism." *Cuban Studies* 41 (2010): 85-104.

Feinsilver, Julie. *Healing the Masses: Cuban Health Politics at Home and Abroad*. Berkeley: University of California Press, 1993.

Feltrim, Luciana da Conceição. "Perseguição da Delegacia de Ordem Política e Social (DOPS/SP): As Personalidades Políticas no Governo JK." *SINAIS—Revista Eletrônica. Ciências Sociais* 7, 1 (2010): 105-22.

Fernandez, Ronald. *Los Macheteros: The Wells Fargo Robbery and the Violent Struggle for Puerto Rican Independence*. New York: Prentice Hall, 1987.

Fernández Martí, Juan J. "Comentarios sobre los Problemas Transferenciales en los Esquizofrénicos." *Revista del Hospital Psiquiátrico de la Habana* 4, 2 (1963): 414-16.

Ferrao, Luis. *Pedro Albizu Campos y el Nacionalismo Puertorriqueño*. San Juan, PR: Cultural, 1990.

Few, Martha. *Women Who Live Evil Lives: Gender, Religion and the Politics of Power in Colonial Guatemala*. Austin: University of Texas Press, 2002.

Field, Thomas C., Jr. *From Development to Dictatorship: Bolivia and the Alliance for Progress in the Kennedy Era*. Ithaca, NY: Cornell University Press, 2014.

Field, Thomas C., Jr. "Ideology as Strategy: Military-Led Modernization and the Origins of the Alliance for Progress in Bolivia." *Diplomatic History* 36, 1 (2012): 147-83.

Field, Thomas C., Jr., Stella Krepp, and Vanni Pettinà, eds. *Latin America and the Third World: An International History*. Chapel Hill: University of North Carolina Press, 2020.

Filerman, Gary Lewis. "An Exploratory Field Study of the National Health Service of Chile: Health Services Organization in Two Communities." PhD diss., University of Minnesota, 1970.

Filho, Claudio Bertolli. "Uma Outra Modernidade: Médicos Brasileiros na União Soviética." *Anos 90* 10 (1998): 102–21.

Fink, Carole. *Cold War: An International History*. Boulder, CO: Westview, 2017.

"Fiscal Ordena Acusar a Fujimori y Tres Exministros por Caso de Esterilizaciones." *La República*, April 26, 2018.

Fitzgerald, Deborah. "Exporting American Agriculture: The Rockefeller Foundation in Mexico." In *Missionaries of Science: The Rockefeller Foundation in Latin America*, edited by Marcos Cueto, 72–96. Bloomington: Indiana University Press, 1994.

Fleury, Sonia. "What Kind of Social Protection for What Kind of Democracy? Dilemmas of Social Inclusion in Latin America." *Social Medicine* 5, 1 (2010): 34–49.

"Florencio Villa Landa: El Psiquiatra Rojo que Seguía a Pavlov." *Público*, October 23, 2011. http://www.publico.es/402899/el-psiquiatra-rojo-que-seguia-a-pavlov.

Fontes, Virginia, and Ana Garcia. "Brazil's New Imperial Capitalism." *Socialist Register* 50 (2014): 300–320.

Foote, Nicola, and Michael Goebel, eds. *Immigration and National Identities in Latin America*. Gainesville: University Press of Florida, 2014.

Ford, Eileen. *Childhood and Modernity in Cold War Mexico City*. London: Bloomsbury Academic, 2018.

Fortes, Jacqueline, and Larissa Adler Lomnitz. *Becoming a Scientist in Mexico: The Challenge of Creating a Scientific Community in an Underdeveloped Country*. University Park: Pennsylvania State University Press, 1994.

Fosdick, Raymond. *The Story of the Rockefeller Foundation*. New Brunswick, NJ: Transaction, 1989.

Fox, Soledad. "Memory and History: The Autobiographies of Constancia de la Mora and María Teresa León." *Moenia* 10 (2004): 375–88.

Fox, T. F. "Russia Revisited: Impressions of Soviet Medicine." *The Lancet* 267, 6842 (1954): 803–7.

Franco, Saúl. "Entre los Negocios y los Derechos." *Revista Cubana de Salud Pública* 39 (2013): 268–84.

Friedman, Jeremy. *Shadow Cold War: The Sino-Soviet Competition for the Third World*. Chapel Hill: University of North Carolina Press, 2015.

Frugoni, Emilio. *De Montevideo a Moscú*. Buenos Aires, Argentina: Claridad, 1945.

Funes Monzote, Reinaldo. *El Despertar del Asociacionismo Científico en Cuba (1876–1920)*. Madrid: Consejo Superior de Investigaciones Científicas, 2004.

Gacetilla. "Diciembre 21: La Política y la Sanidad Son Incompatibles." *Archivo y Revista de Hospitales* 11, 53 (1940): 41.

Gaddis, John Lewis. *We Now Know: Rethinking Cold War History*. New York: Oxford University Press, 1997.

Gadnitskaia, Marina A., and Tatyana A. Samsonenko. "Meditsinskoe Obsluzhivanie v Povsednevnosti Lolkhoznoi Derevni 1930-kh gg." *Vlast'* 5 (2017): 192–97.

Galán Rubí, Fermín. "Ideología y Salud Mental." In *Memoria de la Primera Jornada Nacional de Psiquiatría, 1975,* 80–84. Havana: Orbe, 1977.

Galeano, Eduardo. *Open Veins of Latin America: Five Centuries of the Pillage of a Continent.* New York: Monthly Review Press, 1973.

Galeano, Eduardo. *Las Venas Abiertas de América Latina.* Madrid: Siglo XXI, 2009.

Garcia, Gabriel. "The Rise of the Global South, the IMF and the Future of Law and Development." *Third World Quarterly* 37, 2 (2016): 191–208.

García, Luciano. "La Recepción de la Psicología Soviética en la Argentina: Lecturas y Apropiaciones en la Psicología, Psiquiatría y Psicoanálisis (1936–1991)." PhD diss., Universidad de Buenos Aires, 2012.

García, Roberto, and Arturo Taracena Arriola, eds. *La Guerra Fría y el Anticomunismo en Centroamérica.* Guatemala City, Guatemala: FLACSO, 2017.

Gardner, Lytt I. "Progress Report on the 'Health for Peace' Bill of 1959 (Senate Joint Resolution 41)." *Pediatrics* 25, 1 (1960): 145–50.

Garfield, Richard, and Sarah Santana. "The Impact of the Economic Crisis and the U.S. Embargo on Health in Cuba." *American Journal of Public Health* 87, 1 (1997): 15–20.

Garfield, Richard, and Glen Williams. *Health Care in Nicaragua: Primary Care under Changing Regimes.* New York: Oxford University Press, 1992.

Garrard-Burnett, Virginia, Mark Atwood Lawrence, and Julio Moreno, eds. *Beyond the Eagle's Shadow: New Histories of Latin America's Cold War.* Albuquerque: University of New Mexico Press, 2013.

Garrison, Dorotha J. "Reclamation Project of the Papaloapan River Basin in Mexico." *Economic Geography* 26, 1 (1950): 59–64.

Geidel, Molly. *Peace Corps Fantasies: How Development Shaped the Global Sixties.* Minneapolis: University of Minnesota Press, 2016.

Geidel, Molly. "'Sowing Death in Our Women's Wombs': Modernization and Indigenous Nationalism in the 1960s Peace Corps and Jorge Sanjinés' 'Yawar Mallku.'" *American Quarterly* 62, 3 (2010): 763–86.

Gerbi, Antonello. *The Dispute of the New World: The History of a Polemic, 1750–1900.* Translated by Jeremy Moyle. Pittsburgh: University of Pittsburgh Press, 2010.

Gereffi, Gary. *The Pharmaceutical Industry and Dependency in the Third World.* Princeton, NJ: Princeton University Press, 1983.

Geselbracht, Raymond. *The Civil Rights Legacy of Harry S. Truman.* Kirksville, MO: Truman State University Press, 2007.

Gideonse, Harry D. "A Congressional Committee's Investigation of the Foundations." *Journal of Higher Education* 25, 9 (1954): 457–63.

Gill, Lesley. *The School of the Americas: Military Training and Political Violence in the Americas.* Durham, NC: Duke University Press, 2004.

Gill, Timothy. "Possibilities and Pitfalls of Left-Wing Populism in Socialist Venezuela." *Journal of World-Systems Research* 24, 2 (2018): 304–13.

Gill, Tom. *Land Hunger in Mexico.* Washington, DC: Charles Lathrop Pack Forestry Foundation, 1951.

Gil-Riaño, Sebastián. "Relocating Anti-Racist Science: The 1950 UNESCO Statement on Race and Economic Development in the Global South." *British Journal for the History of Science* 51, 2 (2018): 281–303.

Gilroy, Paul. *The Black Atlantic: Modernity and Double Consciousness.* Cambridge, MA: Harvard University Press, 1993.

G. J. B. "Politics and Economies in Chile." *World Today* 9, 2 (1953): 81–92.

Gleijeses, Piero. *Conflicting Missions: Havana, Washington, and Africa, 1959–1976.* Chapel Hill: University of North Carolina Press, 2002.

Gleijeses, Piero. *Shattered Hope: The Guatemalan Revolution and the United States, 1944–1954.* Princeton, NJ: Princeton University Press, 1992.

Gobat, Michel. "The Invention of Latin America: A Transnational History of Anti-Imperialism, Democracy, and Race." *American Historical Review* 118, 5 (2013): 1345–75.

Golcman, Aída Alejandra. "The Experiment of the Therapeutic Communities in Argentina: The Case of the Hospital Estévez." *Psychoanalysis and History* 14, 2 (2012): 269–84.

Golder, Mario. *Reportajes Contemporáneos a la Psicología Soviética.* Buenos Aires, Argentina: Cartago, 1986.

Golder, Mario, and Alejandro González. *Freud en Vigotsky: Inconsciente y Lenguaje.* Buenos Aires: Ateneo Vigotskiano de la Argentina, 2006.

Goldsmith, Alfredo, Héctor Gutiérrez, and Hernán Sanhueza. *Country Profiles, Chile.* New York: Population Council and Columbia University, 1970.

Goldstein, Alyosha. "The Attributes of Sovereignty: The Cold War, Colonialism, and Community Education in Puerto Rico." In *Imagining our Americas: Toward a Transnational Frame,* edited by Sandhya Shukla and Heidi Tinsman, 313–37. Durham, NC: Duke University Press, 2007.

Gómez, Amparo, Antonio Canales, and Brian Balmer, eds. *Science Policies and Twentieth-Century Dictatorships: Spain, Italy and Argentina.* Farnham, UK: Routledge, 2016.

Gómez, Pablo. *The Experiential Caribbean: Creating Knowledge and Healing in the Early Modern Atlantic.* Chapel Hill: University of North Carolina Press, 2017.

Gómez-Dantés, Héctor, and Anne-Emanuelle Birn. "Malaria and Social Movements in Mexico: The Last 60 Years." *Parassitologia* 42, 1–2 (2000): 69–85.

Góngora, Mario. *Ensayo Histórico sobre la Noción de Estado en Chile en los Siglos XIX y XX.* Santiago, Chile: La Ciudad, 1981.

González, Alex. "Diego Rivera en la Unión Soviética: Una Exposición en la Ciudad de México." World Socialist Web Site, January 22, 2018. https://www.wsws.org/es/articles/2018/01/22/rive-j22.html.

González, Elisa. "Nurturing the Citizens of the Future: Milk Stations and Child Nutrition in Puerto Rico, 1929–60." *Medical History* 59, 2 (2015): 177–98.

González Canosa, Mara. "Los Antecedentes de las 'Fuerzas Armadas Revolucionarias': Acerca del Itinerario Político-Ideológico de Uno de Sus Grupos Fundadores." Paper presented at the Third Conference on Politics in Buenos Aires in the Twentieth Century, La Plata, Argentina, August 28–29, 2008. http://cedinpe.unsam.edu.ar/sites/default/files/pdfs/gonzalez_canosa_m-antecedentes_far_cish_2008.pdf.

González Martín, Diego. "Algunas Consideraciones Críticas sobre la Teoría Freudiana." *Cuba Socialista* 5, 43 (1965): 76.

González Martín, Diego. "Desarrollo de las Ideas Neurofisiológicas en Cuba en el Curso del Proceso Revolucionario." In *Jornada Científica Internacional: 30 Aniversario del Asalto al Cuartel Moncada,* edited by María Salomé Morales and Gaspar Quintana, 658–74. Havana: Editorial de Ciencias Sociales, 1986.

González Martín, Diego. *Experimentos e Ideología: Bases de una Teoría Psicológica.* Mérida, Venezuela: Talleres Gráficos Universitarios, 1960.

González Martín, Diego. "Grandes de la Medicina Cubana. Profesor Rodolfo J. Guiral, Destacado Neuropsiquiatra." *Bohemia* 44, 10 (1952): 25.

González Serra, Diego Jorge. "González Martín: Marxismo y Ciencias del Psiquismo." *Revista Cubana de Psicología* 15, 1 (1998): 74–75.

Goodsell, Charles. *Administration of a Revolution: Executive Reform in Puerto Rico under Governor Tugwell, 1941–1946.* Cambridge, MA: Harvard University Press, 1965.

Gordin, Michael D., Karl Hall, and Alexei Kojevnikov, eds. "Intelligentsia Science: The Russian Century, 1860–1960." *Osiris* 23 (special issue, 2008).

Gordon, Todd, and Jeffery R. Webber. *Blood of Extraction: Canadian Imperialism in Latin America.* Winnipeg, MB: Fernwood, 2016.

Gorry, Conner. "Your Primary Care Doctor May Have an MD from Cuba: Experiences from the Latin American Medical School." *MEDICC Review* 20, 2 (2018): 11–16.

Gorsky, Martin, and Christopher Sirrs. "World Health by Place: The Politics of International Health System Metrics, 1924–c. 2010." *Journal of Global History* 12, 3 (2017): 361–85.

Gorsuch, Anne E. "'Cuba, My Love': The Romance of Revolutionary Cuba in the Soviet Sixties." *American Historical Review* 120, 2 (2015): 497–526.

Goschler, Constantin. "Wahrheit zwischen Seziersaal und Parlament: Rudolf Virchow und der kulturelle Deutungsanspruch der Naturwissenschaften." *Geschichte und Gesellschaft* 30 (2004): 219–49.

Gotkowitz, Laura. "Commemorating the Heroínas: Gender and Civic Ritual in Early-Twentieth-Century Bolivia." In *Hidden Histories of Gender and the State in Latin America,* edited by Elizabeth Dore and Maxine Molyneux, 215–37. Durham, NC: Duke University Press, 2000.

Gotkowitz, Laura. *A Revolution for Our Rights: Indigenous Struggles for Land and Justice in Bolivia, 1880–1952.* Durham, NC: Duke University Press, 2007.

Goure, Leon. "Latin America." In *The Soviet Impact on World Politics,* edited by Kurt London, 182–210. New York: Hawthorn, 1974.

Graboyes, Melissa. *The Experiment Must Continue: Medical Research and Ethics in East Africa, 1940–2014.* Athens: Ohio University Press, 2015.

Granda, Edmundo. "Algunas Reflexiones a los Veinticuatro años de la ALAMES." *Medicina Social* 3, 2 (2008): 217–25.

Grandin, Greg. *Empire's Workshop: Latin America, the United States, and the Rise of the New Imperialism.* New York: Metropolitan, 2006.

Grandin, Greg. *The Last Colonial Massacre: Latin America in the Cold War.* Chicago: University of Chicago Press, 2004.

Greene, Jeremy A. *Prescribing by Numbers: Drugs and the Definition of Disease*. Baltimore, MD: Johns Hopkins University Press, 2008.

Greene, Jeremy A. "Releasing the Flood Waters: Diuril and the Reshaping of Hypertension." *Bulletin of the History of Medicine* 79, 4 (2005): 749–94.

Grimson, Wilbur R. *Sociedad de Locos: Experiencia y Violencia en un Hosptial Psiquiátrico*. Buenos Aires, Argentina: Nueva Visión, 1972.

Guerra, Lillian. *Visions of Power: Revolution and Redemption in Cuba, 1959-1971*. Chapel Hill: University of North Carolina Press, 2011.

Guevara, Ernesto. "At the Afro-Asian Conference in Algeria, February 24, 1965." In *The Che Reader*. North Melbourne, Australia: Ocean Press, 2005. https://www.marxists.org/archive/guevara/1965/02/24.htm.

Guevara, Ernesto. "Discurso a los Estudiantes de Medicina y Trabajadores de la Salud, 1960." In *Che Guevara Presente: Una Antología Mínima*, edited by María del Carmen Ariet García and David Deutschmann, 119. Melbourne, Australia: Ocean Press, 2004.

Guevara, Ernesto. "El Socialismo y el Hombre en Cuba." *La Rosa Blindada* 1, 6 (1965): 4–10.

Guevara, Juan. "Mesa Redonda. Repesando la Historia: A Diez Años del Primer Encuentro entre Psicoanalistas y Psicólogos Marxistas." *Revista Cubana de Psicología* 14, 1 (1997): 23–39.

Guiral, Rodolfo J. "Medicina Psicosomática." *Anales de la Academia de Ciencias Físicas, Médicas y Naturales* 92, 2 (1953–54): 131.

Guy, Donna. "The Pan American Child Congresses, 1916 to 1942: Pan-Americanism, Child Reform, and the Welfare State in Latin America." *Journal of Family History* 23, 3 (1998): 272–91.

Hall, Marie-Françoise. "Los Hombres y la Educación en Planificación de la Familia." *Cuadernos Médico Sociales* 10, 2 (1969): 5–15.

Hankinson, R. K. B., and International Planned Parenthood Federation. *Proceedings of the Eighth International Conference of the International Planned Parenthood Federation, Santiago, Chile, April 9-15, 1967*. London: IPPF, 1967.

Harmer, Tanya. *Allende's Chile and the Inter-American Cold War*. Chapel Hill: University of North Carolina Press, 2011.

Harmer, Tanya. "The Cold War in Latin America." In *The Routledge Handbook of the Cold War*, edited by Artemy M. Kalinovsky and Craig Daigle, 133–48. Abingdon, UK: Routledge, 2014.

Harmer, Tanya, and Alfredo Riquelme Segovia, eds. *Chile y la Guerra Fría Global*. Santiago, Chile: RIL Editores, 2014.

Hartmann, Betsy. *Reproductive Rights and Wrongs: The Global Politics of Population Control*. Boston: South End, 1995.

Hatt, Paul. *Backgrounds of Human Fertility in Puerto Rico: A Sociological Survey*. Princeton, NJ: Princeton University Press, 1952.

Hatzky, Christine. *Cubans in Angola: South-South Cooperation and Transfer of Knowledge, 1976-1991*. Madison: University of Wisconsin Press, 2015.

Hecht, Gabrielle. *Entangled Geographies: Empire and Technopolitics in the Global Cold War*. Cambridge, MA: MIT Press, 2011.

Hernández, Mario, and Diana Obregón. *La OPS y el Estado Colombiano: Cien Años de Historia, 1902-2002*. Bogotá, Colombia: OPS, 2002.

Herrera González, Patricio. "La Confederación de Trabajadores de América Latina y la Implementación de Su Proyecto Sindical Continental (1938-1941)." *Trashumante, Revista Americana de Historia Social* 2 (2013): 136-64.

Herrero, María Belén, and Diana Tussie. "UNASUR Health: A Quiet Revolution in Health Diplomacy in South America." *Global Social Policy* 15, 3 (2015): 261-77.

Heyck, Denis. *Life Stories of the Nicaraguan Revolution*. New York: Routledge, 1990.

Hickling-Hudson, Anne, Jorge Corona González, and Rosemary Preston, eds. *The Capacity to Share: A Study of Cuba's International Cooperation in Educational Development*. New York: Palgrave Macmillan, 2012.

Hill, Reuben, Joseph Stycos, and Kurt Back. *The Family and Population Control: A Puerto Rican Experiment in Social Change*. Chapel Hill: University of North Carolina Press, 1959.

Hirschfeld, Katherine. *Health, Politics, Revolution in Cuba since 1898*. New Brunswick, NJ: Transaction, 2007.

Hochman, Gilberto. "'O Brasil Não é Só Doença': O Programa de Saúde Pública de Juscelino Kubitschek." *Historia, Ciências, Saúde-Manguinhos* 16 (2009): 313-31.

Hochman, Gilberto. "Cambio Político y Reformas de la Salud Pública en Brasil: El Primer Gobierno Vargas (1930-1945)." *Dynamis: Acta Hispanica ad Medicinae Scientiarumque Historiam Illustrandam* 25 (2005): 199-226.

Hochman, Gilberto. "From Autonomy to Partial Alignment: National Malaria Programs in the Time of Global Eradication, Brazil, 1941-1961." *Canadian Bulletin of Medical History* 25, 1 (2008): 161-92.

Hochman, Gilberto. *The Sanitation of Brazil: Nation, State, and Public Health, 1889-1930*. Urbana: University of Illinois Press, 2016.

Hochman, Gilberto. "Vigiar e, Depois de 1964, Punir: Sobre Samuel Pessoa e o Departamento Vermelho da USP." *Ciência e Cultura* 66, 4 (2014): 26-31.

Hochman, Gilberto, María Silvia di Liscia, and Steven Palmer. *Patologías de la Patria: Enfermedades, Enfermos y Nación en América Latina*. Buenos Aires, Argentina: Lugar, 2012.

Hoffman, Beatrix. "Health Care Reform and Social Movements in the United States." *American Journal of Public Health* 93, 1 (2003): 75-85.

Holanda, Nestor de. *Como Seria o Brasil Socialista?* Rio de Janeiro: Editôra Civilização Brasileira, 1963.

Hollander, Nancy Caro. *Love in a Time of Hate: Liberation Psychology in Latin America*. New Brunswick, NJ: Rutgers University Press, 1997.

Hollander, Nancy Caro. *Uprooted Minds: Surviving the Politics of Terror in the Americas*. New York: Routledge, 2010.

Hong, Young-Sun. *Cold War Germany, the Third World, and the Global Humanitarian Regime*. Cambridge: Cambridge University Press, 2015.

Hornstein, Luis. "Un Paseíto por Villa Freud." Paper presented at the Grupo de Saberes-Psi workshop, Buenos Aires, Argentina, December 12, 2014.

"Las Huellas de la Antipsiquiatría." *Panorama*, October 20, 1970.

"Hugo Chavez Kicks Off Russia Visit with Emotional Speech at a Moscow University." RT, September 9, 2009. https://www.rt.com/news/chavez-russia-emotional-speech.

Huneeus, Carlos. *La Guerra Fría Chilena: Gabriel González Videla y la Ley Maldita*. Santiago, Chile: Random House Mondadori, 2009.

Huneeus, Carlos, and María Paz Lanas. "Ciencia Política e Historia: Eduardo Cruz Coke y el Estado de Bienestar en Chile, 1937–1938." *Historia (Chile)* 35 (2002): 151–86.

Hunt, Michael. *Ideology and U.S. Foreign Policy*. New Haven, CT: Yale University Press, 1987.

Iacob, Bogdan C. "Socialist Health Transfers in Africa during the 1970s: Shifting Geographies and Values." In *Jahrbuch für Historische Kommunismusforschung*, 139–57. Berlin, Germany: Metropol, 2019.

Iber, Patrick. "Managing Mexico's Cold War: Vicente Lombardo Toledano and the Uses of Political Intelligence." *Journal of Iberian and Latin American Research* 19, 1 (2012): 11–19.

Iber, Patrick. *Neither Peace nor Freedom: The Cultural Cold War in Latin America*. Cambridge, MA: Harvard University Press, 2015.

Igual, Miguel Marco. "Florencio Villa Landa." Accessed February 27, 2019. http://www.todoslosnombres.org/php/verArchivo.php?id=80.

Igual, Miguel Marco. "Los Médicos Republicanos Españoles Exiliados en la Unión Soviética." *Medicina & Historia* 1 (2009): 1–16.

Igual, Miguel Marco. "Las Neurociencias y los Desvaríos de la Epoca Soviética: Los Médicos Republicanos Españoles, Testigos de Excepción." *Revista de Neurología* 53, 4 (2011): 233–44.

Illanes, María Angélica. *"En el Nombre del Pueblo, del Estado y de la Ciencia . . .": Historia Social de la Salud Pública, Chile, 1880-1973*. Santiago, Chile: Colectivo de Atención Primaria de Salud, 1993.

Illanes, María Angélica. *Historia del Movimiento Social y de la Salud Pública en Chile, 1885-1920: Solidaridad, Ciencia y Caridad*. Santiago, Chile: Colectivo de Atención Primaria, 1989.

Illich, Ivan. "Medical Nemesis." *The Lancet* 303, 7863 (1974): 918–21.

Illich, Ivan. *Medical Nemesis: The Expropriation of Health*. New York: Pantheon, 1976.

Immerwahr, Daniel. *Thinking Small: The United States and the Lure of Community Development*. Cambridge, MA: Harvard University Press, 2015.

"Información del Grupo Plataforma." *Los Libros* 25 (1972): 8.

"In Memoriam: Leo H. Bartemeier, M.D., 1895-1982." *American Journal of Psychiatry* 140, 5 (1983): 630.

Innis, Nancy K. "Lessons from the Controversy over the Loyalty Oath at the University of California." *Minerva* 30, 3 (1992): 337–65.

Iriart, Celia, Emerson Elías Merhy, and Howard Waitzkin. "Managed Care in Latin America: The New Common Sense in Health Policy Reform." *Social Science and Medicine* 52, 8 (2001): 1243–53.

Iriart, Celia, Howard Waitzkin, Jaime Breilh, Alfredo Estrada, and Emerson Elías Merhy. "Medicina Social Latinoamericana: Aportes y Desafíos." *Revista Panamericana de Salud Pública* 12, 2 (2002): 128–36.

Izaguirre, Marcelo. *Jacques Lacan: El Anclaje de Su Enseñanza en la Argentina*. Buenos Aires, Argentina: Catálogos, 2009.

Janer, José, Guillermo Arbona, and J. S. McKenzie-Pollock. "The Place of Demography in Health and Welfare Planning in Latin America." *Milbank Memorial Fund Quarterly* 42, 2 (1964): 328-45.

Jeifets, Víctor L., and Lazar S. Jeifets. "La Comintern y la Formación de Militantes Comunistas Latinoamericanos." *Izquierdas* 31 (2016): 130-61.

Jesualdo. *Mi Viaje a la U.R.S.S.* Montevideo, Uruguay: Pueblos Unidos, 1952.

Jiles Moreno, Ximena, and Claudia Rojas Mira. *De la Miel a los Implantes: Historia de las Políticas de Regulación de la Fecundidad en Chile*. Santiago, Chile: Corporación de Salud y Políticas Sociales, 1992.

John, S. Sándor. *Bolivia's Radical Tradition: Permanent Revolution in the Andes*. Tucson: University of Arizona Press, 2009.

Johns Hopkins Medicine. "Peripheral Nerve Injury." Accessed December 17, 2019. https://www.hopkinsmedicine.org/health/conditions-and-diseases/peripheral-nerve-injury.

Jones, Esyllt. *Radical Medicine: The International Origins of Socialized Health Care in Canada*. Winnipeg, Canada: ARP, 2019.

Joseph, Gilbert M. "Border Crossings and the Remaking of Latin American Cold War Studies." *Cold War History* 19, 1 (2019): 141-70.

Joseph, Gilbert M. "What We Now Know and Should Know: Bringing Latin America More Meaningfully into Cold War Studies." In *In from the Cold: Latin America's New Encounters with the Cold War*, edited by Gilbert Joseph and Daniela Spenser, 3-46. Durham, NC: Duke University Press, 2008.

Joseph, Gilbert M., and Greg Grandin, eds. *A Century of Revolution: Insurgent and Counterinsurgent Violence during Latin America's Long Cold War*. Durham, NC: Duke University Press, 2010.

Joseph, Gilbert M., Catherine LeGrand, and Ricardo Salvatore, eds. *Close Encounters of Empire: Writing the Cultural History of U.S.-Latin American Relations*. Durham, NC: Duke University Press, 1998.

Joseph, Gilbert M., and Daniela Spenser, eds. *In from the Cold: Latin America's New Encounter with the Cold War*. Durham, NC: Duke University Press, 2008.

Kapelusz-Poppi, Ana María. "Physician Activists and the Development of Rural Health in Postrevolutionary Mexico." *Radical History Review* 80 (2001): 35-50.

Kapelusz-Poppi, Ana María. "Rural Health and State Construction in Post-Revolutionary Mexico: The Nicolaita Project for Rural Medical Services." *Americas* 58, 2 (2004): 261-83.

Karl, Robert A. "Reading the Cuban Revolution from Bogotá, 1957-62." *Cold War History* 16, 4 (2016): 337-58.

Katsakioris, Constantin. "The Lumumba University in Moscow: Higher Education for a Soviet–Third World Alliance, 1960-91." *Journal of Global History* 14, 2 (2019): 281-300.

Katsakioris, Constantin. "The Soviet-South Encounter: Tensions in the Friendship with Afro-Asian Partners, 1945-1965." In *Cold War Crossings: International Travel and*

Exchanges across the Soviet Bloc, 1940s–1960s, edited by Patryk Babiracki and Kenyon Zimmer, 134–65. College Station: Texas A&M University Press, 2014.

Keller, Renata. "A Foreign Policy for Domestic Consumption: Mexico's Lukewarm Defense of Castro, 1959–1969." *Latin American Research Review* 47, 2 (2012): 100–119.

Keller, Renata. *Mexico's Cold War: Cuba, the United States, and the Legacy of the Mexican Revolution*. New York: Cambridge University Press, 2015.

Kershaw, Angela. "French and British Female Intellectuals and the Soviet Union: The Journey to the USSR, 1929–1942." *E-rea* 4, 2 (2006). http://journals.openedition.org /erea/250.

Kesselman, Hernán. "Salud Mental y Neocolonialismo." In *Psicología Argentina Hoy*, by R. Bohoslavsky, R. Chevalier, S. Dubcovsky, W. Grimson, H. Kesselman, P. O'Donnell, S. De Pravaz, J. Salvarezza, and F. Ulloa, 111–12. Buenos Aires, Argentina: Búsqueda, 1973.

Kingsbury, Donald. *Only the People Can Save the People: Constituent Power, Revolution, and Counterrevolution in Venezuela*. Albany: State University of New York Press, 2018.

Kinoshita, Dina L. "Organização Comunista na América Latina no pós II Guerra Mundial: Rastros do Comintern." *Revista iZQUIERDAS* 3, 7 (2010): 1–12.

Kinsella, Arianna. "Philanthropy during the Cold War, 1958–1985: A Case Study for Brazilian History in the United States and the Social Sciences in Brazil." PhD diss., University of Paris IV, Paris–Sorbonne, 2013.

Kinsey, Alfred, Wardell Pomeroy, and Clyde Martin. *Sexual Behavior in the Human Male*. Philadelphia: Saunders, 1948.

Kinzer, Stephen. *Blood of Brothers: Life and War in Nicaragua*. Cambridge, MA: Harvard University Press, 1991.

Kirillova, Liana. "Soviet Internationalism: Cultural Diplomacy in Latin America and Peoples' Friendship University." *Bulletin of Udmurt University* 2 (2017): 221–30.

Kirk, John. *Healthcare without Borders: Understanding Cuban Medical Internationalism*. Gainesville: University Press of Florida, 2015.

Kirk, John, and H. Michael Erisman. *Cuban Medical Internationalism: Origins, Evolution, and Goals*. New York: Palgrave Macmillan, 2009.

Kirkendall, Andrew J. *Paulo Freire and the Cold War Politics of Literacy*. Chapel Hill: University of North Carolina Press, 2010.

Klein, Herbert. *Bolivia: The Evolution of a Multi-Ethnic Society*. New York: Oxford University Press, 1992.

Knaul, Felicia Marie, Héctor Arreola-Ornelas, Oscar Méndez-Carniado, and Martha Miranda-Muñoz. *Preventing Impoverishment, Promoting Equity and Protecting Households from Financial Crisis: Universal Health Insurance through Institutional Reform in Mexico*. Mexico City: FUNSALUD–Instituto Nacional de Salud Pública, 2006.

Knoblauch, Heidi Katherine. "'A Campaign Won as a Public Issue Will Stay Won': Using Cartoons and Comics to Fight National Health Care Reform, 1940s and Beyond." *American Journal of Public Health* 104, 2 (2014): 227–36.

Kofas, Jon. "The Politics of Foreign Debt: The IMF, the World Bank, and U.S. Foreign Policy in Chile, 1946–1952." *Journal of Developing Areas* 31, 2 (1997): 157–82.

Krementsov, Nikolai. *The Cure: A Story of Cancer and Politics from the Annals of the Cold War*. Chicago: University of Chicago Press, 2002.

Krementsov, Nikolai. "'In the Shadow of the Bomb': U.S.-Soviet Biomedical Relations in the Early Cold War, 1944–1948." *Journal of Cold War Studies* 9, 4 (2007): 41–67.

Krementsov, Nikolai. "The Promises, Realities, and Legacies of the Bolshevik Revolution, 1917–2017." *American Journal of Public Health* 107, 11 (2017): 1693–94.

Krementsov, Nikolai. *Revolutionary Experiments: The Quest for Immortality in Bolshevik Science and Fiction*. New York: Oxford University Press, 2013.

Krementsov, Nikolai. *Stalinist Science*. Princeton, NJ: Princeton University Press, 1996.

Krementsov, Nikolai, and Anne-Emanuelle Birn. "The Hall of Distorting Mirrors." Review of Anna Geltzer, "In a Distorted Mirror: The Cold War and U.S.-Soviet Biomedical Cooperation and (Mis)Understanding, 1956–1977." June 6, 2013. https://lists.h-net.org/cgi-bin/logbrowse.pl?trx=vx&list=h-diplo&month=1306&week=a&msg=a8zb3Zq3c4dx4HZiYoaoOQ&user=&pw=.

Krementsov, Nikolai, and Susan Gross Solomon. "Giving and Taking across Borders: The Rockefeller Foundation and Russia, 1919–1928." *Minerva* 39, 3 (2001): 265–98.

Krige, John. *American Hegemony and the Postwar Reconstruction of Science in Europe*. Cambridge, MA: MIT Press, 2006.

Krige, John, and Helke Rausch, eds. *American Foundations and the Coproduction of World Order in the Twentieth Century*. Göttingen, Germany: Vandenhoeck & Ruprecht, 2012.

Kumar, Prakash, Timothy Lorek, Tore C. Olsson, Nicole Sackley, Sigrid Schmalzer, and Gabriela Soto Laveaga. "Roundtable: New Narratives of the Green Revolution." *Agricultural History* 91, 3 (2017): 397–422.

Kuznick, Peter J. *Beyond the Laboratory: Scientists as Political Activists in 1930s America*. Chicago: University of Chicago Press, 1987.

La Botz, Dan. "The Communist International, the Soviet Union, and their Impact on the Latin America Workers' Movement." *World Tensions/Tensões Mundiais* 13, 24 (2017): 67–106.

Labra, Maria Eliana. "Medicina Social en Chile: Propuestas y Debates (1920–1950)." *Cuadernos Médico Sociales* 44, 4 (2004): 207–21.

Labra, Maria Eliana. "Poder Médico y Políticas de Salud en Chile: Reflexiones para la Coyuntura." *Salud y Cambio* 6, 21 (1996): 5–14.

Lack, Walter. *Alexander von Humboldt and the Botanical Exploration of the Americas*. Munich: Prestel, 2009.

LaFeber, Walter. *Inevitable Revolutions: The United States in Central America*. New York: Norton, 1983.

Lagos Escobar, Ricardo, ed. *Cien Años de Luces y Sombras*. Santiago, Chile: Taurus, 2010.

Lambe, Jennifer. *Madhouse: Psychiatry and Politics in Cuban History*. Chapel Hill: University of North Carolina Press, 2017.

Landy, David. *Tropical Childhood: Cultural Transmission and Learning in a Rural Puerto Rican Village*. Chapel Hill: University of North Carolina Press, 1959.

Langer, Marie, ed. *Cuestionamos*. Buenos Aires, Argentina: Granica, 1971.

Lapp, Michael. "The Rise and Fall of Puerto Rico as a Social Laboratory, 1945–1965." *Social Science History* 19, 2 (1995): 169–99.

Larionova, Marina, Mark Rakhmangulov, and Marc Berenson. "Russia: A Re-emerging Donor." In *The BRICS in International Development*, edited by Jing Gu, Alex Shankland, and Anuradha Chenoy, 63–92. London: Palgrave Macmillan 2016.

Larraín, Camilo. *La Sociedad Médica de Santiago y el Desarrollo Histórico de la Medicina en Chile*. Santiago: Sociedad Médica de Chile, 2002.

Larrañaga Jiménez, Osvaldo. "El Estado Bienestar en Chile: 1910–2010." In *Cien Años de Luces y Sombras*, edited by Ricardo Lagos Escobar, 178–83. Santiago, Chile: Taurus, 2010.

Latham, Michael E. *The Right Kind of Revolution: Modernization, Development, and U.S. Foreign Policy from the Cold War to the Present*. Ithaca, NY: Cornell University Press, 2011.

Laurell, Asa Cristina. "Health System Reform in Mexico: A Critical Review." *International Journal of Health Services* 37, 3 (2007): 515–35.

Laurell, Asa Cristina, and Oliva Lopez Arellano. "Market Commodities and Poor Relief: The World Bank Proposal for Health." *International Journal of Health Services* 26, 1 (1996): 1–18.

Lear, Walter J. "American Medical Support for Spanish Democracy, 1936–1938." In *Comrades in Health: U.S. Health Internationalists, Abroad and at Home,* edited by Anne-Emanuelle Birn and Theodore Brown, 65–81. New Brunswick, NJ: Rutgers University Press, 2013.

Leffler, Melvyn, and David Painter, eds. *Origins of the Cold War: An International History*. London: Routledge, 1994.

Lehman, Kenneth. *Bolivia and the United States: A Limited Partnership*. Athens: University of Georgia Press, 1999.

Lehman, Kenneth. "Revolutions and Attributions: Making Sense of Eisenhower Administration Policies in Bolivia and Guatemala." *Diplomatic History* 21, 2 (1997): 185–213.

Leitenberg, Milton. "False Allegations of U.S. Biological Weapons Use during the Korean War." In *Terrorism, War, or Disease? Unraveling the Use of Biological Weapons*, edited by Anne L. Clunan, Peter R. Lavoy, and Susan B. Martin, 120–43. Stanford, CA: Stanford University Press, 2008.

Lema, V. Zito. *Conversaciones con Enrique Pichon-Rivière sobre el Arte y la Locura*. Buenos Aires, Argentina: Cinco, 1980.

Lenin, Vladimir. *Imperialism: The Highest Stage of Capitalism*. London: Lawrence and Wishart, 1948.

León-Manríquez, José Luis. "Power Vacuum or Hegemonic Continuity? The United States, Latin America, and the 'Chinese Factor' after the Cold War." *World Affairs* 179, 3 (2016): 59–81.

Leontiev, A. N. *Problemas del Desarrollo del Psiquismo*. Havana: Instituto Cubano del Libro, 1974.

Leopold, Ellen. *Under the Radar: Cancer and the Cold War*. New Brunswick, NJ: Rutgers University Press, 2009.

Leslie, Stuart W. *The Cold War and American Science: The Military-Industrial-Academic Complex at MIT and Stanford*. New York: Columbia University Press, 1993.

Lewis, Stephen. "Indigenista Dreams Meet Sober Realities: The Slow Demise of Federal Indian Policy in Chiapas, Mexico, 1951–1970." *Latin American Perspectives* 39, 5 (2012): 63–79.

Light, Jennifer. *From Warfare to Welfare: Defense Intellectuals and Urban Problems in Cold War America*. Baltimore, MD: Johns Hopkins University Press, 2003.

Lima, Nísia T., Silvia Gerschman, Flavio Coelho Edler, and Julio Manuel Suárez. *Saúde e Democracia: História e Perspectivas do SUS*. Rio de Janeiro, Brazil: Editora Fiocruz, 2005.

Lima, Nísia T., and Gilberto Hochman. "'Condenado pela Raça, Absolvido pela Medicina': O Brasil Descoberto pelo Movimento Sanitarista da Primeira República." In *Raça, Ciência e Sociedade*, edited by Marcos Chor Maio and Ricardo V. Santos, 23–40. Rio de Janeiro, Brazil: Editora Fiocruz/CCBB, 1996.

Lima, Nísia T., and Marcos Chor Maio. "Ciências Sociais e Educação Sanitária: A Perspectiva da Seção de Pesquisa Social do Serviço Especial de Saúde Pública na Década de 1950." *História, Ciências, Saúde-Manguinhos* 17 (2010): 511–26.

Lima, Nísia T., and José Paranaguá de Santana, eds. *Saúde Coletiva como Compromisso: A Trajetória da Abrasco*. Rio de Janeiro, Brazil: Editora Fiocruz, 2006.

Limongi, Fernando P. "Marxismo, Nacionalismo e Cultura: Caio Prado Junior e a Revista Brasiliense." *Revista Brasileira de Ciências Sociais* 2 (1987): 27–46.

Lira, Elizabeth, and Eugenia Weinstein. *Psicoterapia y Represión Política*. Mexico City: Siglo Veintiuno, 1984.

Lobato, Milton, and Reinaldo Machado. *Médicos Brasileiros na U.R.S.S.: Impressões de Viagem e Aspectos da Medicina Soviética*. Rio de Janeiro, Brazil: Vitória, 1955.

Lopez, Iris. *Matters of Choice: Puerto Rican Women's Struggle for Reproductive Freedom*. New Brunswick, NJ: Rutgers University Press, 2008.

López Orozco, Leticia, Mauricio César Ramírez Sánchez, and Dafne Cruz Porchini. "Siqueiros y la Victoria de la Medicina sobre el Cáncer." *Crónicas Revista UNAM* 10–11 (2006): 73–98.

Lora, Guillermo. *A History of the Bolivian Labour Movement*. Edited and abridged by Laurence Whitehead. Translated by Christine Whitehead. Cambridge: Cambridge University Press, 1977.

"Lou Stoumen Is Dead: Photographer Was 75." *New York Times*, October 9, 1991.

Loureiro, Felipe Pereira. "The Alliance for Progress and President João Goulart's Three-Year Plan: The Deterioration of U.S.-Brazilian Relations in Cold War Brazil (1962)." *Cold War History* 17, 1 (2017): 61–79.

Loveman, Brian. *For La Patria: Politics and the Armed Forces in Latin America*. Wilmington, DE: SR, 1999.

Lowen, Rebecca. *Creating the Cold War University: The Transformation of Stanford*. Berkeley: University of California Press, 1997.

Luykx, Aurolyn. *The Citizen Factory: Schooling and Cultural Production in Bolivia*. Albany: State University of New York Press, 1999.

"MacArthur and National Purpose." *Fortune*, May 1951.

Macdonald, Dwight, and Francis Sutton. *The Ford Foundation: The Men and the Millions*. New Brunswick, NJ: Transaction, 2011.

Macekura, Stephen, and Erez Manela, eds. *The Development Century: A Global History*. Cambridge: Cambridge University Press, 2018.

Maguiña, Ciro. *Ser Médico en el Perú: Vivencias y Algo Más*. Huaraz, Peru: Dijaes, 2005.

Mahmood, Qamar, and Carles Muntaner. "Politics, Class Actors, and Health Sector Reform in Brazil and Venezuela." *Global Health Promotion* 20, 1 (2013): 59–67.

Mahmood, Qamar, Carles Muntaner, Rosicar del Valle Mata León, and Ramón Ernesto Perdomo. "Popular Participation in Venezuela's Barrio Adentro Health Reform." *Globalizations* 9, 6 (2012): 815–33.

Maio, Marcos Chor. "O Contraponto Paulista: Florestan Fernandes, Oracy Nogueira e o Projeto Unesco de Relações Raciais." *Antíteses* 7, 13 (2014): 10–39.

Maio, Marcos Chor. "O Projeto Unesco e a Agenda das Ciências Sociais no Brasil dos Anos 40 e 50." *Revista Brasileira de Ciências Sociais* 14, 41 (1999): 141–58.

Maio Marcos Chor, and Magali Romero Sá. "Ciência na Periferia: A Unesco, a Proposta de Criação do Instituto Internacional da Hiléia Amazônica e as Origens do Inpa." *História Ciências Saúde-Manguinhos* 6 (2000): 975–1017.

Maio, Marcos Chor, and Ricardo Ventura Santos. "Antiracism and the Uses of Science in the Post–World War II: An Analysis of UNESCO's First Statements on Race (1950 and 1951)." *Vibrant: Virtual Brazilian Anthropology* 12, 2 (2015): 1–26.

Makari, George. *The Revolution in Mind: The Creation of Psychoanalysis*. New York: HarperCollins, 2008.

Maldonado Denis, Manuel. *Puerto Rico: Una Interpretación Histórico-Social*. Mexico City: Siglo XXI, 1969.

Malloy, James M. *Bolivia: The Uncompleted Revolution*. Pittsburgh: University of Pittsburgh Press, 1970.

Manela, Erez. "A Pox on Your Narrative: Writing Disease Control into Cold War History." *Diplomatic History* 34, 2 (2010): 299–323.

Manke, Albert, Kateřina Březinová, and Laurin Blecha. "Conceptual Readings into the Cold War: Towards Transnational Approaches from the Perspective of Latin American Studies in Eastern and Western Europe." *Estudos Históricos (Rio de Janeiro)* 30, 60 (2017): 203–18.

Manríquez, Germán. "Professor Max Westenhöfer (1871–1957) in Chile." *Revista Médica de Chile* 123, 10 (1995): 1313–17.

Manzano, Valeria. *The Age of Youth in Argentina: Culture, Politics, and Sexuality from Perón to Videla*. Chapel Hill: University of North Carolina Press, 2014.

Mao Zedong. *Obras Escogidas I*. Buenos Aires, Argentina: Rosa Blindada, 1973.

Marcuse, Herbert. *Eros and Civilization: A Philosophical Inquiry into Freud*. Boston: Beacon Press, 1974.

Mardones Restat, Francisco, and Antonio Carlos de Azevedo. "The Essential Health Reform in Chile: A Reflection on the 1952 Process." *Salud Pública de México* 48, 6 (2006): 504–11.

Margulies, Sylvia R. *The Pilgrimage to Russia; the Soviet Union and the Treatment of Foreigners, 1924–1937*. Madison: University of Wisconsin Press, 1968.

Marinho, Maria Gabriela. *Norte-Americanos no Brasil: Uma História da Fundação Rockefeller na Universidade de São Paulo (1934–1952)*. São Paulo, Brazil: Fapesp-Autores Associados–Universidade de São Francisco, 2001.

Marks, Lara. *Sexual Chemistry: A History of the Contraceptive Pill*. New Haven, CT: Yale University Press, 2001.

Marks, Sarah, and Mat Savelli. "Communist Europe and Transnational Psychiatry." In *Psychiatry in Communist Europe*, edited by Mat Savelli and Sarah Marks, 7–10. London: Palgrave Macmillan, 2015.

Marmor, Theodore. "The Right to Health Care: Reflections on Its History and Politics." In *Rights to Health Care*, edited by Thomas Bole III and William Bondeson, 23–49. Norwell, MA: Kluwer Academic, 1991.

Marqués, René. *El Puertorriqueño Dócil*. Barcelona, Spain: Antillana, 1967.

Marques, Rita C. "A Filantropia Científica nos Tempos da Romanização: A Fundação Rockefeller em Minas Gerais (1916–1928)." *Horizontes* 22, 2 (2004): 175–89.

Marqués de Armas, Pedro. *Ciencia y Poder en Cuba: Racismo, Homofobia, Nación (1790–1970)*. Madrid: Verbum, 2014.

Martín-Baro, Ignacio. "Hacia una Psicología de la Liberación." *Boletín de Psicología* 22 (1986): 219–31.

Martínez, Jorge. *Situación y Tendencias de la Migración Internacional en Chile*. Accessed December 23, 2019. https://repositorio.cepal.org/bitstream/handle/11362/7388/S9700062_es.pdf?sequence=1&isAllowed=y.

Mateos, Gisela, and Edna Suárez-Díaz. "'We Are Not a Rich Country to Waste Our Resources on Expensive Toys': Mexico's Version of Atoms for Peace." *History and Technology* 31, 3 (2015): 243–58.

Mauldin, W. Parker, Nazli Choucri, Frank Notestein, and Michael Teitelbaum. "A Report on Bucharest." *Studies in Family Planning* 5, 12 (1974): 357–95.

Mayer, David. "À la fois influente et marginale: L'Internationale Communiste et l'Amérique Latine." *Monde(s)* 2, 10 (2016): 109–28.

McMahon, Robert J. *The Cold War in the Third World*. New York: Oxford University Press, 2013.

McSherry, J. Patrice. *Incomplete Transition: Military Power and Democracy in Argentina*. New York: St. Martin's, 1997.

Medeiros, Maurício de. *Rússia: Notas de Viagem, Impressões, Entrevistas, Observações sobre o Regimen Sovietico*. Rio de Janeiro, Brazil: Calvino, 1931.

Medina, Eden. *Cybernetic Revolutionaries: Technology and Politics in Allende's Chile*. Cambridge, MA: MIT Press, 2011.

Meisler, Stanley. "Argument over Role of CIA in Mexico Reveals Feelings of Annoyance at U.S." *Los Angeles Times*, March 22, 1975.

Mello, Guilherme Arantes. "Pensamento Clássico da Saúde Pública Paulista na Era dos Centros de Saúde e Educação Sanitária." *Revista de Saúde Pública* 46 (2012): 747–50.

Méndez, José Luis. *Las Ciencias Sociales y el Proceso Político Puertorriqueño*. San Juan, PR: Puerto, 2005.

Mendizábal Lozano, Gregorio. *Historia de la Salud Pública en Bolivia: De las Juntas de Sanidad a los Directorios Locales de Salud*. La Paz, Bolivia: Prisa, 2002.

Metzi, Francisco. *Por los Caminos de Chaletenango con la Salud en la Mochila*. San Salvador, El Salvador: UCA, 2003.

"Mexican Hormones." *Fortune*, May 1951.

"México Expulsa a 40 Extranjeros Agitadores de los Disturbios." *Excelsior*, September 12, 1958.

Michaels, Paula A. *Lamaze: An International History*. New York: Oxford University Press, 2014.

Mikkonen, Simo, and Pia Koivunen, eds. *Beyond the Divide: Entangled Histories of the Cold War*. New York: Berghahn, 2015.

Milanich, Nara B. *Children of Fate: Childhood, Class, and the State in Chile, 1850-1930*. Durham, NC: Duke University Press, 2009.

Miller, Francesca. *Latin American Women and the Search for Social Justice*. Hanover, NH: University Press of New England, 1991.

Miller, Martin. *Freud and the Bolsheviks: Psychoanalysis in Imperial Russia and the Soviet Union*. New Haven, CT: Yale University Press, 1998.

Mintz, Sidney. "The People of Puerto Rico Half a Century Later: One Author's Recollections." *Journal of Latin American Anthropology* 6, 2 (2001): 74–83.

Miranda, Mario G. *La Educación y Servicios Médicos en la Unión Soviética*. San José: Universidad de Costa Rica, 1964.

Mitchell, Sean T. *Constellations of Inequality: Space, Race, and Utopia in Brazil*. Chicago: University of Chicago Press, 2018.

Moffatt, Alfredo. *Psicoterapia del Oprimido: Ideología y Técnica de la Psiquiatría Popular*. Buenos Aires, Argentina: Humanitas, 1974.

Molina, Carlos. "Antecedentes del Servicio Nacional de Salud: Historia de Debates y Contradicciones, 1932-1952." *Cuadernos Médico Sociales* 46, 2 (2006): 284-304.

Molina, Carlos. *Institucionalidad Sanitaria Chilena 1889-1989*. Santiago, Chile: LOM, 2010.

Molina, Carlos. "Orígenes de la Asociación Médica de Chile: Una Mirada Crítica." *Polis* 12 (2005). https://journals.openedition.org/polis/5663.

Monckeberg, María Olivia. *El Imperio del Opus Dei en Chile*. Santiago: Penguin Random House, Grupo Editorial Chile, 2016.

Montenegro, Antônio T. "Ligas Camponesas e Sindicatos Rurais em Tempo de Revolução." In *O Brasil Republicano: O Tempo da Experiência Democrática (1945-1964)*, edited by Jorge Ferreira and Lucilia A. N. Delgado, 241-71. Rio de Janeiro: Civilização Brasileira, 2003.

Mor, Jessica Stites. *Human Rights and Transnational Solidarity in Cold War Latin America*. Madison: University of Wisconsin Press, 2013.

Morley, Jefferson. *Our Man in Mexico: Winston Scott and the Hidden History of the CIA*. Lawrence: University Press of Kansas, 2008.

Morley, Morris. *Washington, Somoza, and the Sandinistas: State and Regime in U.S. Policy Toward Nicaragua, 1969-1981*. New York: Cambridge University Press, 1994.

Morris, James Oliver. *Elites, Intellectuals, and Consensus: A Study of the Social Question and the Industrial Relations System in Chile*. Ithaca: New York State School of Industrial and Labor Relations, Cornell University, 1966.

Motta, Rodrigo Patto Sá. *As Universidades e o Regime Militar: Cultura Política Brasileira e Modernização Autoritária*. Rio de Janeiro, Brazil: Jorge Zahar Editor, 2014.

Mueller, Tim B. "The Rockefeller Foundation, the Social Sciences, and the Humanities in the Cold War." *Journal of Cold War Studies* 15, 3 (2013): 108-35.

Musto, Ryan. "'A Desire So Close to the Hearts of all Latin Americans': Utopian Ideals and Imperfections behind Latin America's Nuclear Weapon Free Zone." *Bulletin of Latin American Research* 37, 2 (2018): 160–74.

Nair, Rahul. "The Construction of a 'Population Problem' in Colonial India 1919–1947." *Journal of Imperial and Commonwealth History* 39, 2 (2011): 227–47.

Namikas, Lise. *Battleground Africa: Cold War in the Congo, 1960–1965.* Stanford, CA: Stanford University Press, 2012.

National Security Archive. "Interview with E. Howard Hunt." Accessed March 4, 2019. http://www.gwu.edu/~nsarchiv/coldwar/interviews/episode-18/hunt1.html.

Necochea López, Raúl. "Gambling on the Protestants: The Pathfinder Fund and Birth Control in Peru, 1958–1965." *Bulletin of the History of Medicine* 88, 2 (2014): 344–71.

Necochea López, Raúl. *A History of Family Planning in Twentieth-Century Peru.* Chapel Hill: University of North Carolina Press, 2014.

Needell, Allan A. *Science, Cold War and the American State: Lloyd V. Berkner and the Balance of Professional Ideals.* Amsterdam: Harwood Academic, 2000.

Nelson, Erica. "Birth Rights: Bolivia's Politics of Race, Region, and Motherhood, 1964–2005." PhD diss., University of Wisconsin–Madison, 2009.

Nervi, Laura. "Alma Ata y la Renovación de la Atención Primaria de la Salud." Paper presented at Encuentro Regional, Retos para la Revitalización de la APS en las Américas, La Palma, El Salvador, September 22–25, 2008.

Nicogossian, Arnauld E. *The Apollo-Soyuz Test Project Medical Report.* Washington, DC: NASA, 1977.

Nieves Falcón, Luis. "Puerto Rico: A Case Study of Transcultural Application of Behavioral Science." *Caribbean Studies* 10, 4 (1971): 5–17.

Nogueira Rivero, Gerardo. "Psicoterapia y Principales Escuelas Psicológicas." *Revista del Hospital Psiquiátrico de la Habana* 13, 1 (1977): 83–85.

North, Liisa, Timothy David Clark, and Viviana Patroni, eds. *Community Rights and Corporate Responsibility: Canadian Mining and Oil Companies in Latin America.* Toronto: Between the Lines, 2006.

"Nossa Política: As Resoluções de Viena, Instrumento de Luta pela Paz e a Independência Nacional." *Problemas—Revista Mensal de Cultura Política* 44 (January–February 1953): n.p.

"Notas." *Caribbean Business*, September 25, 2003.

Núñez, Manuel, Clemente Justiniano Barbery, Luis Álvarez, Claudio Román, Verónica Bustos, Michèlle Guillou, Luis Carlos Ortiz, Hernando Cubides, Iván Palacios, Mabel Pinto, Hernán García, Raúl Suárez, Pedro Díaz, Wilder Carpio, Donatila Ávila, Oswaldo Salaverry, Domingo Khan, Ricardo Cañizares Fuentes, Caroline Chang, Hernán Sepúlveda, Norbert Dreesch, Myriam Gamboa, Hugo Rivera, Osvaldo Salgado, and Cristina Merino. "Política Andina de Planificación y Gestión de Recursos Humanos en Salud." *Anales de la Facultad de Medicina* 76 (2015): 27–33.

Nussenzweig, Ruth, and Victor Nussenzweig. "Cura do Câncer, Doença de Chagas e o Camarada Stalin." *Ciência Hoje* 33, 193 (2003): 59–63.

O'Brien, Neil. *An American Editor in Early Revolutionary China: John William Powell and the China Weekly/Monthly Review.* New York: Routledge, 2003.

O'Brien, Thomas F. *Making the Americas: The United States and Latin America from the Age of Revolutions to the Era of Globalization*. Albuquerque: University of New Mexico Press, 2007.

Observatory of Economic Complexity. "Venezuela." Accessed April 22, 2019. https://atlas.media.mit.edu/en/profile/country/ven/.

Oliveira, Nilo Dias de. "A Vigilância do DOPS-SP: Vigia-se Tudo e Todos." *História em Reflexão* 4, 7 (2010): 1–23.

Olmstead, Kathryn S. *Red Spy Queen: A Biography of Elizabeth Bentley*. Chapel Hill: University of North Carolina, 2002.

"100 Years: The Rockefeller Foundation, Mexico: Agriculture." Accessed March 1, 2019. http://rockefeller100.org/exhibits/show/agriculture/mexico.

Ordaz, Bernabé. "Editorial." *Revista del Hospital Psiquiátrico de la Habana* 4, 3 (1963): 1.

Oreskes, Naomi, and John Krige, eds. *Science and Technology in the Global Cold War*. Cambridge, MA: MIT Press, 2014.

Organización Panamericana de la Salud. *Cien Años de Cooperación al Perú, 1902–2002*. Lima: OPS, 2002.

Otero, Gerardo. "Neoliberal Globalization, NAFTA, and Migration: Mexico's Loss of Food and Labor Sovereignty." *Journal of Poverty* 15, 4 (2011): 384–402.

Otero Ojeda, Ángel Arturo. "Carlos Acosta Nodal (1921–2010)." In *Antología de Textos Clásicos de la Psiquiatría Latinoamericana*, edited by Sergio J. Villaseñor Bayardo, Carlos Rojas Malpica, and Jean Garrabé de Lara, 255. Guadalajara, Mexico: Amaya, 2011.

Pacino, Nicole. "Stimulating a Cooperative Spirit? Public Health and U.S.-Bolivia Relations in the 1950s." *Diplomatic History* 41, 2 (2018): 305–35.

Packard, Randall. *A History of Global Health: Interventions into the Lives of Other People*. Baltimore, MD: Johns Hopkins University Press, 2016.

Padilla, Tanalís, and Louise E. Walker. "In the Archives: History and Politics." *Journal of Iberian and Latin American Research* 19, 1 (2013): 1–10.

PAHO. *Renewing Primary Health Care in the Americas: A Position Paper of the Pan American Health Organization/World Health Organization*. Washington, DC: PAHO, 2007.

Paige, Jeffrey. *Coffee and Power: Revolution and the Rise of Democracy in Central America*. Cambridge, MA: Harvard University Press, 1997.

Paim, Jairnilson, Claudia Travassos, Celia Almeida, Ligia Bahia, and James Macinko. "The Brazilian Health System: History, Advances, and Challenges." *The Lancet* 377, 9779 (2011): 1778–97.

Paiva, Carlos Henrique Assunção. "Samuel Pessoa: Uma Trajetória Científica no Contexto do Sanitarismo Campanhista e Desenvolvimentista no Brasil." *História, Ciências, Saúde-Manguinhos* 13 (2006): 795–831.

"Palabras de Carolina de la Torre en el Homenaje a los Graduados de los Años 1970 y 1971." April 11, 2009. http://promociondeeventos.sld.cu/psicosalud/palabras-de-carolina-de-la-torre-en-el-homenaje-a-los-graduados-de-los-anos-1970-y-1971.

Palmer, Steven. *Launching Global Health: The Caribbean Odyssey of the Rockefeller Foundation*. Ann Arbor: University of Michigan Press, 2010.

Palmer, Steven. "Toward Responsibility in International Health: Death Following Treatment in Rockefeller Hookworm Campaigns, 1914–1934." *Medical History* 54, 2 (2010): 149–70.

Palyi, Melchior. *Compulsory Medical Care and the Welfare State: An Analysis Based on a Special Study of Governmentalized Medical Care Systems on the Continent of Europe and in England.* Chicago: National Institute of Professional Services, 1950.

Pandolfi, Dulce. *Camaradas e Companheiros: História e Memória do PCB.* Rio de Janeiro, Brazil: Relume Dumará, 1995.

Paniagua, Manuel, Henry Vaillant, and Clarence Gamble. "Field Trial of a Contraceptive Foam in Puerto Rico." *JAMA* 177, 2 (1961): 125–29.

Pantojas-García, Emilio. *Development Strategies as Ideology: Puerto Rico's Export-Led Industrialization Experience.* Boulder, CO: Rienner, 1990.

Pantojas-García, Emilio. "Puerto Rican Populism Revisited: The PPD during the 1940s." *Journal of Latin American Studies* 21, 3 (1989): 521–57.

Paraguassu, Lissandra. "Six South American Nations Suspend Membership of Anti-U.S. Bloc." Reuters, April 20, 2018. https://www.reuters.com/article/us-unasur -membership/six-south-american-nations-suspend-membership-of-anti-u-s-bloc -idUSKBN1HR2P6.

Parker, Jason. *Hearts, Minds, Voices: U.S. Cold War Public Diplomacy and the Formation of the Third World.* Oxford: Oxford University Press, 2016.

Parmar, Inderjeet. *Foundations of the American Century: The Ford, Carnegie, and Rockefeller Foundations in the Rise of American Power.* New York: Columbia University Press, 2012.

Pastor, Robert A., and Tom Long. "The Cold War and Its Aftermath in the Americas: The Search for a Synthetic Interpretation of U.S. Policy." *Latin American Research Review* 45, 3 (2010): 261–73.

Patch, Richard W. "Bolivia: The Restrained Revolution." *Annals of the American Academy of Political and Social Science* 334, 1 (1961): 123–32.

Pavilack, Jody. *Mining for the Nation: The Politics of Chile's Coal Communities from the Popular Front to the Cold War.* University Park: Pennsylvania State University Press, 2011.

Pedemonte, Rafael. "Cuba, l'URSS et le Chili dans la Guerre Froide globale, 1959–1973: Vers une 'histoire triangulaire' des relations internationales." *Bulletin de l'Institut Pierre Renouvin* 1, 45 (2017): 159–65.

Peña, Ligia. "La Salud Pública en Nicaragua y la Fundación Rockefeller, 1915–1928." *Revista de Historia* 22 (2007): 117–36.

Peña, Ligia, and Steven Palmer. "A Rockefeller Foundation Health Primer for US-Occupied Nicaragua, 1914–1928." *Canadian Bulletin of Medical History* 25, 1 (2008): 43–70.

Peña, Rodolfo, Jerker Liljestrand, Elmer Zelaya, and Lars-Åke Persson. "Fertility and Infant Mortality Trends in Nicaragua: The Role of Women's Education." *Journal of Epidemiology and Community Health* 53, 3 (1999): 132–37.

People's Health Movement, Medact, Medico International, Third World Network, Health Action International, ALAMES, and Health Poverty Action. *Global Health Watch 4: An Alternative World Health Report.* London: Zed, 2014.

Pessoa, Samuel B. *Ensaios Médico-Sociais*. Rio de Janeiro, Brazil: Guanabara Koogan, 1960.

Pessoa, Samuel B. *Ensaios Médico-Sociais*. São Paulo, Brazil: Cebes-Hucitec, 1978.

Pessoa, Samuel B. "Estudo dos Componentes de Oleo Essencial de Quenopódio: Sua Aplicação na Profilaxia da Ancilostomose." Thesis, Faculdade de Medicina e Cirurgia de São Paulo, 1922.

Pessoa, Samuel B. *Parasitologia Médica*. São Paulo, Brazil: Renascença, 1946.

Pessoa, Samuel B. *Problemas Brasileiros de Higiene Rural*. São Paulo, Brazil: Indústria Gráfica José Magalhães, 1949.

Pessoa, Samuel B. "As Verminoses na Zona Rural de S. Paulo." *Revista da Sociedade Rural Brasileira* 16, 190 (1936): 14–23.

Petitjean, Patrick, and Heloisa Maria Bertol Domingues. "Paulo Carneiro: Um Cientista Brasileiro na Diplomacia da Unesco (1946–1950)." In *Ciência, Política e Relações Internacionais: Ensaios sobre Paulo Carneiro*, edited by Marcos Chor Maio, 195–214. Rio de Janeiro, Brazil: Editora Fiocruz/Ediçoes Unesco, 2004.

Pettinà, Vanni. "¡Bienvenido Mr. Mikoyan!: Tacos y Tractores a la Sombra del Acercamiento Soviético-Mexicano, 1958–1964." *Historia Mexicana* 66, 2 (2016): 793–852.

Pettinà, Vanni. *Historia Mínima de la Guerra Fría en América Latina*. Mexico City: Colegio de México, 2018.

Pettinà, Vanni. "The Shadows of Cold War over Latin America: The U.S. Reaction to Fidel Castro's Nationalism, 1956–59." *Cold War History* 11, 3 (2011): 317–39.

Pettinà, Vanni, and José Antonio Sánchez Román. "Beyond U.S. Hegemony: The Shaping of the Cold War in Latin America." *Culture and History Digital Journal* 4, 1 (2015). http://cultureandhistory.revistas.csic.es/index.php/cultureandhistory/article/view/65/240.

Petryna, Adriana. *When Experiments Travel: Clinical Trials and the Global Search for Human Subjects*. Princeton, NJ: Princeton University Press, 2009.

Pieper Mooney, Jadwiga. *The Politics of Motherhood: Maternity and Women's Rights in Twentieth Century Chile*. Pittsburgh: University of Pittsburgh Press, 2009.

Pieper Mooney, Jadwiga, and Fabio Lanza, eds. *Decentering Cold War History: Local and Global Change*. London: Routledge, 2013.

Pino, Paulina, and Giorgio Solimano. "The School of Public Health at the University of Chile: Origins, Evolution, and Perspectives." *Public Health Reviews* 33 (2011): 315–22.

Pinto, S. C., A. Francisco, and Benjamín Viel. *Seguridad Social Chilena: Puntos para una Reforma*. Santiago, Chile: Pacífico, 1950.

Pires-Alves, Fernando A., and Marcos Chor Maio. "Health at the Dawn of Development: The Thought of Abraham Horwitz." *História, Ciências, Saúde-Manguinhos* 22 (2015): 69–93.

Pistorius, Robin. *Scientists, Plants, and Politics: A History of the Plant Genetic Resources Movement*. Rome, Italy: International Plant Genetic Resources Institute, 1997.

Plotkin, Mariano Ben. "The Diffusion of Psychoanalysis under Conditions of Political Authoritarianism." In *Psychoanalysis and Politics: Histories of Psychoanalysis under Conditions of Restricted Political Freedom*, edited by Joy Damousi and Mariano Ben Plotkin, 185–211. New York: Oxford University Press, 2012.

Plotkin, Mariano Ben. *Freud in the Pampas: The Emergence and Development of a Psychoanalytic Culture in Argentina*. Stanford, CA: Stanford University Press, 2001.

Plotkin, Mariano Ben. "José Bleger: Jew, Marxist and Psychoanalyst." *Psychoanalysis and History* 13, 2 (2011): 198–201.

Plotkin, Mariano Ben. "Psychoanalysis, Race Relations, and National Identity: The Reception of Psychoanalysis in Brazil, 1910 to 1940." In *Unconscious Dominions: Psychoanalysis, Colonial Trauma, and Global Sovereignties*, edited by Warwick Anderson, Deborah Jenson, and Richard Keller, 113–37. Durham, NC: Duke University Press, 2011.

Poleman, Thomas. *The Papaloapan Project: Agricultural Development in the Mexican Tropics*. Stanford, CA: Stanford University Press, 1964.

Poppino, Rollie E. *International Communism in Latin America: A History of the Movement, 1917–1963*. London: Free Press of Glencoe, 1964.

Population Council. *A Manual for Surveys of Fertility and Family Planning: Knowledge, Attitudes, and Practice*. New York: Population Council, 1970.

Portell Vilá, Herminio. "Politiquería y Medicina." *Bohemia* 42, 39 (1950): 51, 102–4.

Portell Vilá, Juan. "El Psicoanálisis y Su Aplicación al Estudio del Niño." *Revista Bimestre Cubana* 13 (1928): 534–41.

Porter, Cathy. *Alexandra Kollontai: A Biography*. Chicago: Haymarket, 2014.

Portugal, Ana María. "El Retorno de las Brujas." In *Movimiento Feminista en América Latina y el Caribe: Balance y Perpectivas*, 20–24. Santiago, Chile: Isis, 1986.

Portuondo, Juan. "El Diagnóstico a Través del Test de Rorschach." *Revista del Hospital Psiquiátrico de la Habana* 6, 4 (1965): 666.

Potts, Frisso. "Apuntes para una Historia de la Psicoterapia de Grupo." *Sanidad y Beneficencia Municipal* 12, 3 (1952): 65–69.

Potts, Frisso. "Factores Emocionales en los Grupos Humanos." *Sanidad y Beneficencia Municipal* 16, 1–4 (1956): 14–31.

Potts, Frisso. "Patrones de Conducta en los Grupos Terapéuticos." *Sanidad y Beneficencia Municipal* 16, 1–4 (1956): 46–52.

Power, Margaret. *Right-Wing Women in Chile: Feminine Power and the Struggle against Allende, 1964–1973*. University Park: Pennsylvania State University Press, 2002.

Power, Margaret, and Andor Skotnes, eds. *Radical History Review* 128 (2017).

Pradere, Elsa. "El Machóver como Técnica Complementaria del Diagnóstico de Rorschach." *Revista del Hospital Psiquiátrico de la Habana* 6, 3 (1965): 515.

Prashad, Vijay. *The Darker Nations: A People's History of the Third World*. New York: New Press, 2007.

Prebisch, Raúl. *The Economic Development of Latin America and Its Principal Problems*. New York: United Nations, 1950.

Prevost, Gary. "Cuba and Nicaragua: A Special Relationship?" *Latin American Perspectives* 17, 3 (1990): 120–37.

Pribilsky, Jason. "Developing Selves: Photography, Cold War Science and 'Backwards' People in the Peruvian Andes, 1951–1966." *Visual Studies* 30, 2 (2015): 131–50.

"El Psicoanálisis en la Picota." *Somos*, August 22, 1980.

"Psicoanálisis y Antiimperialismo: Plataforma Internacional." *Nuevo Hombre* 1, 6 (1971): 10.

Psicología Soviética: Selección de Artículos Científicos. Havana: Editorial Nacional de Cuba, Editora Universitaria, 1965.

Pujals, Sandra. "Una Perla en el Caribe Soviético: Puerto Rico en los Archivos de la Komintern en Moscú, 1921–1943." *Op. Cit.* 17 (2006–2007): 117–57.

Quadros, Ciro de, and Daniel Epstein. "Health as a Bridge for Peace: PAHO's Experience." *The Lancet* 360 (2002): s25–s26.

Quevedo, Emilio, Catalina Borda, Juan Carlos Eslava, Claudia García, María del Pilar Guzmán, Paola Mejía, and Carlos Noguera. *Café y Gusanos, Mosquitos y Petróleo: El Tránsito desde la Higiene hacia la Medicina Tropical y la Salud Pública en Colombia, 1873–1953.* Bogotá: Universidad Nacional de Colombia, 2004.

"500 Estudiantes en Facultad de Medicina." *La Prensa,* December 2, 1979.

Quintero Rivera, Ángel. *El Liderato Local de los Partidos y el Estudio de la Política Puertorriqueña.* Río Piedras: Universidad de Puerto Rico, Centro de Investigaciones Sociales, 1970.

Quintero Rivera, Ángel. "La Ideología Populista y la Institucionalización de las Ciencias Sociales." In *Del Nacionalismo al Populismo: Cultura y Política en Puerto Rico,* edited by Silvia Alvarez Curbelo and María Elena Rodríguez Castro, 107–45. San Juan, PR: Huracán, 1993.

Quintero Rivera, Ángel. "Luis Nieves Falcón: Maestro de la Investigación Social." 80Grados, March 12, 2014. http://www.80grados.net/luis-nieves-falcon-maestro-de -la-investigacion-social/.

Rabe, Stephen. *Eisenhower and Latin America: The Foreign Policy of Anticommunism.* Chapel Hill: University of North Carolina Press, 1988.

Rabe, Stephen. *The Killing Zone: The United States Wages Cold War in Latin America.* New York: Oxford University Press, 2016.

Raj, Kapil. *Relocating Modern Science: Circulation and the Construction of Knowledge in South Asia and Europe, 1650–1900.* Basingstoke, UK: Palgrave Macmillan, 2007.

Ramírez de Arellano, Annette, and Conrad Seipp. *Colonialism, Catholicism, and Contraception: A History of Birth Control in Puerto Rico.* Chapel Hill: University of North Carolina Press, 1983.

Ramos, Marco. "Psychiatry, Authoritarianism, and Revolution: The Politics of Mental Illness during Military Dictatorships in Argentina, 1966–1983." *Bulletin of the History of Medicine* 87, 2 (2013): 250–78.

Rasmussen, Nicholas. *On Speed: The Many Lives of Amphetamines.* New York: New York University Press, 2008.

Raymond, Edward. "US-USSR Cooperation in Medicine and Health." *Russian Review* 32, 3 (1973): 229–40.

Reagan, Ronald. "Remarks and a Question-and-Answer Session with the Students and Faculty at Moscow State University, May 31, 1988." https://www.reaganlibrary.gov /research/speeches/053188b.

Recalde, Héctor. *La Higiene y el Trabajo: 1870–1930.* Buenos Aires, Argentina: Centro Editor de América Latina, 1988.

Reece, B. Carroll. "Tax-Exempt Subversion." *American Mercury*, July 1957.

Reeves, Michelle Denise. "Extracting the Eagle's Talons: The Soviet Union in Cold War Latin America." PhD diss., University of Texas at Austin, 2014.

Reinaga, Fausto. *El Sentimiento Mesiánico del Pueblo Ruso*. La Paz, Bolivia: Sindicato de Escritores Revolucionarios, 1960.

Reinhardt, Bob. *The End of a Global Pox: America and the Eradication of Smallpox in the Cold War Era*. Chapel Hill: University of North Carolina Press, 2015.

Ribeiro, Jayme. "Os 'Combatentes da Paz': A Participação dos Comunistas Brasileiros na Campanha pela Proibição das Armas Atômicas (1950)." *Estudos Históricos* 21 (2008): 261–83.

Richardson, William. "The Dilemmas of a Communist Artist: Diego Rivera in Moscow, 1927–1928." *Mexican Studies/Estudios Mexicanos* 3, 1 (1987): 49–69.

Richardson, William Harrison. *Mexico through Russian Eyes, 1806–1940*. Pittsburgh: University of Pittsburgh Press, 1988.

Rico, José Antonio. *En los Dominios del Kremlin (8 Años y Medio en Rusia)*. Mexico City: Atlántico, 1951.

Ridenti, Marcelo S. "Brasilidade Vermelha: Artistas e Intelectuais Comunistas nos Anos 1950." In *O Moderno em Questão: A Década de 1950 no Brasil*, eds. André Bastos Botelho, Elide Rugai, and Glaucia Villas Bôas, 169–209. Rio de Janeiro, Brazil: Topbooks, 2008.

Riggirozzi, Pía, and Jean Grugel. "Políticas de Salud en UNASUR: Legitimidad, Democracia y Legitimidad de Resultado." *Pensamiento Propio* 43 (2016): 173–200.

Rivera Cusicanqui, Silvia. *Oppressed but Not Defeated: Peasant Struggles among the Aymara and Qhechwa in Bolivia, 1900–1980*. Geneva: UNRISD, 1987.

Rivera Núñez, Gregorio. "Estudio Clínico de la Angustia." *Revista del Hospital Psiquiátrico de la Habana* 8, 1 (1967): 95.

Rockefeller Foundation, *Annual Reports*. 1948, 1949, 1951–59. New York.

Rodrigues, Leôncio Martins. "O PCB: Os Dirigentes e a Organização." In *História Geral da Civilização Brasileira, O Brasil Republicano*, edited by Boris Fausto, 3:1–43. São Paulo, Brazil: Difel, 1983.

Rodríguez, Daniel. "'To Fight These Powerful Trusts and Free the Medical Profession': Medicine, Class Formation, and Revolution in Cuba, 1925–1935." *Hispanic American Historical Review* 95, 4 (2015): 595–629.

Rodríguez, Daniel. *The Right to Live in Health: Medical Politics in Postcolonial Havana*. Chapel Hill: University of North Carolina Press, forthcoming.

Rodríguez Mesa, Reina. "Recorrido Histórico de los Modelos de Psicoterapia Utilizadas [sic] en Cuba." Interpsiquis, 9º Congreso Virtual de Psiquiatría, February 2008. http://www.psiquiatria.com/bibliopsiquis/handle/10401/3939.

Rojas Mira, Claudia. "Lo Global y lo Local en los Inicios de la Planificación Familiar en Chile." *Estudios Avanzados* 2 (2009): 7–27.

Romero, Hernán. "Hitos Fundamentales de la Medicina Social en Chile." In *Medicina Social en Chile*, edited by Jorge Jiménez de la Jara, 11–18. Santiago, Chile: Aconcagua, 1977.

Romero, Hernán, E. Medina, and J. Vildósola. "Aportes al Conocimiento de la Procreación." *Revista Chilena de Higiene y Medicina Preventiva* 15, 3–4 (1953): 73–90.

Rose, Kenneth W., Erwin Levold, and Lee R. Hiltzik. "Ivan Pavlov on Communist Dogmatism and the Autonomy of Science in the Soviet Union in the Early 1920s." *Minerva* 29, 4 (1991): 463–75.

Rosemblatt, Karin. "Charity, Rights, and Entitlement: Gender, Labor, and Welfare in Early-Twentieth-Century Chile." *Hispanic American Historical Review* 81, 3–4 (2001): 555–85.

Rosselot, Jorge. "Regulación de la Natalidad en el Servicio Nacional de Salud de Chile." *Cuadernos Médico Sociales* 7, 2 (1966): 16–22.

Rosselot, Jorge. "Reseña Histórica de las Instituciones de Salud en Chile." *Cuadernos Médico Sociales* 24, 1 (1993): 7–20.

Rostow, Walt. *The Stages of Economic Growth: A Non-Communist Manifesto*. Cambridge: Cambridge University Press, 1961.

Rothwell, Matthew. *Transpacific Revolutionaries: The Chinese Revolution in Latin America*. New York: Routledge, 2012.

Rubinstein, S. L. *El Ser y la Conciencia*. Translated by Augusto Vidal Roget. Havana: Editorial Nacional de Cuba, Editora Universitaria, 1965.

Rudolph, John L. *Scientists in the Classroom: The Cold War Reconstruction of American Science Education*. New York: Palgrave, 2002.

Ruilova, Eduardo. *China Popular en America Latina*. Quito, Ecuador: ILDIS, 1978.

Ruperthuz Honorato, Mariano. "El 'Retorno de lo Reprimido': El Papel de la Sexualidad en la Recepción del Psicoanálisis en el Círculo Médico Chileno, 1910–1940." *História, Ciências, Saúde-Manguinhos* 22 (2015): 1173–97.

Rupprecht, Tobias. "Globalisation and Internationalism beyond the North Atlantic: Soviet-Brazilian Encounters and Interactions during the Cold War." In *Internationalism, Imperialism and the Formation of the Contemporary World: The Pasts of the Present*, edited by Miguel Bandeira Jerónimo and José Pedro Monteiro, 327–52. Cham, Switzerland: Palgrave Macmillan, 2018.

Rupprecht, Tobias. *Soviet Internationalism after Stalin: Interaction and Exchange between the USSR and Latin America during the Cold War*. Cambridge: Cambridge University Press, 2015.

"Russia's Industrial Expansion." *Fortune*, May 1951.

Russo, Jane A. "The Social Diffusion of Psychoanalysis during the Brazilian Military Regime: Psychological Awareness in an Age of Political Repression." In *Psychoanalysis and Politics: Histories of Psychoanalysis under Conditions of Restricted Political Freedom*, edited by Joy Damousi and Mariano Ben Plotkin, 165–84. New York: Oxford University Press, 2012.

Saavedra, Angelina. *El Espiritismo como una Religión*. Río Piedras, PR: CIS, 1970.

Sagarra, J. Solé. "La Psiquiatría en Cuba y Otros Países Socialistas. (Impresiones de un Viaje)." *Archivos de Neurobiología* 37, 6 (1974): 581.

Sagredo Acebal, Oscar. "Tratamiento Somatopsíquico de una Neurosis Obsesiva." *Sanidad y Beneficencia Municipal* 12, 3 (1952): 76–81.

Saítta, Sylvia, ed. *Hacia la Revolución: Viajeros Argentinos de Izquierda*. Buenos Aires, Argentina: Fondo de Cultura Económica, 2007.

Salinas, René. "Salud, Ideología y Desarrollo Social en Chile, 1830–1950." *Cuadernos de Historia* 3 (1983): 99–126.

Salomón Rex, Carlos. "Organización y Funcionamiento de una Unidad Sanitaria." *Revista Chilena de Higiene y Medicina Preventiva* 8, 3 (1946): 137–98.

Samsonenko, Tatyana A. *Kollektivizatsiia i Zdravookhranenie na Iuge Rossii 1930-kh gg.* Novocherkassks, Russia: IuRGTU, 2011.

Samsonenko, Tatyana A. "Staffing and Efficiency of Medical Personnel in Rural Healthcare Institutions of Don, Kuban and Stavropol Territories in the 1930s." *European Journal of Social and Human Sciences* 4, 4 (2014): 216–20.

Santos, Luiz A. Castro. "A Reforma Sanitária 'Pelo Alto': O Pioneirismo Paulista no Início do Século XX." *Dados—Revista de Ciências Sociais* 36, 3 (1993): 361–92.

Schlesinger, Stephen, and Stephen Kinzer. *Bitter Fruit: The Untold Story of the American Coup in Guatemala.* Garden City, NY: Anchor Press/Doubleday, 1983.

Schmidt, Elizabeth. *Foreign Intervention in Africa: From the Cold War to the War on Terror.* Cambridge: Cambridge University Press, 2013.

Schöpp-Schilling, Hanna, and Cees Flinterman. *Circle of Empowerment: Twenty-Five Years of the UN Committee on the Elimination of Discrimination against Women.* New York: Feminist Press, 2007.

Schoultz, Lars. *Beneath the United States: A History of U.S. Policy toward Latin America.* Cambridge, MA: Harvard University Press, 1998.

Schoultz, Lars. "Latin America." In *The Oxford Handbook of the Cold War*, edited by Richard H. Immerman and Petra Goedde, 190–210. Oxford: Oxford University Press, 2013.

Schreiber, Rebecca M. *Cold War Exiles in Mexico: U.S. Dissidents and the Culture of Critical Resistance.* Minneapolis: University of Minnesota Press, 2008.

Schuler, Friedrich E. "Mexico and the Outside World." In *The Oxford History of Mexico*, edited by Michael C. Meyer and William H. Beezley, 503–31. New York: Oxford University Press, 2000.

Secord, James A. "Knowledge in Transit." *Isis* 95, 4 (2004): 654–72.

Seda Bonilla, Eduardo. *Interacción Social y Personalidad en una Comunidad de Puerto Rico.* San Juan, PR: Juan Ponce de León, 1964.

Seda Bonilla, Eduardo. *Requiem por una Cultura.* Río Piedras, PR: Edil, 1970.

Segatto, José A. "PCB: A Questão Nacional e a Democracia." In *O Brasil Republicano*, vol. 3, *O Tempo da Experiência Democrática, da Democratização de 1945 ao Golpe Civil-Militar de 1964*, edited by Jorge Ferreira and Lucília de Almeida Neves, 217–40. Rio de Janeiro: Civilização Brasileira, 2003.

Seigel, Micol. "Beyond Compare: Comparative Method after the Transnational Turn." *Radical History Review* 91 (2005): 63–90.

"Seminario Psicoanalítico." *Diario de la Marina*, February 22, 1955.

"Sesión Ordinaria el 2 de Agosto de 1956." *Revista Archivos de Neurología y Psiquiatría* 7, 2 (1956): 53.

Shabanov, A. N. *La Enseñanza Médica en la Unión Soviética.* Havana: Páginas, 1947.

Sharpless, John. "Population Science, Private Foundations, and Development Aid: The Transformation of Demographic Knowledge in the United States, 1945-1965." In *International Development and the Social Sciences*, edited by Frederick Cooper and Randall Packard, 176–202. Berkeley: University of California Press, 1997.

Shchepin, O. P., ed. *Aktual'nye Problemy Zarubezhnogo Zdravookhranenniia.* Moscow: Minzdrav, 1978.

Shchepin, O. P. *Problemy Zdrabookhraneniia Razvivaiushchikhsia Stran (po Materialam Afrikanskogo Kontinenta).* Moscow: Meditsina, 1976.

Siddiqi, Javed. *World Health and World Politics: The World Health Organization and the UN System.* Columbia: University of South Carolina Press, 1995.

Siegel, Morris. *Un Pueblo Puertorriqueño.* Hato Rey, PR: Publicaciones Puertorriqueñas, 2005.

Siekmeier, James. *The Bolivian Revolution and the United States, 1952 to the Present.* University Park: Pennsylvania State University Press, 2011.

Siekmeier, James. "'The Most Generous Assistance': U.S. Economic Aid to Guatemala and Bolivia, 1944–1959." *Journal of American and Canadian Studies* 11 (1994): 1–46.

Siekmeier, James. "Trailblazer Diplomat: Bolivian Ambassador Víctor Andrade Uzquiano's Efforts to Influence U.S. Policy, 1944–1962." *Diplomatic History* 28, 3 (2004): 385–406;

Sigal, Silvia. *Intelectuales y Poder en Argentina: La Década del Sesenta.* Buenos Aires, Argentina: Siglo XXI, 2002.

Sigerist, Henry E. *Socialized Medicine in the Soviet Union.* New York: Norton, 1937.

Silva, Fernando Teixeira da, and Marco Aurélio Santana. "O Equilibrista e a Política: O 'Partido da Classe Operária' (PCB) na Democratização (1945–1964)." In *Nacionalismo e Reformismo Radical (1945–1965): As Esquerdas no Brasil,* edited by Jorge Ferreira and Daniel Aarão Reis, 2:103–40. Rio de Janeiro: Civilização Brasileira, 2007.

Silva, Raul Ribeiro da. *A Rússia Vista por um Médico Brasileiro.* Rio de Janeiro: Civilização Brasileira, [1953?].

Silvestrini, Blanca. *Los Trabajadores Puertorriqueños y el Partido Socialista, 1932–1940.* Río Piedras, PR: Universitaria, 1978.

Sinke, Suzanne M. *Dutch Immigrant Women in the United States, 1880–1920.* Urbana: University of Illinois Press, 2002.

Sivasundaram, Sujit. "Sciences and the Global: On Methods, Questions, and Theory." *Isis* 101, 1 (2010): 146–58.

Smillie, W. G., and S. B. Pessoa. "Treatment of Hookworm Disease with a Mixture of Carbon Tetrachloride and Ascaridol." *American Journal of Tropical Medicine* 5, 1 (1925): 71–80.

Smith, Arthur K., Jr. "Mexico and the Cuban Revolution: Foreign Policy–Making in Mexico under President Adolfo López Mateos (1958–1964)." PhD diss., Cornell University, 1970.

Smith, Christian. *Resisting Reagan: The U.S. Central America Peace Movement.* Chicago: University of Chicago Press, 1996.

Solomon, Susan Gross, ed. *Doing Medicine Together: Germany and Russia between the Wars.* Toronto: University of Toronto Press, 2006.

Solomon, Susan Gross. "The Perils of Unconstrained Enthusiasm: John Kingsbury, Soviet Public Health, and 1930s America." In *Comrades in Health: U.S. Health Internationalists, Abroad and at Home,* edited by Anne-Emanuelle Birn and Theodore M. Brown, 45–64. New Brunswick, NJ: Rutgers University Press, 2013.

Solomon, Susan Gross. "Thinking Internationally, Acting Locally: Soviet Public Health as Cultural Diplomacy in the 1920s." In *Russian and Soviet Health Care from an International Perspective: Comparing Professions, Practice and Gender, 1880–1960*, ed. Susan Grant, 193–216. Cham, Switzerland: Palgrave Macmillan, 2017.

Solomon, Susan Gross, and Nikolai Krementsov. "Giving and Taking across Borders: The Rockefeller Foundation and Russia, 1919–1928." *Minerva* 39, 3 (2001): 265–98.

Solomon, Susan Gross, Lion Murard, and Patrick Zylberman, eds. *Shifting Boundaries of Public Health: Europe in the Twentieth Century*. Rochester, NY: University of Rochester Press, 2008.

Solovey, Mark. "Project Camelot and the 1960s Epistemological Revolution: Rethinking the Politics-Patronage-Social Science Nexus." *Social Studies of Science* 31, 2 (2001): 171–206.

Solovey, Mark. "Science and the State during the Cold War: Blurred Boundaries and a Contested Legacy." *Social Studies of Science* 31, 2 (2001): 165–70.

Solovey, Mark. *Shaky Foundations: The Politics-Patronage-Social Science Nexus in Cold War America*. New Brunswick, NJ: Rutgers University Press, 2013.

Solovey, Mark, and Hamilton Cravens, eds. *Cold War Social Science: Knowledge Production, Liberal Democracy and Human Nature*. New York: Palgrave Macmillan, 2012.

Sorhegui, Roberto. "Algunas Correlaciones Psicoanalítico-Físicas en la Estructuración de la Personalidad." *Revista Archivos de Neurología y Psiquiatría* 10, 4 (1960): 226.

Soto Laveaga, Gabriela. "Bringing the Revolution to Medical Schools: Social Service and a Rural Health Emphasis in 1930s Mexico." *Estudios Mexicanos/Mexican Studies* 29, 2 (2013): 397–427.

Soto Laveaga, Gabriela. "Building the Nation of the Future, One Waiting Room at a Time: Hospital Murals in the Making of Modern Mexico." *History and Technology* 31, 3 (2015): 275–94.

Soto Laveaga, Gabriela. *Jungle Laboratories: Mexican Peasants, National Projects, and the Making of the Pill*. Durham, NC: Duke University Press, 2009.

Soto Laveaga, Gabriela. "*Largo Dislocare*: Connecting Microhistories to Remap and Recenter Histories of Science." *History and Technology* 34, 1 (2018): 21–30.

Soto Laveaga, Gabriela. "Medicamentos Milagrosos: Embajadas y Enfermedades en el México de la Guerra Fría." In *Aproximaciones a lo Local y lo Global: América Latina en la Historia de la Ciencia Contemporanea*, edited by Gisela Mateos and Edna Suárez-Díaz, 243–67. Mexico City: UNAM, 2016.

Souza, Letícia Pumar Alves de. "Between National and International Science and Education: Miguel Ozório de Almeida and the League of Nations' Intellectual Co-operation Project." In *Beyond Geopolitics: New Histories of Latin America at the League of Nations*, edited by Alan McPherson and Yannick Wehrli, 169–84. Albuquerque: University of New Mexico Press, 2015.

Spenser, Daniela, ed. *Espejos de la Guerra Fría: México, América Central y el Caribe*. Mexico City: Ciesas/Porrua, 2004.

Spenser, Daniela. *Impossible Triangle: Mexico, Soviet Russia, and the United States in the 1920s*. Durham, NC: Duke University Press, 1999.

Starks, Tricia. *The Body Soviet: Propaganda, Hygiene, and the Revolutionary State*. Madison: University of Wisconsin Press, 2008.

Starr, Paul. *The Social Transformation of American Medicine: The Rise of a Sovereign Profession and the Making of a Vast Industry*. New York: Basic Books, 1982.

Stein, Stanley, and Barbara Stein. *The Colonial Heritage of Latin America: Essays on Economic Dependence in Perspective*. New York: Oxford University Press, 1970.

Stepan, Nancy Leys. *Eradication: Ridding the World of Diseases Forever?* London: Reaktion, 2013.

Stern, Alexandra. *Eugenic Nation: Faults and Frontiers of Better Breeding in Modern America*. Berkeley: University of California Press, 2016.

Stern, Steve. *Battling for Hearts and Minds: Memory Struggles in Pinochet's Chile, 1973–1988*. Durham, NC: Duke University Press, 2006.

Sternbach, Nancy Saporta, Marysa Navarro-Aranguren, Patricia Chuchryk, and Sonia Alvarez. "Feminisms in Latin America: From Bogotá to San Bernardo." *Signs* 17, 2 (1992): 393–434.

Sternsher, Bernard. *Rexford Tugwell and the New Deal*. New Brunswick, NJ: Rutgers University Press, 1964.

Steward, Julian, Robert Manners, Eric Wolf, Elena Padilla, Sidney Mintz, and Raymond Scheele. *The People of Puerto Rico: A Study in Social Anthropology*. Urbana: University of Illinois Press, 1956.

Stites, Richard. *Revolutionary Dreams: Utopian Vision and Experimental Life in the Russian Revolution*. New York: Oxford University Press, 1988.

Studer, Brigitte. "Le voyage en URSS et son 'retour.'" *Le Mouvement Social* 4, 205 (2003): 3–8.

Stycos, Joseph. *Family and Fertility in Puerto Rico: A Study of the Lower Income Group*. New York: Columbia University Press, 1955.

Stycos, Joseph. "Further Observations on the Recruitment and Training of Interviewers in Other Cultures." *Public Opinion Quarterly* 19, 1 (1955): 68–78.

Stycos, Joseph. *Human Fertility in Latin America: Sociological Perspectives*. Ithaca, NY: Cornell University Press, 1968.

Stycos, Joseph. "Interviewer Training in Another Culture." *Public Opinion Quarterly* 16, 2 (1952): 236–46.

Stycos, Joseph, and Reuben Hill. "The Prospects of Birth Control in Puerto Rico." *Annals of the American Academy of Political and Social Science* 285 (1953): 137–44

Suárez-Díaz, Edna. "Indigenous Populations in Mexico: Medical Anthropology in the Work of Rubén Lisker in the 1960s." *Studies in History and Philosophy of Biological and Biomedical Sciences* 47 (2014): 108–17.

Suárez-Díaz, Edna. "The Molecular Basis of Evolution and Disease: A Cold War Alliance." *Journal of the History of Biology* 52, 2 (2017): 325–46.

Szreter, Simon. "The Idea of Demographic Transition and the Study of Fertility Change: A Critical Intellectual History." *Population and Development Review* 19, 4 (1993): 659–701.

Taffet, Jeffrey. *Foreign Aid as Foreign Policy: The Alliance for Progress in Latin America*. New York: Routledge, 2007.

Taiana, Cecilia. "Transatlantic Migration of the Disciplines of the Mind: Examination of the Reception of Wundt's and Freud's Theories in Argentina." In *Internationaliz-*

ing the History of Psychology, edited by Adrian C. Brock, 34–55. New York: New York University Press, 2006.

Tajer, Débora. "Latin American Social Medicine: Roots, Development during the 1990s, and Current Challenges." American Journal of Public Health 93, 12 (2003): 2023–27.

Tamagno, Carla, and Norma Velásquez. "Dinámicas de las Asociaciones Chinas en Perú: Hacia una Caracterización y Tipología." Migración y Desarrollo 14, 26 (2016): 145–66.

Tedeschi, Sara, Theodore Brown, and Elizabeth Fee. "Salvador Allende: Physician, Socialist, Populist, and President." American Journal of Public Health 93, 12 (2003): 2014–15.

Terry, Michael, and Laura Turiano. "Brigadistas and Revolutionaries: Health and Social Justice in El Salvador." In Comrades in Health: U.S. Health Internationalists, Abroad and at Home, edited by Anne-Emanuelle Birn and Theodore Brown, 221–37. New Brunswick, NJ: Rutgers University Press, 2013.

Testa, Mario. "¿Atención Primaria o Primitiva? de Salud." In Pensar en Salud, 125–37. Buenos Aires, Argentina: Organización Panamericana de la Salud, 1989.

Tobbell, Dominique A. Pills, Power, and Policy: The Struggle for Drug Reform in Cold War America and Its Consequences. Berkeley: University of California Press, 2012.

Tobbell, Dominique A. "'Who's Winning the Human Race?' Cold War as Pharmaceutical Political Strategy." Journal of the History of Medicine and Allied Sciences 64, 4 (2009): 429–73.

Todes, Daniel. Pavlov's Physiology Factory: Experiment, Interpretation, Laboratory. Baltimore, MD: Johns Hopkins University Press, 2002.

"Torres Bodet in Warning." New York Times, November 5, 1952.

Tôrres, Raquel Mundim. "O Inferno e o Paraíso se Confundem: Viagens de Brasileiros à URSS (1928–1933)." Master's thesis, Universidade Estadual de Campinas, 2013.

Tôrres, Raquel Mundim. "Relatos de Viagem de Brasileiros à URSS na Guerra Fria: Por uma Tipologia Possível (1950–1963)." In Anais do XXIX Simpósio Nacional de História, 2017. https://www.snh2017.anpuh.org/resources/anais/54/1502852280_ARQUIVO_R elatosdeviagemdebrasileirosaURSSnaGuerraFria.pdf.

Tôrres, Raquel Mundim. "Visões do 'Extraordinário': O Cotidiano Soviético aos Olhares de Viajantes Brasileiros no Primeiro Plano Quinquenal (1929–1933)." In Anais do XXVI Simpósio Nacional de História 2011, 1–18. São Paulo: ANPUH, 2011.

Torres-Goitia Torres, Javier. "Visión Médica y Sanitaria de China." Boletín Médico 3, 28 (1959): 21–25.

Torres-Goitia Torres, Javier, Javier Torres-Goitia Caballero, and Mario Lagrava Burgoa. La Salud como Derecho: Conquista y Evolución en Bolivia. La Paz, Bolivia: Plural, 2015.

Torroella, Gustavo. "Estado de la Psicometría en la URSS." Revista del Hospital Psiquiátrico de la Habana 9, 2 (1968): 297.

Torroella, Gustavo. "Situación Actual de las Pruebas o Exámenes Psicológicos en los Países Socialistas." Revista del Hospital Psiquiátrico de la Habana 8, 3 (1967): 436.

Totton, Nick. The Politics of Psychotherapy: New Perspectives. London: McGraw-Hill Education, 2006.

Tournès, Ludovic, and Giles Scott-Smith, eds. *Global Exchanges: Scholarships and Transnational Circulations in the Modern World*. New York: Berghahn, 2017.

"Town Topics." *Excelsior*, September 9, 1958.

Triana Noa, Pedro. "Diego González Martín y las Raíces de la Psicología Marxista Leninista en Cuba." *Revista Cubana de Psicología* 9, 3 (1992): 213–22.

Truman, Harry S. *Strictly Personal and Confidential: The Letters Harry Truman Never Mailed*. Edited by Monte M. Poen. Boston: Little, Brown, 1982.

Tugwell, Rexford. *The Stricken Land: The Story of Puerto Rico*. New York: Praeger, 1968.

Twigg, Judyth, ed. *Russia's Emerging Global Health Leadership*. Washington, DC: Center for Strategic and International Studies, 2012.

UN General Assembly. "Treaty on the Prohibition of Nuclear Weapons." Accessed July 7, 2017. http://undocs.org/A/CONF.229/2017/8.

Urquidi Morales, Arturo. *El Feudalismo en América y la Reforma Agraria Boliviana*. Cochabamba, Bolivia: Los Amigos del Libro, 1966.

Urquidi Morales, Arturo. *Labor Universitaria*. Cochabamba, Bolivia: Imprenta Universitaria, 1955.

U.S. Congress. *Hearings before the Committee on Un-American Activities House of Representatives, June 27 and 28, 1955*. Washington DC: U.S. Government Printing Office, 1955.

U.S. Congress. *Tax-Exempt Foundations: Hearings before the Select Committee to Investigate Tax-Exempt Foundations and Comparable Organizations, House of Representatives, 82nd Congress, 2nd sess., on H.Res. 561, November 18–21, 24–25, December 2–3, 5–11, 15, 22–23, and 30, 1952*. Washington, DC: U.S. Government Printing Office, 1953.

"U.S.-Cuba Health and Science Cooperation: They Persisted." *MEDICC Review* 20, 2 (2018): 1–5.

U.S. Department of Justice, Federal Bureau of Investigation. "A Brief History." Accessed March 1, 2019. http://www.fbi.gov/about-us/history/brief-history.

U.S. Department of State. *Foreign Relations of the United States, 1955–1957*. Vol. 7, *American Republics: Central and South America, 1955–1957*. Washington, DC: Government Printing Office, 1988.

U.S. House of Representatives, History, Art and Archives. "Puerto Rico." Accessed June 22, 2017. http://history.house.gov/Exhibitions-and-Publications/HAIC/Historical-Essays/Foreign-Domestic/Puerto-Rico/.

U.S.-Soviet Cooperation in Space. Washington, DC: U.S. Congress, Office of Technology Assessment, 1985.

Valcárcel, Gustavo. *Medio Siglo de Revolución Invencible: Segunda Parte de "Reportaje al Futuro."* Lima, Peru: Unidad, 1967.

Valcárcel, Gustavo. *Reportaje al Futuro: Crónicas de un Viaje a la URSS*. Lima: Perú Nuevo, 1963.

Valdivia Ortiz de Zárate, Verónica. *La Milicia Republicana: Los Civiles en Armas, 1932–1936*. Santiago, Chile: Dirección de Bibliotecas, Archivos y Museos, 1992.

Valenstein, Elliot. *Great and Desperate Cures: The Rise and Decline of Psychosurgery and Other Radical Treatments for Mental Illness*. New York: Basic Books, 1986.

Varas, Augusto. *Documento de Trabajo Programa*. Santiago, Chile: FLACSO, 1984.

Varela, Alfredo. *Un Periodista Argentino en la Unión Soviética*. Buenos Aires, Argentina: Viento, 1950.

Vargha, Dóra. "A Forgotten Episode of International Health." History of Medicine in Ireland, March 13, 2017. https://historyofmedicineinireland.blogspot.ca/2017/03/a -forgotten-episode-of-international.html.

Vargha, Dóra. *Polio across the Iron Curtain: Hungary's Cold War with an Epidemic*. Cambridge: Cambridge University Press, 2018.

Vargha, Dóra. "The Roots of Socialist International Health: View from Eastern Europe." Paper presented at the annual meeting of the American Association for the History of Medicine, Los Angeles, May 10–13, 2018.

Vargha, Dóra. "The Socialist World in Global Polio Eradication." *Revue d'Études Comparatives Est-Ouest* 49, 1 (2018): 71–94.

Vargas, Carlos, Cristina Sarmento, and Patricia Oliveira. "Cultural Networks between Portugal and Brazil: A Postcolonial Review." *International Journal of Cultural Policy* 23, 3 (2017): 300–311.

Vargas, Virginia. "Los Feminismos Peruanos: Breve Balance de Tres Décadas." In *25 Años de Feminismo en el Perú: Historia, Confluencias y Perspectivas*, edited by Gaby Cevasco, 15–28. Lima, Peru: Flora Tristán, 2005.

Vargas Cariola, Juan Eduardo. "Los Médicos, entre la Clientela Particular y los Empleos del Estado (1870–1951)." *Boletín de la Academia Chilena de Historia* III (2002): 133–65.

Vargas Catalá, Nelson. *Historia de la Pediatría Chilena: Crónica de una Alegría*. Santiago, Chile: Editorial Universitaria, 2002.

Vatlin, Aleksandr. *Komintern: Idei, Resheniia, Sud'by*. Moscow: Rosspen, 2009.

Vaughan, Mary Kay. "Nationalizing the Countryside: Schools and Rural Communities in Mexico in the 1930s." In *The Eagle and the Virgin: Nation and Cultural Revolution in Mexico*, edited by Mary Kay Vaughan and Stephen Lewis, 157–75. Durham, NC: Duke University Press, 2006.

Vázquez Calzada, José. *La Población de Puerto Rico y Su Trayectoria Histórica*. Río Piedras: Escuela Graduada de Salud Pública, Recinto de Ciencias Médicas, Universidad de Puerto Rico, 1988.

Venediktov, D. D. *Mezhdunarodnye Problemy Zdravookhraneniia*. Moscow: Meditsina, 1977.

Venegas Valdebenito, Hernán. "Anticomunismo y Control Social en Chile: La Experiencia de los Trabajadores del Carbón en Lota y Coronel a Mediados del siglo XX." *Revista de Historia Social y de las Mentalidades* 16, 2 (2012): 79–106.

Venegas Valdebenito, Hernán. "La 'Ley Maldita': El Parlamento Chileno y sus Planteamientos frente a la Exclusión del Partido Comunista de Chile." In *Fragmentos de una Historia: El Partido Comunista de Chile en el Siglo XX, Democratización, Clandestinidad, Rebelión, 1912–1994*, edited by Rolando Alvarez Vallejos, Augusto Samaniego M., and Hernán Venegas Delgado, 117–34. Santiago, Chile: ICAL, 2008.

Verbitsky, B., et al., eds. *Israel: Un Tema para la Izquierda*. Buenos Aires, Argentina: Nueva Sion, 1968.

Vezzetti, Hugo. *Aventuras de Freud en el País de los Argentinos*. Buenos Aires, Argentina: Paidós, 1996.

Vezzetti, Hugo. "Psicoanálisis y Revolución: Vieja y Nueva Izquierda en las Fracturas del Psicoanálisis en los Setenta." In *Política y Violencia: Lucha Armada en la Argentina*, 58–78. Buenos Aires, Argentina: Ejercitar la Memoria Editores, 2011.

Vezzetti, Hugo, and Guillermo Pecheny. "Standard Electric: Trabajo y Represión." *Los Libros* 37 (1974): 3–6.

Victorov, I. T. "Análisis de las Bases Teóricas del Freudismo." *Revista del Hospital Psiquiátrico de la Habana* 4, 3 (1963): 485–88.

Victorov, I. T. "El Carácter Idealista y Reaccionario de las Ideas Fundamentales de la Psicología Social Burguesa Contemporánea." *Revista del Hospital Psiquiátrico de la Habana* 6, 2 (1965): 229.

Victorov, I. T. "Exposición de las Relaciones Mutuas entre la Teoría de la Actividad Nerviosa Superior, la Psicología y la Psiquiatría." *Revista del Hospital Psiquiátrico de la Habana* 4, 4 (1963): 733.

Victorov, I. T. "Patofisiología de la Esquizofrenia y su Patogénesis según Autores Soviéticos." *Revista del Hospital Psiquiátrico de la Habana* 6, 3 (1965): 399.

Victorov, I. T. "Pensamiento Autista, Autismo y Delirio Autista a la Luz de la Teoría de la Reflexión Marxista-Leninista." *Revista del Hospital Psiquiátrico de la Habana* 5, 4 (1964): 584–87.

Victorov, I. T. "El Trastorno del Pensamiento y de la Inteligencia en la Esquizofrenia y su Esencia desde un Punto de Vista de la Teoría Marxista-Leninista." *Revista del Hospital Psiquiátrico de la Habana* 7, 3 (1966): 414.

Viel, Benjamín. *The Demographic Explosion: The Latin American Experience*. New York: Irvington, 1976.

Viel, Benjamín. *La Explosión Demográfica: ¿Cuántos Son Demasiados?* Santiago: Ediciones de la Universidad de Chile, 1966.

Viel, Benjamín. "Family Planning in Chile." *Journal of Sex Research* 3, 4 (1967): 284–91.

Viel, Benjamín. *La Medicina Socializada y Su Aplicación en Gran Bretaña, Unión Soviética y Chile*. Santiago: Editorial Universidad de Chile, 1961.

Viel, Benjamín. "Medicina y Calidad de Vida: Memorias de un Salubrista." *Revista Médica de Chile* 113 (1985): 595.

Viel, Benjamín. "The Population Explosion in Latin America." *Proceedings of the Academy of Political Science* 30, 4 (1972): 42–49.

Villarroel, Emilio, and Gabriela Venturini. "La Contribución del Colegio Médico a la Educación Médica Chilena." *Revista Médica de Chile* 100, 7 (1979): 844–52.

Virchow, Rudolf. "Excerpts from 'Report on the Typhus Epidemic in Upper Silesia.'" *American Journal of Public Health* 96, 12 (2006): 2102–5.

Virreira Sánchez, Efraín, ed. *Bibliografía del Doctor Arturo Urquidi Morales: Maestro de la Juventud Boliviana*. Cochabamba, Bolivia: Editorial Universitaria, 1980.

"Vows to Oust Red Agitators from Mexico." *Chicago Tribune*, September 12, 1958.

Waitzkin, Howard. "Commentary: Salvador Allende and the Birth of Latin American Social Medicine." *International Journal of Epidemiology* 34, 4 (2005): 739–41.

Waitzkin, Howard. "Social Medicine Then and Now: Lessons from Latin America." *American Journal of Public Health* 91, 10 (2001): 1592–1601.

Waitzkin, Howard, Celia Iriart, Alfredo Estrada, and Silvia Lamadrid. "Social Medicine in Latin America: Productivity and Dangers Facing the Major National Groups." *The Lancet* 358, 9278 (2001): 315–23.

Wallerstein, Immanuel. *World-Systems Analysis: An Introduction.* Durham, NC: Duke University Press, 2004.

Wang, Jessica. *American Science in an Age of Anxiety: Scientists, Anticommunism, and the Cold War.* Chapel Hill: University of North Carolina Press, 1999.

Wang, Jessica. "Science, Security, and the Cold War: The Case of E. U. Condon." *Isis* 83, 22 (1992): 238–69.

Wang, Zuoyue. *In Sputnik's Shadow: The President's Science Advisory Committee and Cold War America.* New Brunswick, NJ: Rutgers University Press, 2008.

Weaver, Karol K. *Medical Revolutionaries: The Enslaved Healers of Eighteenth-Century Saint Domingue.* Urbana: University of Illinois Press, 2006.

Weindling, Paul. "'Out of the Ghetto': The Rockefeller Foundation and German Medicine after the Second World War." In *Rockefeller Philanthropy and Modern Biomedicine: International Initiatives from World War I to the Cold War,* edited by William H. Schneider, 208–22. Bloomington: Indiana University Press, 2002.

Wells, Harry K. *Sigmund Freud: A Pavlovian Critique.* New York: International, 1960.

Werthein, Silvia. "Palabras en la Mesa de Apertura, VI Encuentro de Psicoanalistas y Psicólogos Marxistas, La Habana, Cuba, Febrero 1996)." *Revista Cubana de Psicología* 14, 1 (1997): 19–22.

Westad, Odd Arne. *The Global Cold War: Third World Interventions and the Making of Our Times.* Cambridge: Cambridge University Press, 2005.

Whitaker, Reg, and Gary Marcuse. *Cold War Canada: The Making of a National Insecurity State, 1945–1957.* Toronto: University of Toronto Press, 1996.

Whitehead, Laurence. "The Bolivian National Revolution: A Twenty-First Century Perspective." In *Proclaiming Revolution: Bolivia in Comparative Perspective,* edited by Merilee Grindle and Pilar Domingo, 25–53. Cambridge, MA: Harvard University Press, 2003.

Wilkie, James W. *The Bolivian Revolution and U.S. Aid since 1952: Financial Background and Context of Political Decisions.* Los Angeles: University of California Latin American Center, 1969.

Winnie, William W., Jr. "The Papaloapan Project: An Experiment in Tropical Development." *Economic Geography* 34, 3 (1958): 227–48.

Wolfe, Audra J. *Competing with the Soviets: Science, Technology, and the State in Cold War America.* Baltimore, MD: Johns Hopkins University Press, 2013.

Wolikow, Serge. *L'Internationale Communiste (1919–1943): Le Komintern ou le rêve déchu du parti mondial de la révolution.* Ivry-sur-Seine, France: l'Atelier, 2010.

World Bank. *World Development Report 1993: Investing in Health.* New York: Oxford University Press, 1993.

World Health Organization. *Declaration of Alma-Ata: International Conference on Primary Health Care.* Geneva, Switzerland: WHO, 1978.

"Ya Expulsaron a Nueve de los Agitadores Extranjeros." *Excelsior*, September 11, 1958.

Young, Glennys. "To Russia with 'Spain': Spanish Exiles in the USSR and the Longue Durée of Soviet History." *Kritika: Explorations in Russian and Eurasian History* 15, 2 (2014): 395–419.

Zajicek, Benjamin. "Insulin Coma Therapy and the Construction of Therapeutic Effectiveness in Stalin's Soviet Union, 1936–1953." In *Psychiatry in Communist Europe*, edited by Mat Savelli and Sarah Marks, 50–72. London: Palgrave Macmillan, 2015.

Zajicek, Benjamin. "Scientific Psychiatry in Stalin's Soviet Union: The Politics of Modern Medicine and the Struggle to Define 'Pavlovian' Psychiatry, 1939–1953." PhD diss., University of Chicago, 2009.

Zapata, Carlos. *De Independentista a Autonomista: La Transformación del Pensamiento Político de Luis Muñoz Marín, 1931–1949*. San Juan, PR: Fundación Luis Muñoz Marín, 2003.

Zárate, María Soledad. *Dar a Luz en Chile, Siglo XIX: De la "Ciencia de Hembra" a la Ciencia Obstétrica*. Santiago, Chile: Universidad Alberto Hurtado, 2007.

Zárate, María Soledad, and Maricela González Moya. "Planificación Familiar en la Guerra Fría Chilena: Política Sanitaria y Cooperación Internacional." *Historia Crítica* 55 (2015): 207–30.

Zaretsky, Eli. *Political Freud*. New York: Columbia University Press, 2015.

Zeno, Lelio. *La Medicina en Rusia, con un Prefacio del Profesor Sergio Judine*. Buenos Aires, Argentina: Anaconda, 1933.

Zimmerman, Matilde. *Sandinista: Carlos Fonseca and the Nicaraguan Revolution*. Durham, NC: Duke University Press, 2000.

Zolov, Eric. "Cuba Sí, Yanquis No! The Sacking of the Instituto Cultural México-Norteamericano in Morelia, Michoacán, 1961." In *In from the Cold: Latin America's New Encounters with the Cold War*, edited by Gilbert Joseph and Daniela Spenser, 214–52. Durham, NC: Duke University Press, 2008.

Zolov, Eric. "Expanding our Conceptual Horizons: The Shift from an Old to a New Left in Latin America." *A Contracorriente: Revista de Historia Social y Literatura en América Latina* 5, 2 (2008): 47–73.

Zulawski, Ann. "The National Revolution and Bolivia in the 1950s: What Did Che See?" In *Che's Travels: The Making of a Revolutionary in 1950s Latin America*, edited by Paulo Drinot, 181–209. Durham, NC: Duke University Press, 2010.

Zulawski. Ann. *Unequal Cures: Public Health and Political Change in Bolivia, 1900–1950*. Durham, NC: Duke University Press, 2007.

Cheasty Anderson received her PhD in History from the University of Texas, Austin in 2014. Her essay "Doctors within Borders: Cuban Medical Diplomacy to Sandinista Nicaragua, 1979–1990" appears in *Beyond the Eagle's Shadow: New Histories of Latin America's Cold War* (2013). She currently works as the Director of Immigration, Policy, and Advocacy at the Children's Defense Fund–Texas.

Anne-Emanuelle Birn is Professor of Critical Development Studies and of Global Health at the University of Toronto. Her research explores the history, politics, and political economy of international/global health, focusing on Latin American health and social justice movements, with emphases ranging from the scatological to the ideological. Her work has appeared in Latin American, African, Asian, North American, and European journals and presses. Her books include *Marriage of Convenience: Rockefeller International Health and Revolutionary Mexico* (2006); *Comrades in Health: U.S. Health Internationalists, Abroad and at Home* (2013); the *Textbook of International Health: Global Health in a Dynamic World* (2009); and the *Textbook of Global Health* (2017).

Katherine E. Bliss is a Senior Fellow in the Global Health Policy Center at the Center for Strategic and International Studies (CSIS). She received her PhD in History from the University of Chicago. She is particularly interested in how political and cultural perspectives shape approaches to such global health challenges as HIV/AIDS, vaccine-preventable diseases, and access to safe drinking water and sanitation. Her publications include *Compromised Positions: Prostitution, Public Health, and Gender Politics in Revolutionary Mexico City* (2001) and *Key Players in Global Health: How Brazil, Russia, India, China, and South Africa Are Influencing the Game* (2010).

Gilberto Hochman is a Researcher and Professor in the History of Science and Health Unit, Oswaldo Cruz Foundation (Fiocruz). His research interests span the history of public health in modern Brazil; health, democracy, and development in Brazil; and science, health, and the Cold War in Latin America. He is the author of *Sanitation of Brazil: Nation, State, and Public Health, 1889–1930* (2016) and coeditor of *História da Saúde no Brasil* (2018), *Médicos Intérpretes do Brasil* (2015), and *Patologías de la Patria: Enfermedades, Enfermos y Nación en América Latina* (2012).

Jennifer Lynn Lambe is Associate Professor of History at Brown University. She is the author of *Madhouse: Psychiatry and Politics in Cuban History* (2017) and coeditor of *The Revolution from Within: Cuba, 1959–1980* (2019).

Raúl Necochea López is Associate Professor of Social Medicine and Adjunct Associate Professor of History at the University of North Carolina–Chapel Hill. He is the author of *A History of Family Planning in Twentieth-Century Peru* (2014), translated as *La Planificación Familiar en el Perú del Siglo XX* (2016). His research spans sexual and reproductive health, migrant health, and the social/ethical implications of HIV/AIDS cure research. His current project is a history of cervical cancer care in Latin America from the late nineteenth century to the age of HPV.

Nicole L. Pacino is Associate Professor of History at the University of Alabama in Huntsville. Her research on the aftermath of the 1952 revolution in Bolivia explores how health, hygiene, and sanitation became an integral part of postrevolutionary conversations about national economic, political, and social transformation. This research draws on archival collections located both in Bolivia and in the United States. Her published articles can be found in journals based in the United States, the United Kingdom, and Latin America, including the *Journal of Women's History*, the *Bulletin of Latin American Research*, *Diplomatic History*, and *História, Ciências, Saúde–Manguinhos*.

Carlos Henrique Assunção Paiva holds master's and doctoral degrees in Public Health from the Institute of Social Medicine, Rio de Janeiro State University, and a bachelor's degree in History from Rio de Janeiro State University. He is a Professor of the History of Science and Health, Oswaldo Cruz Foundation (Fiocruz). He has published papers in Brazilian and international journals, including *Reports in Public Health*; *História, Ciências, Saúde–Manguinhos*; and the *Pan American Journal of Public Health*.

Jadwiga E. Pieper Mooney is Associate Professor of History at the University of Arizona. She specializes in Latin American and gender history with an interest in the politics of health and rights in the twentieth century. Her publications include *The Politics of Motherhood: Maternity and Women's Rights in Twentieth-Century Chile* (2009) as well as articles on histories of feminism, gender and activism, and forced sterilization campaigns. She has coedited *Decentering Cold War History: Local and Global Change* (2013) and *The Global Sixties: Convention, Contest and Counterculture* (2017).

Marco Ramos is a historian and resident psychiatrist at Yale University. His research explores how mental health has operated as both a source of postcolonial power and control in Latin America and a platform for political justice and protest during the twentieth century. He is currently adapting his dissertation on mental health activism in Cold War Argentina into a book. An essay based on his dissertation won the Shryock Medal from the American Association for the History of Medicine. He has published in historical and clinical journals, including *Bulletin of the History of Medicine* and *The Lancet*.

Gabriela Soto Laveaga is Professor of the History of Science and Antonio Madero Professor for the Study of Mexico at Harvard University. Her first book, *Jungle Laboratories: Mexican Peasants, National Projects, and the Making of the Pill* (2009) won the

Robert K. Merton Best Book Prize in Science, Knowledge, and Technology Studies from the American Sociological Association. Her current research interests and recent publications interrogate knowledge production and circulation between Mexico and India; medical professionals and social movements; and science and development projects in the twentieth century. Her next monograph, *Sanitizing Rebellion: Physician Strikes, Public Health, and Repression in Twentieth Century Mexico*, is forthcoming.